New Advance in Cardiovascular Drugs: In Celebration of the 90th Birthday of Professor Akira Endo

New Advance in Cardiovascular Drugs: In Celebration of the 90th Birthday of Professor Akira Endo

Guest Editor

Alfredo Caturano

MDPI

Basel • Beijing • Wuhan • Barcelona • Belgrade • Novi Sad • Cluj • Manchester

Guest Editor
Alfredo Caturano
Department of Advanced Medical and
Surgical Sciences
University of Campania Luigi Vanvitelli
Naples
Italy

Editorial Office
MDPI AG
Grosspeteranlage 5
4052 Basel, Switzerland

This is a reprint of the Special Issue, published open access by the journal *Biomedicines* (ISSN 2227-9059), freely accessible at: https://www.mdpi.com/journal/biomedicines/special_issues/G07Y28OV35.

For citation purposes, cite each article independently as indicated on the article page online and as indicated below:

Lastname, A.A.; Lastname, B.B. Article Title. *Journal Name* **Year**, *Volume Number*, Page Range.

ISBN 978-3-7258-7432-3 (Hbk)
ISBN 978-3-7258-7433-0 (PDF)
https://doi.org/10.3390/books978-3-7258-7433-0

Contents

About the Editor

Alfredo Caturano

Alfredo Caturano, MD, PhD, graduated in Medicine and Surgery from the Second University of Naples (SUN) in 2016. He achieved a Specialization Degree in Internal Medicine in 2021 at the University of Campania "Luigi Vanvitelli". His specialization thesis, concerning the impact of glycemic control on cardiovascular outcomes and mortality in a cohort of patients with type 2 diabetes mellitus in a multifactorial randomized controlled trial, was awarded the 2021 Annapaola Braggio prize by the Italian Society of Diabetology as the best specialization thesis on topics related to insulin resistance. He defended his PhD in *Clinical and Experimental Medicine* in January 2025, earning the title of Doctor Europaeus. His doctoral thesis focused on the cardiometabolic and hepatic effects of innovative glucose-lowering strategies in patients with type 2 diabetes. Since November 2024, he has served as Assistant Professor of Internal Medicine at San Raffaele Roma University.

biomedicines

MDPI

Editorial

New Advances in Cardiovascular Drugs: A Celebration of the 90th Birthday of Professor Akira Endo

Alfredo Caturano

Department of Human Sciences and Promotion of the Quality of Life, San Raffaele Roma Open University, 00166 Rome, Italy; alfredo.caturano@virgilio.it; Tel.: +39-3338616985

1. Introduction: Professor Endo's Journey and Revolutionary Discoveries

In this Special Issue, we celebrate a giant of cardiovascular pharmacology, Professor Akira Endo, on the occasion of his 90th birthday. Professor Endo's journey to improve cardiovascular research was driven by curiosity and a dedication to innovation. Born on November 14, 1933, in Higashiyuri, Northern Japan, he developed a deep interest in the natural world, particularly fungi, which led him to the field of biochemistry. Inspired by the transformative work of Alexander Fleming, Professor Endo pursued his studies at Tokohu University, graduating from the Faculty of Agriculture in 1957 [1]. After completing his Ph.D., he joined Sankyo Pharmaceuticals in Tokyo, where he initially focused on developing fungal enzymes for juice production. However, a turning point came when he theorized that certain fungi might produce compounds that inhibit the enzyme 3-hydroxy-3-methyl-glutaryl (HMG)-CoA reductase—the rate-limiting enzyme in cholesterol biosynthesis. His hypothesis laid the foundation for the development of statins, a class of drugs that would prove essential in lowering cholesterol and reducing cardiovascular risk [1]. In 1971, Professor Endo embarked on this ambitious exploration, sifting through nearly 6000 fungal compounds. His perseverance paid off with the discovery of mevastatin (ML-236B, compactin) in 1973, marking the inception of statin therapy. However, at that time, the significance of this discovery was not immediately apparent. Only in the ensuing years did researchers, including the Nobel laureates Michael Brown and Joseph Goldstein, begin to unravel the role of low-density lipoprotein (LDL) in atherosclerosis, providing context for the groundbreaking nature of Professor Endo's work [1]. Despite various challenges and skepticism from some sectors, statins gained traction, culminating in the development and eventual approval of lovastatin in the United States in 1987. Since then, statins have become a cornerstone in the prevention of cardiovascular disease (CVD), significantly lowering the risk of myocardial infarction, stroke, and other cardiovascular events.

2. The Legacy of Statins and Their Broad Impact

The impact of statins on public health cannot be overstated. Statins have proven invaluable in CVD prevention by lowering cholesterol levels and addressing a primary driver of atherosclerosis. Numerous studies over the last several decades have demonstrated their efficacy in the primary and secondary prevention of cardiovascular events, transforming the treatment landscape for conditions once deemed inexorably progressive [2]. Beyond their cholesterol-lowering effects, statins have shown potential benefits in various other fields, including anti-inflammatory properties, and emerging research has explored possible anticancer benefits [3,4]. This broad therapeutic versatility reflects the profound impact of Professor Endo's work, which has fundamentally reshaped our understanding and management of cardiovascular risk factors [5,6]. Today, millions of patients benefit from statins and their life-saving properties, and this is directly attributable to Professor Endo's tenacity and vision. By reducing global cardiovascular mortality and morbidity rates, statins exemplify the ideal of translating scientific discovery into societal benefits, demonstrating the power of curiosity-driven research in tackling some of humanity's most pressing health issues.

3. Expanding Horizons in Cardiovascular Risk Management: From Singular Targets to Multifactorial Strategies

Professor Endo's pioneering work on statins marked a turning point in cardiovascular medicine, demonstrating the power of targeted pharmacological interventions in lowering cholesterol and, ultimately, reducing the risk of cardiovascular events. However, as the understanding of CVD advanced, so did the recognition that its underlying drivers extend beyond cholesterol alone. Today, cardiovascular risk is understood as a complex, multifactorial process influenced by metabolic, genetic, and environmental factors, as well as lifestyle and social determinants [7]. This broader view has led to a paradigm shift in risk management, where single-target therapies like statins are now combined with additional treatments and approaches that address the diverse contributors to CVD [5,6]. Building on the foundation established by statins, the introduction of novel therapies such as PCSK9 inhibitors, SGLT2 inhibitors, and GLP-1 receptor agonists has further transformed the landscape of cardiovascular prevention. Each of these agents targets distinct mechanisms, from improving glucose metabolism and reducing body weight to providing direct cardiovascular protection, particularly in high-risk groups like those with diabetes and chronic kidney disease [5,6]. This multimodal approach aligns with the current emphasis on precision medicine, where the goal is to provide tailored interventions based on a patient's unique risk profile rather than a one-size-fits-all solution [8–10].

In addition to pharmacological advancements, the importance of lifestyle modifications and social determinants of health has become increasingly clear. Diet, physical activity, smoking cessation, and weight management remain essential pillars of CVD prevention and are now often prescribed alongside drug therapies [11]. This holistic approach underscores the evolving role of clinicians, who must not only prescribe medications but also guide patients in modifying their behaviors to address these lifestyle factors. Public health strategies have also shifted toward more comprehensive risk-reduction models, incorporating community-based interventions that promote healthier living environments, especially in underserved populations, where CVD risk remains disproportionately high [12].

4. Overview of Published Articles

Building on Professor Endo's legacy, the field of cardiovascular pharmacology has continued to evolve, propelled by discoveries that extend and refine our approach to managing CVD. This Special Issue brings together contributions from leading researchers in this field, each exploring a facet of cardiovascular drug development that holds promise for future clinical practice.

Josipa Radić et al. (contribution 1) investigated the relationship between arterial stiffness, measured by pulse wave velocity (PWV), and various factors in a study in hypertensive patients. They found that older patients with poorly controlled blood pressure exhibited higher PWV, influenced by systolic blood pressure and certain medications. Their research highlights the connections between arterial stiffness, blood pressure control, and body composition.

Iida Tuunanen et al. (contribution 2) explored the association between prediagnostic metformin and statin use and the prognosis of patients with hepatocellular carcinoma (HCC) and type 2 diabetes. They found that metformin use was linked to reduced overall mortality (hazard ratio 0.84) compared to no use. The study concluded that while metformin users showed slightly reduced HCC and other-cause mortality, statin use did not significantly impact mortality outcomes in this population.

Jan Kyselovic et al. (contribution 3) investigated outcomes and predictive factors in autologous bone marrow cell (BMC) therapy in patients with "no-option" critical limb ischemia (CLI). They identified baseline C-reactive protein (CRP) and transcutaneous oxygen pressure (TcPO2) as prognostic factors in treatment response, with atorvastatin use associated with improved TcPO2 and reduced pain post-treatment. The study concluded that the prior use of statin and renin–angiotensin system (RAS)-acting agents positively correlated with treatment outcomes, indicating a potential role for these agents in enhancing the efficacy of BMC therapy.

Peter Stanko et al. (contribution 4) investigated the protective effects of angiotensin receptor-neprilysin inhibitors (ARNIs) in a model of hypertension-induced heart disease using Wistar rats. They found that ARNI treatment, similarly to captopril, reduced systolic blood pressure and alleviated left-ventricular (LV) hypertrophy and fibrosis, preventing systolic and diastolic dysfunction. This study concluded that ARNIs may offer significant protection against structural remodeling and functional impairment in hypertensive heart disease.

Nanami Irie et al. (contribution 5) investigated the efficacy of a statin–dipyridamole combination treatment in metastatic melanoma, focusing on its effects in both human and canine melanoma cell lines. They found that combining atorvastatin with dipyridamole significantly reduced the half-maximal inhibitory concentration (IC50) by 68–92%, with some cell lines showing nearly complete inhibition of proliferation. The study concluded that this combination therapy could enhance melanoma treatment, particularly in patients with the BRAF V600E mutation, and suggested potential new developments in melanoma therapy based on the concordant findings in both canine and human models.

Olena Popazova et al. (contribution 6) assessed the cardioprotective effects of nitric oxide (NO) system modulators, including L-arginine, Thiotriazoline, Angiolin, and Mildronate, in newborn rats following intrauterine hypoxia. This study involved 50 female rats, with offspring divided into groups based on treatment after prenatal hypoxia. The results indicated that Angiolin enhanced eNOS mRNA expression and activity in the myocardium, while L-arginine and Thiotriazoline helped restore normal cardiac nitroxidergic system parameters, and Mildronate increased iNOS mRNA levels while reducing nitrotyrosine levels, highlighting its antioxidative properties.

Ying Jie Chee and Rinkoo Dalan (contribution 7) review the increasing incidence of CVD and kidney disease in T2DM and emphasized that a solely glucose-centric approach is inadequate in mitigating cardiovascular risks. They highlight recent advancements in pharmaceutical options, particularly sodium-glucose cotransporter type 2 inhibitors and glucagon-like peptide receptor agonists, which show strong cardiorenal protective effects. The review also discusses emerging combinatorial therapies to enhance patient adherence and improve glycemic control, as well as exploring mechanisms of cardiorenal protection and summarizing upcoming agents in early-phase trials.

Inês Henriques Vieira et al. (contribution 8) review the relationship between T2DM and stroke risk, noting that while strict glycemic control benefits microvascular complications, its role in reducing macrovascular complications such as stroke is less established. They report that current risk reduction strategies focus on multiple factors, including hypertension and dyslipidemia, and that novel T2DM therapies have been the subject of cardiovascular safety trials since 2008. The review highlights the potential stroke prevention benefits of glucagon-like peptide 1 receptor agonists, while the findings regarding sodium-glucose cotransporter type 2 inhibitors remain controversial and dipeptidyl peptidase 4 inhibitors appear neutral regarding stroke prevention.

Andrea Mormone et al. (contribution 9) explored the significance of hypercholesterolemia in the development of lipid plaques, emphasizing the role of elevated low-density lipoprotein cholesterol (LDL-C) in increasing the risk of cardiovascular, cerebrovascular, and peripheral arterial diseases. They report that the control of LDL-C levels is a critical modifiable risk factor in reducing the morbidity and mortality associated with cardiovascular conditions. The review highlights the historical effectiveness of statins, which inhibit the enzyme HMG-CoA reductase, but also introduces newer non-statin agents that offer a favorable cost–benefit ratio as alternative treatments for hypercholesterolemia.

Janette Alejandra Gamiño-Gutiérrez et al. (contribution 10) discuss the significant impact of cardiovascular diseases on global morbidity and mortality. They focus on the renin–angiotensin system (RAS), noting that the overactivation of the classical RAS contributes to disease progression. In contrast, the counter-regulatory RAS produces peptides like Angiotensin-(1-7), which activate cardioprotective mechanisms through receptors such as AT2R, MasR, and MrgD. These mechanisms include reducing cardiac fibrosis, promoting vasodilation, and lowering blood pressure. This review highlights the therapeutic potential of these counter-regulatory peptides in mitigating cardiovascular disease progression.

5. The Future of Cardiovascular Pharmacotherapy

As we look to the future, cardiovascular pharmacology stands on the brink of unprecedented advancements. Emerging research into gene editing and RNA interference offers promising avenues for more precise and effective treatments [13]. Gene editing, utilizing technologies like CRISPR-Cas9, allows for the direct modification of specific genes associated with cardiovascular diseases, potentially correcting genetic defects or altering disease pathways at their source [14]. This could lead to targeted therapies that address the underlying causes of conditions such as familial hypercholesterolemia or other genetic disorders impacting cardiovascular health. RNA interference (RNAi) involves the use of small RNA molecules to silence the expression of specific genes. By targeting and degrading messenger RNA (mRNA) associated with disease pathways, RNAi can effectively reduce the production of harmful proteins implicated in cardiovascular conditions. Both gene editing and RNAi hold the potential to revolutionize treatment approaches, offering tailored interventions that align with individual patient profiles. In addition to exploring new mechanisms of action, researchers are increasingly investigating ways of optimizing the delivery and efficacy of existing drugs [14]. These efforts have the potential to provide more personalized, effective care for patients with cardiovascular disease [15,16]. By combining established drugs like statins with newer therapies, we aim to further improve outcomes for high-risk patients, opening up new avenues for the prevention and management of cardiovascular disease.

6. Tribute to Professor Endo and Closing Reflections

Finally, we would like to pay tribute to Professor Akira Endo, whose life's work exemplifies the profound impact that one individual can have on global health. Although he passed away in June 2024, Professor Endo's discovery of statins continues to save countless lives and remains an enduring source of inspiration for generations of researchers dedicated to advancing scientific knowledge. His contributions extend far beyond cardiovascular pharmacology, standing as a powerful testament to the transformative power of curiosity, innovation, and perseverance in the pursuit of scientific progress. For instance, statins have not only significantly reduced rates of myocardial infarction and stroke but have also transformed clinical guidelines and practices worldwide, leading to more proactive approaches to managing cholesterol levels and cardiovascular risk factors. Millions of patients currently benefit from statins, showcasing how a single discovery can ripple through healthcare systems, influencing treatment paradigms and improving patient outcomes.

As we celebrate Professor Endo's legacy on what would have been his 90th birthday, we recognize his influence on the life-saving therapies now accessible to patients worldwide. Looking ahead, we are inspired to carry forward his work, embracing the same spirit of inquiry that propelled his pioneering research. Through ongoing dedication to research and innovation, we strive to honor Professor Endo's memory by advancing cardiovascular pharmacotherapy. Like a spark igniting a torch, a true teacher leaves aspects of themselves along every path that they illuminate, so that their legacy shines on long after their journey has ended. Professor Endo was such a light, illuminating a path that has profoundly transformed cardiovascular medicine—a path that will continue to guide us toward a healthier future for generations to come.

Funding: The author received no financial support for the research, authorship, and/or publication of this article.

Institutional Review Board Statement: The author has reviewed the literature data and has reported results coming from studies approved by local ethics committee.

Informed Consent Statement: Not applicable.

Data Availability Statement: No dataset was generated for the publication of this article.

Conflicts of Interest: The author declares no conflicts of interest.

List of Contributions:

1. Radić, J.; Vučković, M.; Đogaš, H.; Gelemanović, A.; Belančić, A.; Radić, M. Is Arterial Stiffness Interconnected with Cardiovascular Drug Prescription Patterns, Body Composition Parameters, and the Quality of Blood Pressure Regulation in Hypertensive Patients? *Biomedicines* **2024**, *12*, 2062. https://doi.org/10.3390/biomedicines12092062
2. Tuunanen, I.; Hautakoski, A.; Huhtamäki, H.; Arffman, M.; Sund, R.; Puistola, U.; Karihtala, P.; Jukkola, A.; Urpilainen, E. The Association of Metformin, Other Antidiabetic Medications, and Statins with the Prognosis of Hepatocellular Carcinoma in Patients with Type 2 Diabetes: A Retrospective Cohort Study. *Biomedicines* **2024**, *12*, 1654. https://doi.org/10.3390/biomedicines12081654
3. Kyselovic, J.; Adamičková, A.; Gažová, A.; Valášková, S.; Chomaničová, N.; Červenák, Z.; Madaric, J. Atorvastatin Treatment Significantly Increased the Concentration of Bone Marrow-Derived Mononuclear Cells and Transcutaneous Oxygen Pressure and Lowered the Pain Scale after Bone Marrow Cells Treatment in Patients with "No-Option" Critical Limb Ischaemia. *Biomedicines* **2024**, *12*, 922. https://doi.org/10.3390/biomedicines12040922
4. Stanko, P.; Repova, K.; Baka, T.; Krajcirovicova, K.; Aziriova, S.; Barta, A.; Zorad, S.; Adamcova, M.; Simko, F. Sacubitril/Valsartan Alleviates Cardiac Remodeling and Dysfunction in L-NAME-Induced Hypertension and Hypertensive Heart Disease. *Biomedicines* **2024**, *12*, 733. https://doi.org/10.3390/biomedicines12040733
5. Irie, N.; Mizoguchi, K.; Warita, T.; Nakano, M.; Sasaki, K.; Tashiro, J.; Osaki, T.; Ishikawa, T.; Oltvai, Z.N.; Warita, K. Repurposing of the Cardiovascular Drug Statin for the Treatment of Cancers: Efficacy of Statin–Dipyridamole Combination Treatment in Melanoma Cell Lines. *Biomedicines* **2024**, *12*, 698. https://doi.org/10.3390/biomedicines12030698
6. Popazova, O.; Belenichev, I.; Bukhtiyarova, N.; Ryzhenko, V.; Oksenych, V.; Kamyshnyi, A. Cardioprotective Activity of Pharmacological Agents Affecting NO Production and Bioavailability in the Early Postnatal Period after Intrauterine Hypoxia in Rats. *Biomedicines* **2023**, *11*, 2854. https://doi.org/10.3390/biomedicines11102854
7. Chee, Y.J.; Dalan, R. Novel Therapeutics for Type 2 Diabetes Mellitus—A Look at the Past Decade and a Glimpse into the Future. *Biomedicines* **2024**, *12*, 1386. https://doi.org/10.3390/biomedicines12071386
8. Vieira, I.H.; Carvalho, T.S.; Saraiva, J.; Gomes, L.; Paiva, I. Diabetes and Stroke: Impact of Novel Therapies for the Treatment of Type 2 Diabetes Mellitus. *Biomedicines* **2024**, *12*, 1102. https://doi.org/10.3390/biomedicines12051102
9. Mormone, A.; Tortorella, G.; Esposito, F.; Caturano, A.; Marrone, A.; Cozzolino, D.; Galiero, R.; Marfella, R.; Sasso, F.C.; Rinaldi, L. Advances in Pharmacological Approaches for Managing Hypercholesterolemia: A Comprehensive Overview of Novel Treatments. *Biomedicines* **2024**, *12*, 432. https://doi.org/10.3390/biomedicines12020432
10. Gamiño-Gutiérrez, J.A.; Terán-Hernández, I.M.; Castellar-Lopez, J.; Villamizar-Villamizar, W.; Osorio-Llanes, E.; Palacios-Cruz, M.; Rosales, W.; Chang, A.Y.; Díaz-Ariza, L.A.; Ospino, M.C.; et al. Novel Insights into the Cardioprotective Effects of the Peptides of the Counter-Regulatory Renin–Angiotensin System. *Biomedicines* **2024**, *12*, 255. https://doi.org/10.3390/biomedicines12020255

References

1. Endo, A. A historical perspective on the discovery of statins. *Proc. Jpn. Acad. Ser. B Phys. Biol. Sci.* **2010**, *86*, 484–493. [CrossRef] [PubMed]

2. Marx, N.; Federici, M.; Schütt, K.; Müller-Wieland, D.; Ajjan, R.A.; Antunes, M.J.; Christodorescu, R.M.; Crawford, C.; Di Angelantonio, E.; Eliasson, B.; et al. 2023 ESC Guidelines for the management of cardiovascular disease in patients with diabetes. *Eur. Heart J.* **2023**, *44*, 4043–4140. [CrossRef] [PubMed]
3. Khatiwada, N.; Hong, Z. Potential benefits and risks associated with the use of statins. *Pharmaceutics* **2024**, *16*, 214. [CrossRef] [PubMed]
4. Russo, V.; Silverio, A.; Scudiero, F.; Attena, E.; D'Andrea, A.; Nunziata, L.; Parodi, G.; Celentani, D.; Varbella, F.; Albani, S.; et al. Preadmission statin therapy and clinical outcome in hospitalized patients with COVID-19: An Italian multicenter observational study. *J. Cardiovasc. Pharmacol.* **2021**, *78*, e94–e100. [CrossRef] [PubMed]
5. Visseren, F.L.J.; Mach, F.; Smulders, Y.M.; Carballo, D.; Koskinas, K.C.; Bäck, M.; Benetos, A.; Biffi, A.; Boavida, J.M.; Capodanno, D.; et al. 2021 ESC Guidelines on cardiovascular disease prevention in clinical practice. *Eur. Heart J.* **2021**, *42*, 3227–3337. [CrossRef] [PubMed]
6. Writing Committee Members; Virani, S.S.; Newby, L.K.; Arnold, S.V.; Bittner, V.; Brewer, L.C.; Demeter, S.H.; Dixon, L.D.; Fearon, W.F.; Hess, B.; et al. 2023 AHA/ACC/ACCP/ASPC/NLA/PCNA guideline for the management of patients with chronic coronary disease: A report of the American Heart Association/American College of Cardiology Joint Committee on Clinical Practice Guidelines. *J. Am. Coll. Cardiol.* **2023**, *82*, 833–955, Erratum in *J. Am. Coll. Cardiol.* **2023**, *82*, 1808. https://doi.org/10.1016/j.jacc.2023.09.794. [CrossRef] [PubMed]
7. Ojeda-Granados, C.; Campisi, E.; Barchitta, M.; Agodi, A. Genetic, lifestyle and metabolic factors contributing to cardiovascular disease in the Italian population: A literature review. *Front. Nutr.* **2024**, *11*, 1379785. [CrossRef] [PubMed]
8. Adams, S.A.; Petersen, C. Precision medicine: Opportunities, possibilities, and challenges for patients and providers. *J. Am. Med. Inform. Assoc.* **2016**, *23*, 787–790. [CrossRef] [PubMed]
9. Cozzolino, D.; Sessa, G.; Salvatore, T.; Sasso, F.C.; Giugliano, D.; Lefebvre, P.J.; Torella, R. The involvement of the opioid system in human obesity: A study in normal weight relatives of obese people. *J. Clin. Endocrinol. Metab.* **1996**, *81*, 713–718. [PubMed]
10. Di Francia, R.; Rinaldi, L.; Cillo, M.; Varriale, E.; Facchini, G.; D'Aniello, C.; Marotta, G.; Berretta, M. Antioxidant diet and genotyping as tools for the prevention of liver disease. *Eur. Rev. Med. Pharmacol. Sci.* **2016**, *20*, 5155–5163. [PubMed]
11. Ghodeshwar, G.K.; Dube, A.; Khobragade, D. Impact of lifestyle modifications on cardiovascular health: A narrative review. *Cureus* **2023**, *15*, e42616. [CrossRef] [PubMed]
12. Vaduganathan, M.; Mensah, G.A.; Turco, J.V.; Fuster, V.; Roth, G.A. The global burden of cardiovascular diseases and risk: A compass for future health. *J. Am. Coll. Cardiol.* **2022**, *80*, 2361–2371. [CrossRef] [PubMed]
13. Singh, S.; Sarma, D.K.; Verma, V.; Nagpal, R.; Kumar, M. Unveiling the future of metabolic medicine: Omics technologies driving personalized solutions for precision treatment of metabolic disorders. *Biochem. Biophys. Res. Commun.* **2023**, *682*, 1–20. [CrossRef] [PubMed]
14. Verbaanderd, C.; Rooman, I.; Huys, I. Exploring new uses for existing drugs: Innovative mechanisms to fund independent clinical research. *Trials* **2021**, *22*, 322. [CrossRef] [PubMed]
15. Li, T.; Yang, Y.; Qi, H.; Cui, W.; Zhang, L.; Fu, X.; He, X.; Liu, M.; Li, P.F.; Yu, T. CRISPR/Cas9 therapeutics: Progress and prospects. *Signal Transduct. Target. Ther.* **2023**, *8*, 36. [CrossRef] [PubMed]
16. Singh, S.; Kumar, R.; Payra, S.; Singh, S.K. Artificial intelligence and machine learning in pharmacological research: Bridging the gap between data and drug discovery. *Cureus* **2023**, *15*, e44359. [CrossRef] [PubMed]

biomedicines

MDPI

Article

Is Arterial Stiffness Interconnected with Cardiovascular Drug Prescription Patterns, Body Composition Parameters, and the Quality of Blood Pressure Regulation in Hypertensive Patients?

Josipa Radić [1,2], Marijana Vučković [1], Hana Đogaš [2], Andrea Gelemanović [3], Andrej Belančić [4] and Mislav Radić [2,5,*]

1 Department of Internal Medicine, Division of Nephrology and Dialysis, University Hospital of Split, 21000 Split, Croatia; josiparadic1973@gmail.com (J.R.); mavuckovic@kbsplit.hr (M.V.)
2 School of Medicine, University of Split, 21000 Split, Croatia; hana.dogas@gmail.com
3 Mediterranean Institute for Life Sciences (MedILS), 21000 Split, Croatia; andrea.gelemanovic@gmail.com
4 Department of Basic and Clinical Pharmacology with Toxicology, Faculty of Medicine, University of Rijeka, Braće Branchetta 20, 51000 Rijeka, Croatia; andrej.belancic@uniri.hr
5 Department of Internal Medicine, Division of Rheumatology, Allergology and Clinical Immunology, University Hospital of Split, 21000 Split, Croatia
* Correspondence: mislavradic@gmail.com

Abstract: Background: Arterial hypertension (AH) is a significant risk factor for cardiovascular disease and is associated with increased arterial stiffness, particularly as measured by pulse wave velocity (PWV). This study aims to explore the relationships between age groups, antihypertensive and new oral antidiabetic drugs, body composition, and arterial stiffness parameters in hypertensive patients. Methods: A single-center cross-sectional study was conducted including 584 participants who underwent 24 h ambulatory blood pressure monitoring (including central blood pressure (BP) and PWV measurement), body composition analysis, and provided medical history and current pharmacotherapy data. Results: The study found that PWV was significantly higher in patients with poorly regulated BP in those aged 65 years and older. Significant PWV predictors included systolic BP, heart rate, peripheral mean arterial pressure, peripheral pulse pressure, augmentation index, calcium channel blockers, moxonidine, sodium–glucose co-transporter 2 inhibitors, urapidil, and statin prescription. Also, statistically significant negative correlations were found between PWV and visceral fat level, fat-free mass, and the percentage of muscle mass. Conclusions: The findings suggest that arterial stiffness is interconnected with peripheral and central blood pressure parameters, body composition parameters, and prescribed hypertensive and new antidiabetic drugs.

Keywords: arterial hypertension; arterial stiffness; pulse wave velocity; body composition; antihypertensive medication

1. Introduction

Arterial hypertension (AH) is one of the major risk factors for cardiovascular disease (CVD), affecting more than one-third of the population, and accounting for 20.5% of the global burden of CVD. Also, AH is the leading cause of death and disability worldwide [1]. Large artery stiffness is an established biomarker of vascular aging. The progression of artery stiffness is related not only to aging but also to cumulative exposure to many cardiovascular risk factors throughout life [2]. The relationship between AH and arterial stiffness is complex and is probably bidirectional, with high blood pressure stiffening arteries and stiff arteries inducing blood pressure (BP) increase [3].

Arterial stiffness, measured mostly by pulse wave velocity (PWV), is a crucial marker in assessing cardiovascular health. Elevated PWV is linked to worse outcomes in BP control and overall vascular function [4]. In the China Stroke Primary Prevention Trial, which included over 3000 hypertensive subjects, it was found that individuals with higher baseline PWV experienced smaller reductions in BP during short-term antihypertensive treatment. This inverse relationship between PWV and BP reduction was most pronounced for systolic BP, suggesting that arterial stiffness plays a significant role in determining the efficacy of antihypertensive therapy [5].

The results from a recently published meta-analysis support that antihypertensive drugs are a suitable treatment to reduce arterial stiffness in patients with AH. Based on the results, angiotensin-converting enzyme inhibitors (ACEi), angiotensin receptor blockers (ARB), beta-blockers (BB), calcium channel blockers (CCB), renin inhibitors, the thiazide diuretics/ACEi combination, the ARB/CCB combination, and the ACEi/ARB combination could be useful for patients with AH who have higher levels of arterial stiffness [6].

In addition to its role in BP control, PWV is also influenced by other cardiometabolic factors, including insulin resistance (IR) and visceral adipose tissue (VAT). The combination of IR and VAT further exacerbates arterial stiffness and increases the risk of hypertension. Notably, VAT acts as a mediator of IR's effects on arterial stiffness, emphasizing the importance of targeting both IR and visceral fat (VF) in managing cardiovascular risk [7].

Therefore, some data suggest that antidiabetic drugs might influence arterial stiffness measured as PWV. Both glucagon-like peptide-1 receptor agonists (GLP1-RA) and, to a lesser extent, dipeptidyl peptidase 4 inhibitors (DPP4i) significantly decreased PWV [8]. Dapagliflozin can reduce arterial stiffness in people with type 2 diabetes mellitus (T2DM) [9] and is also associated with a significant decrease in BP [10] and a favorable lipid profile [10,11]. In contrast, the results from a recently published meta-analysis showed that there was no evidence of a favorable change in arterial stiffness indices found following the administration of sodium–glucose transport protein 2 inhibitors (SGLT-2i) or GLP1-RA [12].

Body composition, including fat mass (FM) and lean mass (LM), also plays crucial roles in arterial health. Increased FM, particularly in the trunk region, is linked to higher PWV and arterial stiffness. Interestingly, there is an "arterial paradox" where higher FM may sometimes correlate with better arterial function, highlighting the complexity of these relationships [13].

Considering the significant effects arterial stiffness has on overall morbidity and mortality in hypertensive and obese patients, the aim of this study was to evaluate and further explore the interplay between age groups, antihypertensive and new oral antidiabetic drugs, body composition, and arterial stiffness parameters to gain a better understanding of the effects and possible advantages in treating high-risk hypertensive patients.

2. Materials and Methods

2.1. Study Population and Design

A single-center, cross-sectional study was conducted at the Outpatient Clinic for Arterial Hypertension, Nephrology and Dialysis Division, Internal Medicine Department, University Hospital Centre Split, Croatia, between February 2021 and June 2023.

Patients prescribed with antihypertensive medicine/s (AMs) and/or with confirmed AH via 24 h ambulatory blood pressure monitoring (24h-ABPM) (criteria/threshold applied: systolic blood pressure > 130 mmHg and/or diastolic blood pressure > 80 mmHg) were included if they avoided the following exclusion criteria: (i) incomplete or invalid blood pressure measurement, (ii) pregnancy, (iii) immobility, (iv) implanted pacemaker or cardioverter–defibrillator, (v) limb amputation, (vi) existing edema, (vii) existing acute infection, or (viii) active underlying malignant disease. The selection process with the inclusion and exclusion criteria is visually presented in detail in Figure 1.

All the eligible patients performed a 24h-ABPM and body composition analysis. Medical history as well as ambulatory self-reports were used to obtain data on pharmacotherapy.

The participants were informed of the purpose of the study and provided written and verbal consent. This study was conducted in accordance with the guidelines of the latest version of the Declaration of Helsinki, good clinical practice (GCP) standards, and the study protocol was approved by the Ethics Committee of the University Hospital of Split on 27 September 2022 (Class 500-03/22-01/170, Ur.no. 500-03/23-01/84).

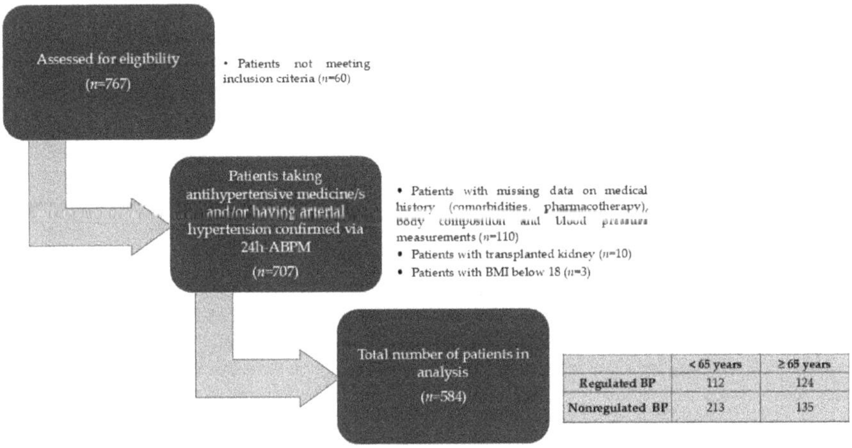

Figure 1. Participant selection process. Abbreviations: 24h-ABPM—24 h ambulatory blood pressure measurement; BMI—body mass index; BP—blood pressure.

2.2. Blood Pressure Measurement

BP measurement was performed based on oscillometry principles using a 24h-ABPM monitor IEM Mobile-O-Graph (IEM GmbH, Stolberg, Germany); its oscillometric cuff was placed on the non-dominant arm. The latter device was programmed to measure BP from 8:01 a.m. to 12:00 p.m. and from 12:01 a.m. to 8:00 a.m. at 15 min and 30 min intervals, respectively. The records having at least 20 ambulatory BP measurements during the day and 10 during the night (which is at least 70% of all the measurements) were considered valid. Instructions from the device manual were fully followed for all the measurements [14]. The following parameters were collected: central systolic blood pressure (cSBP; mmHg), central diastolic blood pressure (cDBP; mmHg), peripheral systolic blood pressure (pSBP; mmHg), peripheral diastolic blood pressure (pDBP; mmHg), peripheral mean arterial pressure (pMAP; mmHg), heart rate (HR; bpm), peripheral pulse pressure (pPP; mmHg), stroke volume (SV; mL/beat), augmentation index normalized to 75 beats per minute (Aix@75), PWV (m/s), and the dipping status of systolic and diastolic BP.

Data on the regulation of BP was collected using 24h-ABPM with the cut-off being systolic BP > 130 mmHg and/or diastolic BP > 80 mmHg in total 24 h average values. The regulation was defined as a good regulation of BP if both systolic and diastolic were below cut-off points, whilst the inadequate regulation of BP was differentiated as inadequate systolic, diastolic, or systolic–diastolic depending on the component/s (systolic, diastolic, or both) with elevated total 24 h average values.

2.3. Body Composition Measurements

On the same day when the 24h-ABPM monitor was placed, the body composition parameters were collected via the MC-780 Multifrequency Segmental Body Mass Analyzer (Tanita, Tokyo, Japan). Prior to the body composition measurements, a stadiometer was used to determine the height of the participants. All the participants were instructed in advance to follow the guidance from the instrument's instruction manual, which are (i) emptying the bladder, (ii) not consuming food or liquid for at least 3 h before the measurement, and (iii) refraining from strenuous physical activity and alcohol consumption for at least one day before the measurement [15]. The scale, using the bioelectrical impedance model, was then used to determine the body mass (kg), body mass index (BMI; kg/m^2), percentage of muscle mass (PMM; %), fat-free mass (FFM; kg), fat mass (FM; kg and %), visceral fat (VF), skeletal muscle index (SMI), and phase angle (PhA; °) for each study participant.

2.4. Medical History and Current Medication Treatment

Medical history/records as well as ambulatory self-reports were used to obtain the following data: the presence of chronic kidney disease (CKD), diabetes mellitus (DM), CVD, cerebrovascular disease (CBD), and a history of malignancy (either currently active or in remission). Additionally, the data on current pharmacotherapy were collected for the following medicine groups: BB, ACEi, ARB, CCB, diuretics, moxonidine, urapidil, α-1 antagonists, aldosterone antagonist (MRA), oral antihyperglycemics in general, SGLT-2i, GLP-1RA, insulin, statins, and uric acid inhibitors. Data on the total number of prescribed medicines as well as antihypertensive fixed-combination prescriptions were also noted.

2.5. Statistical Analysis

To perform descriptive statistical analysis, a Shapiro–Wilk test was first conducted to assess the normality of the numerical variables. These variables were then presented with mean and standard deviation (SD) if they were normally distributed, or with medians and interquartile range (IQR) if they deviated from normality. The categorical variables were presented with frequencies and percentages. To assess the differences between the two groups (those with regulated and nonregulated BP), the chi-square test was used for the categorical variables, and *t*-test or Mann–Whitney U test for the numerical variables depending on the normality distribution. To identify the predictors of PWV, a generalized linear regression model was performed, corrected for the effects of age, sex, the presence of DM and CKD, and BP regulation. Finally, to evaluate the correlation between PWV and visceral fat levels, the Pearson correlation analysis was performed separately. The statistically significant results were those with a p-value < 0.05. The regression results were presented with betas and standard errors (SEs), while the correlation results were presented with Pearson correlation coefficient (R). All the analyses were performed in R v4.3.2 [15].

3. Results

A total of 584 participants (48.6% females) were included in the study, with a median age of 63 years (IQR 19). Table 1 presents the sociodemographic, body composition, and 24h-ABPM parameters. Supplementary Table S1 provides a more comprehensive overview of the general characteristics of the study population. Furthermore, Figure 2 provides a detailed overview of the pharmacotherapy prescriptions among the study participants.

Table 1. General characteristics of study population.

Variable *,**,***		**All (n = 584)**
Sex, n (%)	Male	300 (51.37)
	Female	284 (48.63)
Age (years), median (IQR)		63 (19)
Height (cm), mean (SD)		173.61 (9.75)
Weight (kg), median (IQR)		86 (23.43)
BMI (kg/m^2), median (IQR)		28.75 (6.52)
FM (%), mean (SD)		29.03 (8.69)
FM (kg), median (IQR)		24.9 (13.6)
VF level, median (IQR)		10 (6)
FFM (kg), median (IQR)		61.35 (16.85)
PMM (%), median (IQR)		58.25 (16.05)

Table 1. *Cont.*

Variable *,**,***		All (n = 584)
SMI, median (IQR)		8.42 (2.05)
PhA (°), median (IQR)		5.4 (1)
Smoking, n (%)	Yes	127 (21.75)
	No	457 (78.25)
CKD, n (%)	Yes	243 (41.61)
	No	341 (58.39)
DM, n (%)	Yes	188 (32.19)
	No	396 (67.81)
Malignancies, n (%)	Yes	66 (11.3)
	No	518 (88.7)
CVD, n (%)	Yes	120 (20.55)
	No	464 (79.45)
CBD, n (%)	Yes	16 (2.74)
	No	568 (97.26)
pSBP (mmHg), median (IQR)		129 (17)
pDBP (mmHg), median (IQR)		78 (13)
HR (bpm), median (IQR)		70 (12)
pMAP (mmHg), median (IQR)		101 (14)
pPP (mmHg), median (IQR)		50 (13)
cSBP (mmHg), median (IQR)		118 (15)
cDBP (mmHg), median (IQR)		79.5 (14)
AIx@75, median (IQR)		25 (10)
PWV (m/s), median (IQR)		9 (2.9)
SV (mL/beat), median (IQR)		70 (9)
Dipping systole, n (%)	No	423 (72.43)
	Yes	161 (27.57)
Dipping diastole, n (%)	No	346 (59.25)
	Yes	238 (40.75)

* Formatting of the first column: variable (unit of measurement), type of data provided. Note: in case no unit of measurement is provided, the variable does not require it as it is a number or an index. ** Measuring units in order of appearance: cm—centimeter; kg—kilogram; kg/m^2—kilogram per meter square; %—percentage; °—degree; mmHg—millimeters of mercury; m/s—meter per second; bpm—beats per minute; mL/beat—milliliters per beat. *** Abbreviations in order of appearance: IQR—interquartile range; SD—standard deviation; BMI—body mass index, FM—fat mass; VF—visceral fat; FFM—fat-free mass; PMM—percentage of muscle mass; SMI—skeletal muscle index; PhA—phase angle; CKD—chronic kidney disease; DM—diabetes mellitus, CVD—cardiovascular disease; CBD—cerebrovascular disease; pSBP—peripheral systolic blood pressure; pDBP—peripheral diastolic blood pressure; HR—heart rate; pMAP—peripheral mean arterial pressure; pPP—peripheral pulse pressure; cSBP—central systolic blood pressure; cDBP—central diastolic blood pressure; AIx@75—augmentation index normalized to 75 beats per minute; PWV—pulse wave velocity; SV—stroke volume.

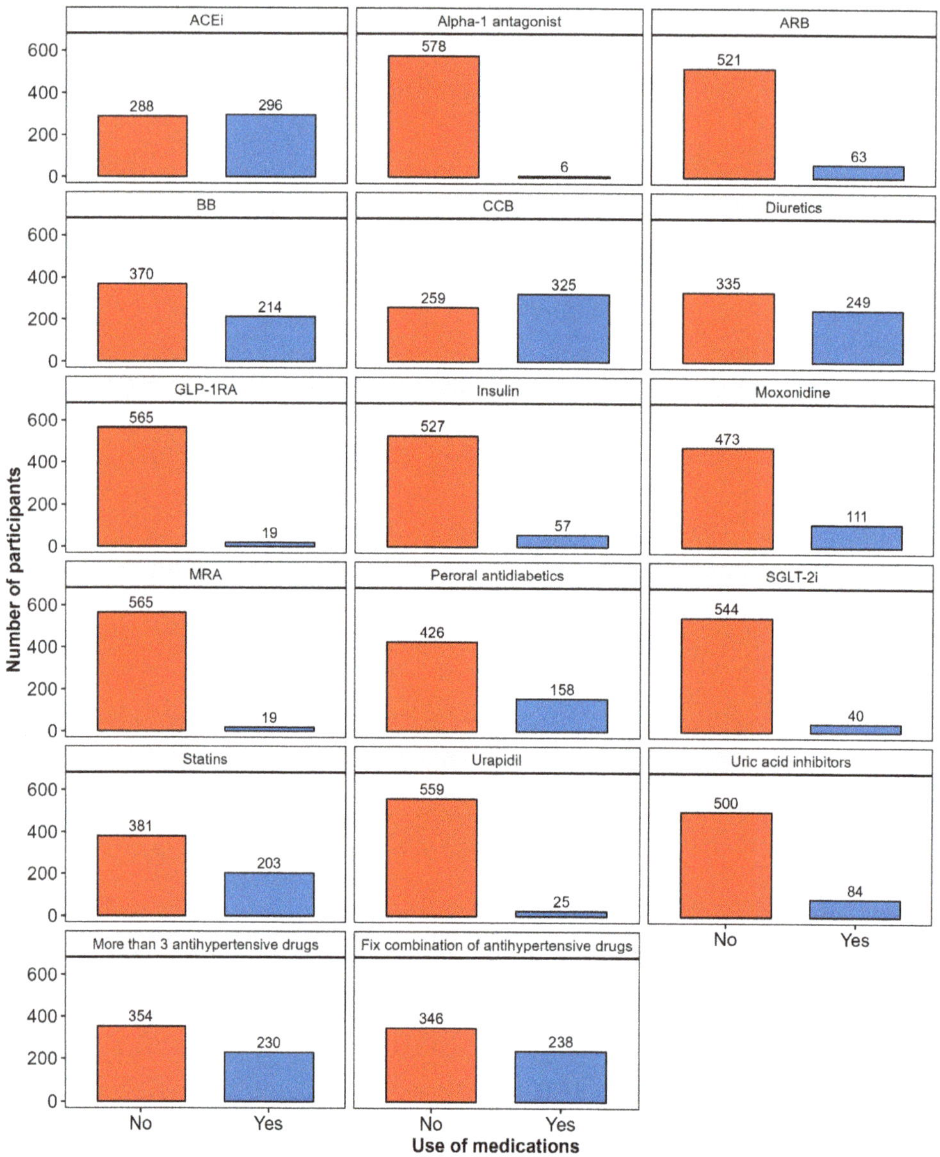

Figure 2. Pharmacotherapy prescription patterns in studied population. Abbreviations: ACEi—angiotensin-converting enzyme inhibitors; ARB—angiotensin receptor blocker; BB—beta-blocker; CCB—calcium channel blockers; GLP-1RA—glucagon-like peptide-1 receptor agonist; MRA—aldosterone antagonist; SGLT-2i—sodium–glucose transport protein 2 inhibitors.

To assess differences in BP regulation, the participants were classified into two groups based on their 24h-ABPM results: those with well-regulated blood pressure (systolic < 130 mmHg and diastolic < 80 mmHg) and those with poorly regulated blood pressure (systolic $\geq$ 130 mmHg and/or diastolic $\geq$ 80 mmHg). Considering age-related variations in blood pressure profiles, the participants were further divided into two subgroups: younger than 65 years and 65 years and older. Table 2 highlights significant differences in the measured parameters between these groups, while Supplementary Table S2 provides a complete overview of all the measured and evaluated parameters. Notably, both age groups exhibited higher FFM and PMM in individuals with poorly regulated blood pressure. Interestingly, PWV, the primary outcome of this study, was significantly elevated only in the older participants (≥65 years) with poorly regulated BP.

Table 2. Significant differences in the measured parameters regarding the age and blood pressure regulation.

Variable *,**,***		Regulated BP < 65 Years (*n* = 112)	Nonregulated BP < 65 Years (*n* = 213)	*p*	Regulated BP ≥ 65 Years (*n* = 124)	Nonregulated BP ≥ 65 Years (*n* = 135)	*p*
Age (years), median (IQR)		55.5 (12.25)	52 (13)	**0.001**	72 (7)	71 (8)	0.591
Height (cm), mean (SD)		173 (12.4)	176 (13)	**0.013**	170.21 (9.15)	171.25 (9.32)	0.367
FFM (kg), median (IQR)		62.25 (17.2)	64.1 (17)	**0.025**	58.2 (13.52)	61.3 (16.5)	**0.039**
PMM (%), median (IQR)		59.15 (16.4)	60.9 (16.2)	**0.025**	55.3 (12.9)	58.2 (15.7)	**0.039**
CVD, *n* (%)	Yes	21 (18.75)	21 (9.86)	**0.036**	37 (29.84)	41 (30.37)	1.000
	No	91 (81.25)	192 (90.14)	**0.036**	87 (70.16)	94 (69.63)	1.000
pSBP (mmHg), median (IQR)		120 (10)	134 (13)	**0.000**	121 (10)	138 (15)	**<0.001**
pDBP (mmHg), median (IQR)		73 (8)	86 (10)	**0.000**	69.52 (5.55)	80.23 (7.43)	**<0.001**
HR (bpm), median (IQR)		70.26 (8.57)	73.95 (9.38)	**0.001**	66.4 (8.92)	67.91 (9.31)	0.183
pMAP (mmHg), median (IQR)		94 (8)	107 (11)	**<0.001**	93.5 (8)	107 (9)	**<0.001**
pPP (mmHg), median (IQR)		47 (9.25)	48 (15)	**0.008**	50 (7)	58 (16)	**<0.001**
cSBP (mmHg), median (IQR)		110 (7.25)	123 (13)	**<0.001**	110 (10)	125 (11.5)	**<0.001**
cDBP (mmHg), median (IQR)		75 (8.25)	87 (9)	**<0.001**	71.5 (8)	82 (10.5)	**<0.001**
AIx@75, median (IQR)		22.05 (7.55)	23.39 (7.59)	0.132	26 (10)	28 (8)	0.001
PWV (m/s), median (IQR)		7.7 (1.63)	7.8 (1.9)	0.198	10.2 (1.1)	10.9 (1.35)	**<0.001**
ACEi, *n* (%)	Yes	73 (65.18)	85 (39.91)	**<0.001**	71 (57.26)	67 (49.63)	0.269
	No	39 (34.82)	128 (60.09)	**<0.001**	53 (42.74)	68 (50.37)	0.269
Statins, *n* (%)	Yes	35 (31.25)	41 (19.25)	0.022	66 (53.23)	61 (45.19)	0.243
	No	77 (68.75)	172 (80.75)	0.022	58 (46.77)	74 (54.81)	0.243
Fixed antihypertensive drugs combinations use, *n* (%)	Yes	60 (53.57)	61 (28.64)	**<0.001**	63 (50.81)	54 (40)	0.105
	No	52 (46.43)	152 (71.36)	**<0.001**	61 (49.19)	81 (60)	0.105

* Formatting of the first column: variable (unit of measurement), type of data provided. Note: in case no unit of measurement is provided, the variable does not require it as it is a number or an index. ** Measuring units in order of appearance: cm—centimeter; kg—kilogram; %—percentage; mmHg—millimeters of mercury; bpm—beats per minute; m/s—meter per secund. *** Abbreviations in order of appearance: IQR—interquartile range; SD—standard deviation; FFM—fat-free mass; PMM—percentage of muscle mass; CVD—cardiovascular disease; pSBP—peripheral systolic blood pressure; pDBP—peripheral diastolic blood pressure; HR—heart rate; pMAP—peripheral mean arterial pressure; pPP—peripheral pulse pressure; cSBP—central systolic blood pressure; cDBP—central diastolic blood pressure; AIx@75—augmentation index normalized to 75 beats per minute; PWV—pulse wave velocity; ACEi—angiotensin-converting enzyme inhibitors.

When analyzing medication use in relation to PWV, the patients using beta-blockers BB, ACEi, and ARB had significantly higher PWV values. Other medications associated with increased PWV included CCB, moxonidine, diuretics, peroral antidiabetics, insulin, statins, and uric acid inhibitors. Additionally, PWV was significantly higher in the patients using more than three antihypertensive drugs or fixed combination drug regimens. Figure 3 presents a comprehensive analysis of the relationship between medication use and PWV.

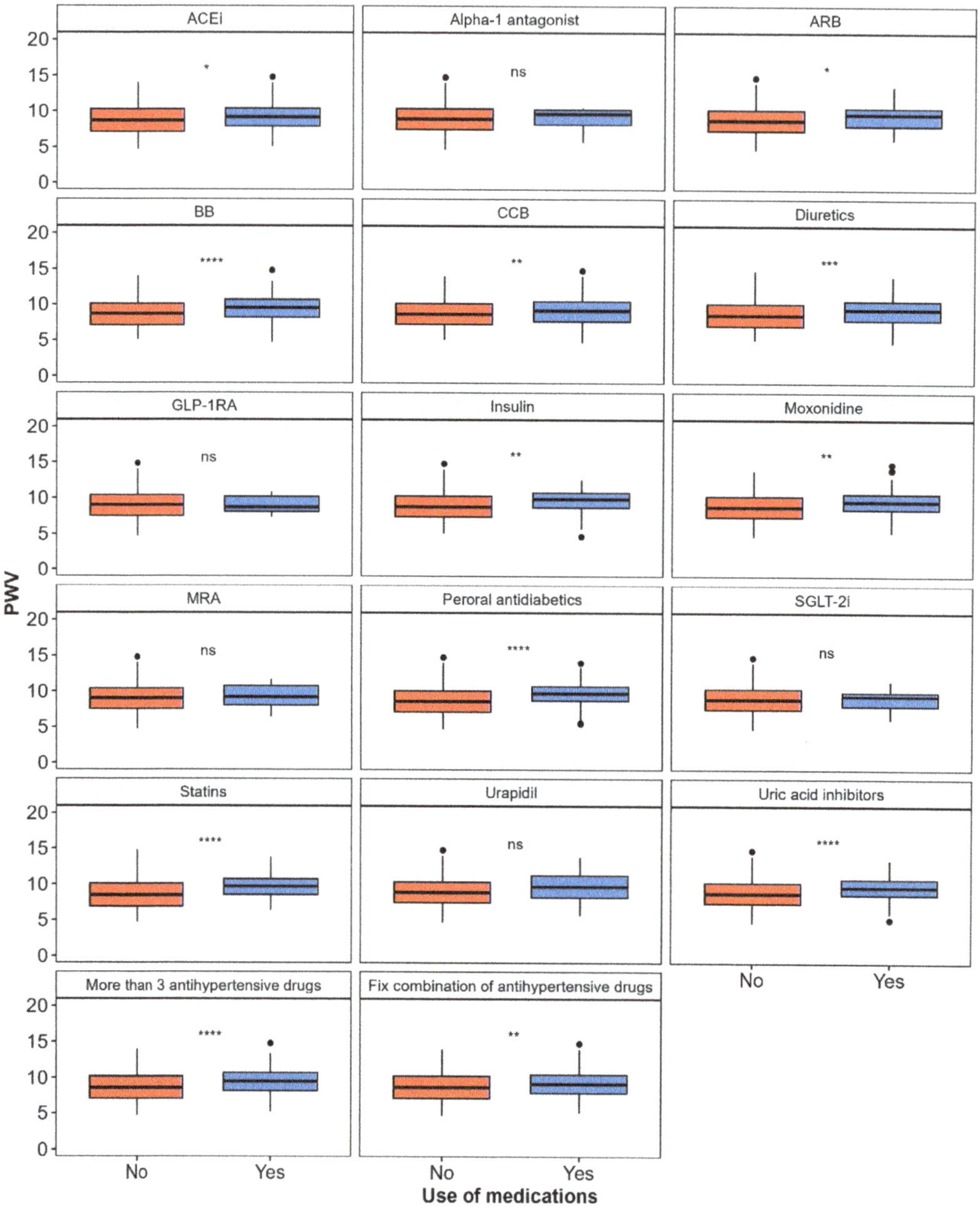

Figure 3. Pulse wave velocity values based on pharmacotherapy prescription patterns. Abbreviations: PWV—pulse wave velocity; ACEi—angiotensin-converting enzyme inhibitors; ARB—angiotensin receptor blocker; BB—beta-blocker; CCBs—calcium channel blockers; GLP-1RA—glucagon-like peptide-1 receptor agonist; MRA—aldosterone antagonist; SGLT-2i—sodium–glucose transport protein 2 inhibitors. p-value labels: **** $p < 0.0001$, *** $p < 0.001$, ** $p < 0.01$, * $p < 0.05$, ns depicts no statistical significance ($p > 0.05$).

As the primary focus of this research was to evaluate arterial stiffness, PWV was further analyzed to identify potential predictors. A generalized linear regression model was used to determine the predictors of PWV among all the study participants, adjusting for age, sex, the presence of DM and CKD, and BP regulation. After adjusting for the mentioned confounders, our regression model revealed that increased pSBP, cSBP, Aix@75, pMAP, pPP, the prescription of CCB, moxonidine, and urapidil were significantly associated with higher PWV.

Conversely, greater height, weight, VF level, FFM, PMM, HR, and the use of SGLT-2i and statins were significantly associated with lower PWV. Table 3 presents the statistically significant predictors of PWV, while Supplementary Table S3 provides a comprehensive analysis of all the predictors.

Table 3. Significant predictors of PWV in all study subjects (generalized linear regression model corrected for age, sex, presence of DM, CKD, and BP regulation).

Variable *	Beta	SE	*p*
Height	−0.01237	0.00407	0.002
Weight	−0.0031	0.00151	0.04
VF level	−0.02303	0.00668	<0.001
FFM	−0.00811	0.00316	0.011
PMM	−0.00851	0.00331	0.011
pSBP	0.03512	0.00193	<0.001
HR	−0.00856	0.0029	0.003
pMAP	0.03299	0.00313	<0.001
pPP	0.04143	0.00202	<0.001
Csbp	0.03213	0.00232	<0.001
AIx@75	0.02005	0.00488	<0.001
CCB use	0.11212	0.05252	0.033
Moxonidine use	0.1839	0.06752	0.007
SGLT-2i use	−0.23252	0.10858	0.033
Statin use	−0.12192	0.05876	0.038
Urapidil use	0.3763	0.12964	0.004

* Abbreviations: PWV—pulse wave velocity; DM—diabetes mellitus; CKD—chronic kidney disease; VF—visceral fat; FFM—fat-free mass; PMM—percentage of muscle mass; pSBP—peripheral systolic blood pressure; HR—heart rate; pMAP—peripheral mean arterial pressure; pPP—peripheral pulse pressure; cSBP—central systolic blood pressure; AIx@75—augmentation index normalized to 75 beats per minute; CCBs—calcium channel blockers; SGLT-2i—sodium–glucose transport protein 2 inhibitors.

To further investigate the relationship between PWV and VF level, we analyzed the correlation between these factors while considering medication use and age. A statistically significant positive correlation between PWV and VF level was observed in the participants not using ACEi, ARB, CCB, moxonidine, SGLT-2i, MRA, diuretics, urapidil, BB, or statins. Additionally, a statistically significant positive correlation between PWV and VF level was found in the participants younger than 65 years old. Conversely, the participants aged 65 years or older exhibited a statistically significant negative correlation between PWV and VF level. Figure 4A,B illustrate these findings.

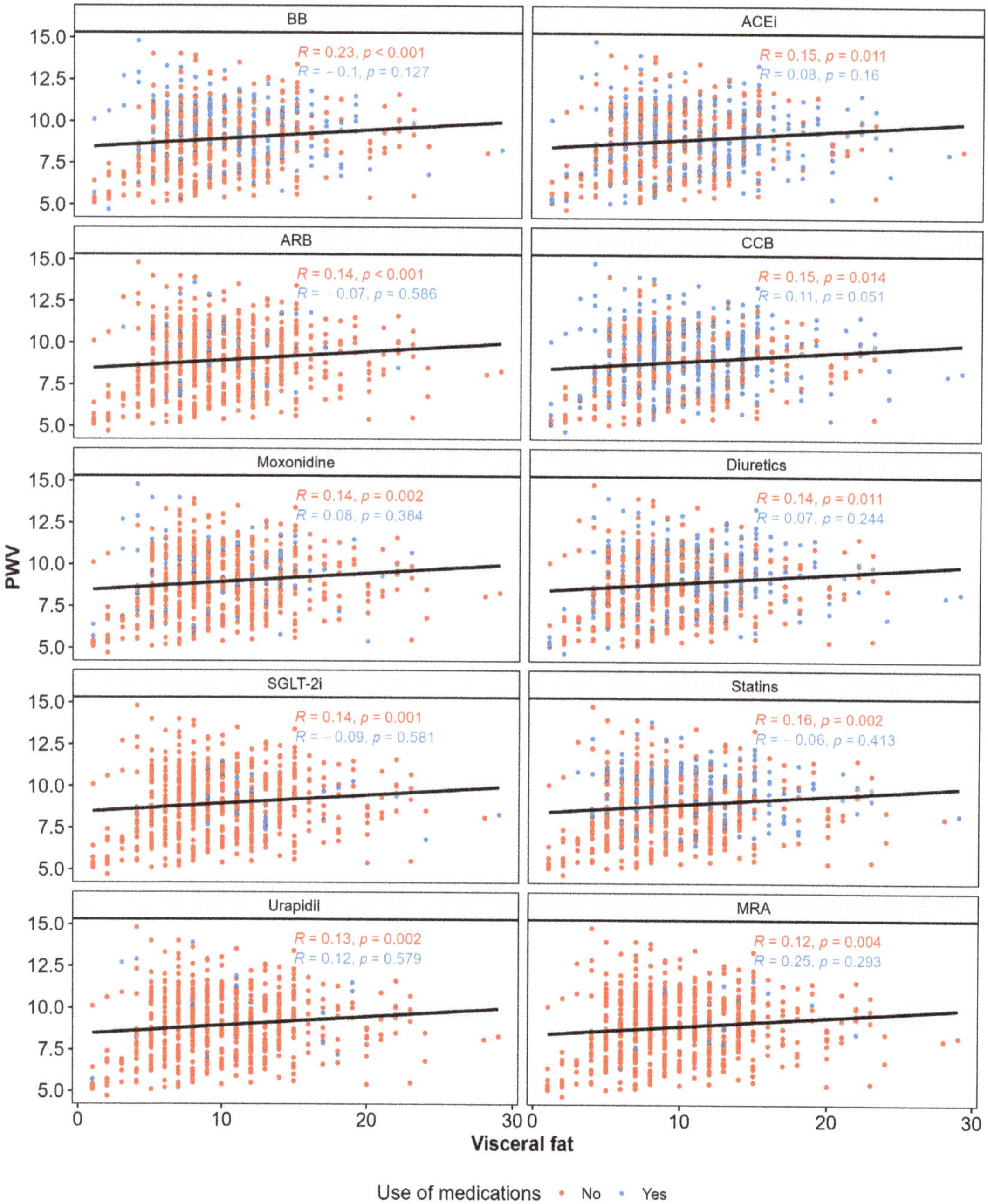

(A)

Figure 4. *Cont.*

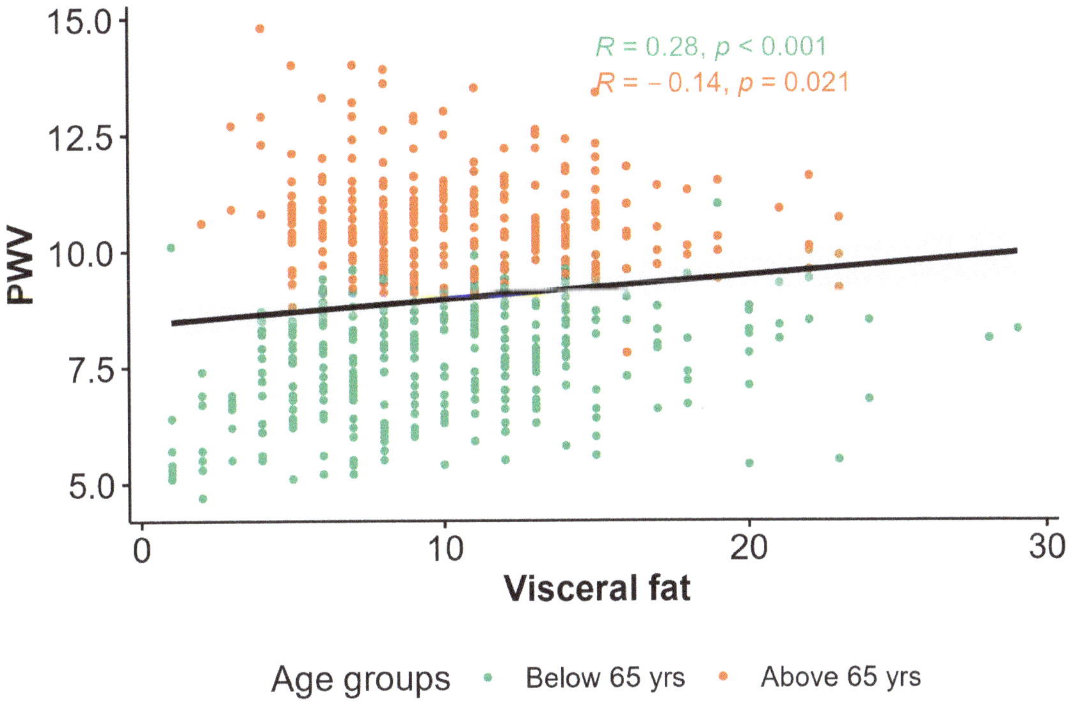

(**B**)

Figure 4. Correlations between PWV and VF level within medication groups (**A**) and age (**B**). Abbreviations: PWV—pulse wave velocity; ACEi—angiotensin-converting enzyme inhibitors; ARB—angiotensin receptor blocker; BB—beta-blocker; CCB—calcium channel blockers; MRA—aldosterone antagonist; SGLT-2i—sodium–glucose transport protein 2 inhibitors; yrs—years.

4. Discussion

Our research offers a thorough examination of the factors contributing to PWV in a group of hypertensive patients and highlights the complex interactions that affect arterial stiffness, including those mediated by pharmaceuticals, body composition, and hemodynamic parameters.

4.1. Pharmacological Therapy and PWV

Our findings suggest that the use of CCB, moxonidine, and urapidil was associated with higher PWV. This observation is particularly interesting, as CCB are generally considered to reduce arterial stiffness through their vasodilatory effects and promote vascular remodeling and improve endothelial function [6,16]. However, it is possible that the prescription of CCB. in this cohort reflects a response to higher baseline arterial stiffness or more severe hypertension or isolated systolic hypertension in this multimorbid population rather than a direct causal relationship. The association with a centrally acting antihypertensive agent moxonidine may be confounded by its use in patients with difficult-to-control AH and CKD. A positive association was also seen between PWV and urapidil, an alpha-1 adrenoceptor antagonist with central sympatholytic effects. This link may have resulted from urapidil's use in patients who needed strong blood pressure control and had established vascular stiffness.

On the other hand, the use of SGLT-2i and statins appeared as significant negative predictors of PWV. SGLT-2i are known to offer multiple cardiorenal benefits and pleiotropic effects such as weight loss, improvement of hyperuricemia, or improvement in hepatic steatosis [17,18]. Its role in the reduction in arterial stiffness is thought to be by reducing BP, inflammation, and oxidative stress; decreasing endothelial cell activation; stimulating direct vasorelaxation; and ameliorating endothelial dysfunction or the expression of pro-atherogenic cells and molecules [18–20]. The negative association with PWV observed in our study adds to the growing body of evidence on SGLT-2i and vascular properties.

Statin prescription was also negatively associated with PWV in this study. Beyond their cholesterol-lowering effects, statins have been shown to exert pleiotropic effects, including anti-inflammatory and endothelial-protective actions, which may contribute to improved arterial stiffness [21]. A recent meta-analysis found that statins had a beneficial effect on aortic arterial stiffness [22]. A study on 5105 Chinese adults with high atherosclerotic risk showed statin use associated with slower progression of arterial stiffness [23]. These findings should be interpreted while keeping in mind the design of the study and sample size.

4.2. Anthropometric Parameters, Body Composition, and PWV

In further analysis, the anthropometric measures of height and weight and the body composition parameters VF level, FFM, and PMM were inversely associated with PWV. Vascular stiffness and body composition have a complicated and diverse interaction. A recent study found short body height significantly associated with increasing BP and PWV measures for central and peripheral arterial stiffness in Chinese adults which is consistent with our findings [24].

The negative association with VF is particularly interesting, as visceral adiposity is typically linked to adverse cardiovascular outcomes [25]. Obesity increases arterial stiffness due to endothelial dysfunction, impaired vascular smooth muscle cell function, IR, elevated cholesterol, C-peptide levels, fat distribution, adipose tissue-related renin-aldosterone-angiotensin system, and increased leptin levels [26]. A cross-sectional population study on 2819 participants who had their VF detected by abdominal CT scan, and PWV detected by brachial ankle PWV showed similar results to ours. They found a very weak inverse association between VF and PWV but only significant in women [27]. It is possible that this finding is a specificity of our population and reflects the interplay between other epigenetic factors such as sarcopenic obesity or perhaps it could be due to the use of SGLT2i or GLP-1RA which have favorable cardiometabolic effects.

The inverse correlation between PWV and both FFM and muscle mass, the indicators of lean body tissue, is consistent with the existing literature [28–30] and highlights the complex interplay between muscle mass and arterial stiffness. Arterial stiffness increases systolic BP and pulse pressure, causing muscle damage and reduced blood supply to the muscle, impairing nutrient supplementation, and leading to muscle death and reduced strength. IR, fat infiltration, inflammation, and oxidative stress contribute to arterial stiffness. Regular physical activity improves endothelial function, reduces oxidative stress, and improves muscle mass and strength, ultimately reducing aortic stiffness [30]. Also, sarcopenic obesity was found to be an even greater risk for arterial stiffness than sarcopenia or visceral obesity alone [31]. Maintaining lean body mass may thus serve as a protective factor against the development of arterial stiffness, which emphasizes the importance of promoting physical activity and resistance training in the treatment of AH.

4.3. Blood Pressure, Hemodynamic Parameters, and PWV

Out of BP and hemodynamic parameters, pSBP, cSBP, AIx@75, pMAP, and pPP were found to be the positive predictors of PWV while AIx@75 was found to be a negative predictor. AH and arterial stiffness are closely related, with each having a major impact on the other [32]. There is a reciprocal association between arterial stiffness and BP. The artery's ability to dilate and constrict in response to changes in BP diminishes as arterial stiffness rises. This decreased elasticity over time may cause pSBP and pPP to rise. This is due to the fact that stiffer arteries have a reduced capacity to expand [32,33].

However, HR was found to be a negative predictor of PWV in our population. On the contrary, in the results of the Corinthia study, HR and PWV show a significant association independent of any confounding variables but only in those individuals with elevated aortic stiffness [34]. The median heart rate in our study was 70/min but we did not assess the heart rate variability which could be a confounding factor.

4.4. Limitations

This study has several limitations that should be considered when interpreting the findings. The primary limitation is a cross-sectional study design which prevents us from drawing causal conclusions. Furthermore, physical activity was not assessed, which is an important factor in arterial stiffness progression and management. Also, given that the study was carried out at an outpatient clinic for AH in a tertiary facility, there is a possibility of recruitment bias as the patients referred typically to a tertiary facility have poorer disease history and risk profiles than those not referred there. Therefore, due to a referral bias, comorbidities and obesity may have an increased prevalence in the outpatient sample compared to general data. As a result, this analysis is specifically suited for the generally high-risk population with AH. These findings are to be noted in agreement with the earlier mentioned. To provide a deeper understanding of metabolic differences and their impact on FFM and PMM variations, including a more comprehensive set of biomarkers (e.g., laboratory indices such as lipid profile), should be a forte of future research.

5. Conclusions

The relationships between PWV and LM demonstrate the possible advantages of lifestyle modifications that enhance physical fitness and metabolic health. The results regarding pharmacotherapy, in particular the inverse relationship between arterial stiffness and SGLT-2i and statins, imply that these medications may have cardiovascular advantages apart from their primary indications.

Our research further emphasizes the importance of an individualized approach to managing arterial stiffness and AH. The variety of the PWV predictors highlights the importance of considering the unique characteristics of each patient as well as their biochemical, hemodynamic, and pharmacological profiles when creating a treatment plan. More prospective studies are needed to determine the causal relationships underlying these associations and to identify potential therapeutic targets for reducing arterial stiffness and improving BP control. Long-term trials are necessary to examine the possibility that the class-specific effects of antihypertensive medicines on PWV could improve over time and be linked to better long-term outcomes.

Furthermore, routine PWV measurement and body composition measurements should be considered in the management of AH in order to improve risk stratification and therapy decisions. Given the significance of PWV in prognosis, it is crucial to conduct further studies to ascertain if antihypertensive medications specifically reduce PWV or if their effects are merely the result of lowering BP, which dilates the artery wall.

Supplementary Materials: The following supporting information can be downloaded at: https://www.mdpi.com/article/10.3390/biomedicines12092062/s1, Table S1: General characteristics of studied population.; Table S2: Differences in the measured parameters regarding the age and blood pressure regulation.; Table S3: Predictors of pulse wave velocity in all study subjects (generalized linear regression model corrected for age, sex, presence of DM and CKD, and BP regulation).

Author Contributions: Conceptualization, J.R. and M.R.; methodology, J.R.; validation, M.R. and A.G.; formal analysis, A.G.; investigation, M.V. and J.R.; resources, M.R.; data curation, A.G. and H.Đ.; writing—original draft preparation, M.V., J.R., H.Đ. and A.B.; writing—review and editing, M.R., J.R., A.G., A.B. and M.V.; visualization, A.G.; supervision, M.R. and J.R.; project administration, M.R. and J.R.; funding acquisition, M.R. and J.R. All authors have read and agreed to the published version of the manuscript.

Funding: This research is funded by the project "Digitalization and improvement of nutritional care for patients with chronic diseases", co-financed by the European Regional Development Fund through the Operational Program "Competitiveness and Cohesion 2014–2020" KK.01.1.1.04.0115., through the acquisition of the devices used in data collection.

Institutional Review Board Statement: The study was conducted in accordance with the Declaration of Helsinki and approved by the Ethics Committee of the University Hospital of Split (Class 500-03/22-01/170, Ur.no. 500-03/23-01/84, date of approval 27 September 2022).

Informed Consent Statement: Informed consent was obtained from all the subjects involved in the study.

Data Availability Statement: The raw data supporting the conclusions of this article will be made available by the corresponding author upon reasonable request.

Acknowledgments: The authors give special thanks to Dora Bučan Nenadić and Ela Kolak for their contribution to technical and administrative support.

Conflicts of Interest: The authors declare no conflicts of interest.

References

1. Cooper, R.S.; Kaufman, J.S.; Bovet, P. Global Burden of Disease Attributable to Hypertension. *JAMA* **2017**, *317*, 2017–2018. [CrossRef]
2. Laurent, S.; Marais, L.; Boutouyrie, P. The Noninvasive Assessment of Vascular Aging. *Can. J. Cardiol.* **2016**, *32*, 669–679. [CrossRef] [PubMed]
3. Nilsson, P.M.; Laurent, S.; Cunha, P.G.; Olsen, M.H.; Rietzschel, E.; Franco, O.H.; Ryliškyte, L.; Strazhesko, I.; Vlachopoulos, C.; Chen, C.H.; et al. Characteristics of Healthy Vascular Ageing in Pooled Population-Based Cohort Studies: The Global Metabolic Syndrome and Artery Research Consortium. *J. Hypertens.* **2018**, *36*, 2340–2349. [CrossRef] [PubMed]
4. Boutouyrie, P.; Chowienczyk, P.; Humphrey, J.D.; Mitchell, G.F. Arterial Stiffness and Cardiovascular Risk in Hypertension. *Circ. Res.* **2021**, *128*, 864–886. [CrossRef] [PubMed]
5. Zheng, M.; Huo, Y.; Wang, X.; Xu, X.; Qin, X.; Tang, G.; Xing, H.; Fan, F.; Li, J.; Zhang, Y.; et al. A Prospective Study on Pulse Wave Velocity (PWV) and Response to Anti-Hypertensive Treatments: PWV Determines BP Control. *Int. J. Cardiol.* **2015**, *178*, 226–231. [CrossRef]
6. Cavero-Redondo, I.; Saz-Lara, A.; Lugones-Sánchez, C.; Pozuelo-Carrascosa, D.P.; Gómez-Sánchez, L.; López-Gil, J.F.; García-Ortiz, L.; Bruno, R.M.; Gómez-Marcos, M.Á. Comparative Effect of Antihypertensive Drugs in Improving Arterial Stiffness in Adults with Hypertension (RIGIPREV Study). A Network Meta-Analysis. *Front. Pharmacol.* **2023**, *14*, 1225795. [CrossRef]
7. Antonio-Villa, N.E.; Bello-Chavolla, O.Y.; Vargas-Vázquez, A.; Mehta, R.; Fermín-Martínez, C.A.; Martagón-Rosado, A.J.; Barquera-Guevara, D.A.; Aguilar-Salinas, C.A.; Arellano-Campos, O.; Gómez-Velasco, D.V.; et al. Increased Visceral Fat Accumulation Modifies the Effect of Insulin Resistance on Arterial Stiffness and Hypertension Risk. *Nutr. Metab. Cardiovasc. Dis.* **2021**, *31*, 506–517. [CrossRef]
8. Batzias, K.; Antonopoulos, A.S.; Oikonomou, E.; Siasos, G.; Bletsa, E.; Stampouloglou, P.K.; Mistakidi, C.V.; Noutsou, M.; Katsiki, N.; Karopoulos, P.; et al. Effects of Newer Antidiabetic Drugs on Endothelial Function and Arterial Stiffness: A Systematic Review and Meta-Analysis. *J. Diabetes Res.* **2018**, *2018*, 1232583. [CrossRef]
9. Hidalgo Santiago, J.C.; Maraver Delgado, J.; Cayón Blanco, M.; López Saez, J.B.; Gómez-Fernández, P. Effect of Dapagliflozin on Arterial Stiffness in Patients with Type 2 Diabetes Mellitus. *Med. Clin.* **2020**, *154*, 171–174. [CrossRef]
10. Sjöström, C.D.; Johansson, P.; Ptaszynska, A.; List, J.; Johnsson, E. Dapagliflozin Lowers Blood Pressure in Hypertensive and Non-Hypertensive Patients with Type 2 Diabetes. *Diab. Vasc. Dis. Res.* **2015**, *12*, 352–358. [CrossRef]
11. Hayashi, T.; Fukui, T.; Nakanishi, N.; Yamamoto, S.; Tomoyasu, M.; Osamura, A.; Ohara, M.; Yamamoto, T.; Ito, Y.; Hirano, T. Dapagliflozin Decreases Small Dense Low-Density Lipoprotein-Cholesterol and Increases High-Density Lipoprotein 2-Cholesterol in Patients with Type 2 Diabetes: Comparison with Sitagliptin. *Cardiovasc. Diabetol.* **2017**, *16*, 1–13. [CrossRef]
12. Rizos, E.C.; Tagkas, C.F.; Asimakopoulos, A.-G.I.; Tsimihodimos, V.; Anastasiou, G.; Rizzo, M.; Agouridis, A.P.; Ntzani, E.E. The Effect of SGLT2 Inhibitors and GLP1 Receptor Agonists on Arterial Stiffness: A Meta-Analysis of Randomized Controlled Trials. *J. Diabetes Complicat.* **2024**, *38*, 108781. [CrossRef] [PubMed]
13. Agbaje, A.O.; Barker, A.R.; Tuomainen, T.P. Cardiorespiratory Fitness, Fat Mass, and Cardiometabolic Health with Endothelial Function, Arterial Elasticity, and Stiffness. *Med. Sci. Sports Exerc.* **2022**, *54*, 141–152. [CrossRef] [PubMed]

14. IEM Mobil-O-Graph User Manual. Available online: https://medaval.ie/docs/manuals/IEM-Mobil-O-Graph-Manual.pdf (accessed on 30 January 2021).
15. R Core Team. *R: A Language and Environment for Statistical Computing*; R Foundation for Statistical Computing: Vienna, Austria, 2015.
16. Dudenbostel, T.; Glasser, S.P. Effects of Antihypertensive Drugs on Arterial Stiffness. *Cardiol. Rev.* **2012**, *20*, 259–263. [CrossRef] [PubMed]
17. Klug, E.; Rayner, B.; Wasserfall, M.; Kok, A.; Mpe, M.; Ruder, S.; Mohamed, N.; Webb, D. Cardiorenal Effects of SGLT2 Inhibitors: Who Might Benefit? *J. Endocrinol. Metab. Diabetes South Afr.* **2024**, *29*, 8–17. [CrossRef]
18. Adam, C.A.; Anghel, R.; Marcu, D.T.M.; Mitu, O.; Roca, M.; Mitu, F. Impact of Sodium–Glucose Cotransporter 2 (SGLT2) Inhibitors on Arterial Stiffness and Vascular Aging—What Do We Know So Far? (A Narrative Review). *Life* **2022**, *12*, 803. [CrossRef]
19. Lopaschuk, G.D.; Verma, S. Mechanisms of Cardiovascular Benefits of Sodium Glucose Co-Transporter 2 (SGLT2) Inhibitors: A State-of-the-Art Review. *JACC Basic Transl. Sci.* **2020**, *5*, 632–644. [CrossRef]
20. Liu, L.; Ni, Y.Q.; Zhan, J.K.; Liu, Y.S. The Role of Sglt2 Inhibitors in Vascular Aging. *Aging Dis.* **2021**, *12*, 1323–1336. [CrossRef]
21. Alidadi, M.; Montecucco, F.; Jamialahmadi, T.; Al-Rasadi, K.; Johnston, T.P.; Sahebkar, A. Beneficial Effect of Statin Therapy on Arterial Stiffness. *Biomed. Res. Int.* **2021**, *2021*, 5548310. [CrossRef]
22. Upala, S.; Wirunsawanya, K.; Jaruvongvanich, V.; Sanguankeo, A. Effects of Statin Therapy on Arterial Stiffness: A Systematic Review and Meta Analysis of Randomized Controlled Trial. *Int. J. Cardiol.* **2017**, *227*, 338–341. [CrossRef]
23. Zhou, Y.F.; Wang, Y.; Wang, G.; Zhou, Z.; Chen, S.; Geng, T.; Zhang, Y.B.; Wang, Y.; Chen, J.X.; Pan, A.; et al. Association between Statin Use and Progression of Arterial Stiffness among Adults with High Atherosclerotic Risk. *JAMA Netw. Open* **2022**, *5*, e2218323. [CrossRef] [PubMed]
24. Qiu, Q.; Meng, X.; Li, Y.; Liu, X.; Teng, F.; Wang, Y.; Zang, X.; Wang, Y.; Liang, J. Evaluation of the Associations of Body Height with Blood Pressure and Early-Stage Atherosclerosis in Chinese Adults. *J. Clin. Hypertens.* **2020**, *22*, 1018–1024. [CrossRef] [PubMed]
25. Huang, Y.; Hu, Y.; Bao, B. Relationship of Body Mass Index and Visceral Fat Area Combination with Arterial Stiffness and Cardiovascular Risk in Cardiovascular Disease-Free People: NHANES (2011–2018). *Endocr. Connect.* **2023**, *12*, e230291. [CrossRef] [PubMed]
26. Seifalian, A.; Filippatos, T.; Joshi, J.; Mikhailidis, D. Obesity and Arterial Compliance Alterations. *Curr. Vasc. Pharmacol.* **2010**, *8*, 155–168. [CrossRef] [PubMed]
27. Ishida, A.; Taira, H.; Shinzato, T.; Ohya, Y. Association between Visceral Fat Mass and Arterial Stiffness among Community-Based Screening Participants. *Hypertens. Res.* **2023**, *46*, 2488–2496. [CrossRef]
28. Rodríguez, A.J.; Karim, M.N.; Srikanth, V.; Ebeling, P.R.; Scott, D. Lower Muscle Tissue Is Associated with Higher Pulse Wave Velocity: A Systematic Review and Meta-Analysis of Observational Study Data. *Clin. Exp. Pharmacol. Physiol.* **2017**, *44*, 980–992. [CrossRef]
29. Dvoretskiy, S.; Lieblein-Boff, J.C.; Jonnalagadda, S.; Atherton, P.J.; Phillips, B.E.; Pereira, S.L. Exploring the Association between Vascular Dysfunction and Skeletal Muscle Mass, Strength and Function in Healthy Adults: A Systematic Review. *Nutrients* **2020**, *12*, 715. [CrossRef]
30. Aminuddin, A.; Noor Hashim, M.F.; Mohd Zaberi, N.A.S.; Zheng Wei, L.; Ching Chu, B.; Jamaludin, N.A.; Salamt, N.; Che Roos, N.A.; Ugusman, A. The Association between Arterial Stiffness and Muscle Indices among Healthy Subjects and Subjects With Cardiovascular Risk Factors: An Evidence-Based Review. *Front. Physiol.* **2021**, *12*, 742338. [CrossRef]
31. Ohara, M.; Kohara, K.; Tabara, Y.; Ochi, M.; Nagai, T.; Igase, M.; Miki, T. Sarcopenic Obesity and Arterial Stiffness, Pressure Wave Reflection and Central Pulse Pressure: The J-SHIPP Study. *Int. J. Cardiol.* **2014**, *174*, 214–217. [CrossRef]
32. Kim, H.L. Arterial Stiffness and Hypertension. *Clin. Hypertens.* **2023**, *29*, 31. [CrossRef]
33. O'Rourke, M.F.; Hashimoto, J. Mechanical Factors in Arterial Aging. A Clinical Perspective. *J. Am. Coll. Cardiol.* **2007**, *50*, 1–13. [CrossRef] [PubMed]
34. Papaioannou, T.G.; Oikonomou, E.; Lazaros, G.; Christoforatou, E.; Vogiatzi, G.; Tsalamandris, S.; Chasikidis, C.; Kalambogias, A.; Mystakidi, V.X.; Galiatsatos, N.; et al. The Influence of Resting Heart Rate on Pulse Wave Velocity Measurement Is Mediated by Blood Pressure and Depends on Aortic Stiffness Levels: Insights from the Corinthia Study. *Physiol. Meas.* **2019**, *40*, 055005. [CrossRef] [PubMed]

biomedicines

MDPI

Article

The Association of Metformin, Other Antidiabetic Medications, and Statins with the Prognosis of Hepatocellular Carcinoma in Patients with Type 2 Diabetes: A Retrospective Cohort Study

Iida Tuunanen [1,2,3], Ari Hautakoski [2,3], Heikki Huhtamäki [4], Martti Arffman [5], Reijo Sund [6], Ulla Puistola [1,2,3], Peeter Karihtala [7], Arja Jukkola [8] and Elina Urpilainen [1,2,3,*]

1 Department of Obstetrics and Gynecology, Oulu University Hospital, Wellbeing Services County of North Ostrobothnia, University of Oulu, 90220 Oulu, Finland
2 Research Unit of Clinical Medicine, University of Oulu, 90220 Oulu, Finland
3 Medical Research Center, Oulu University Hospital, Wellbeing Services County of North Ostrobothnia, University of Oulu, 90220 Oulu, Finland
4 Research Unit of Mathematical Sciences, Faculty of Science, University of Oulu, 90014 Oulu, Finland
5 Department of Public Health and Welfare, Finnish Institute for Health and Welfare, 00271 Helsinki, Finland
6 Institute of Clinical Medicine, University of Eastern Finland, 70029 Kuopio, Finland
7 Department of Oncology, University of Helsinki, Helsinki University Hospital Comprehensive Cancer Center, 00029 Helsinki, Finland
8 Department of Oncology and Radiotherapy, Tays Cancer Center, Tampere University Hospital, Faculty of Medicine and Health Technology, Tampere University, 33521 Tampere, Finland; arja.jukkola@tuni.fi
* Correspondence: elina.urpilainen@gmail.com

Abstract: This study aimed to explore whether the prediagnostic use of metformin and statins is associated with the prognosis of patients with hepatocellular carcinoma (HCC) and type 2 diabetes. We identified 1383 eligible individuals who had both type 2 diabetes and HCC diagnosed between 1998 and 2017 from several Finnish registers. Cox models were fitted for cause-specific and all-cause mortality in relation to the use of antidiabetic medications and statins prior to the HCC diagnosis. Prediagnostic metformin use was associated with decreased overall mortality (hazard ratio 0.84, 95% confidence interval 0.74–0.94) compared with nonuse in patients with type 2 diabetes. Similarly, slightly decreased HCC mortality and other-cause mortality were observed among metformin users. The results were inconclusive regarding metformin use and both overall and HCC mortality among patients with localized HCC. No discernible contrast between statin users and nonusers was found in overall mortality nor HCC mortality in either the whole cohort or patients with localized cancer.

Keywords: diabetes mellitus; epidemiology; liver neoplasms; malignancy; mortality

1. Introduction

Liver cancer is the sixth most commonly diagnosed cancer worldwide, with 866,136 new cases reported in 2022 [1]. It ranked as the third-highest cause of cancer deaths in the same year with 758,725 deaths [1]. According to the Finnish Cancer Registry, there were 513 new cases of liver cancer in Finland in 2022 [2]. The most common type of primary liver cancer is hepatocellular carcinoma (HCC), amounting to approximately 90% of all cases [3]. A major risk factor for HCC is perpetual infection with the hepatitis B or C virus and alcohol abuse [4,5]. Particularly in developed countries, nonalcoholic fatty liver disease and nonalcoholic steatohepatitis may soon replace alcohol- and viral-related liver diseases as the major risk factors for HCC. Nonalcoholic fatty liver disease develops due to metabolic syndrome, which is strongly associated with obesity, dyslipidemia, hypertension, and type 2 diabetes (T2D) [6].

HCC patients with T2D have a lower overall survival (OS) rate and increased mortality compared to HCC patients without T2D [7–10]. Some recent meta-analyses indicate that first-line T2D treatment with metformin is associated with prolonged OS after curative treatments for HCC in both Caucasian and Asian populations [11,12].

People with T2D are often administered statins as the primary prevention of cardiovascular disease and due to diabetes-associated cardiovascular disease [13]. In Finland, 46% of the patients diagnosed with diabetes use lipid-lowering medication within 6–12 months after their T2D diagnosis [14]. Statin use is associated with a reduced risk of HCC, reduced all-cause mortality in the patients with HCC, decreased recurrence of HCC, and reduced incidence of HCC in people with T2D [15–17]. The effect of statin use on the HCC-specific survival of people with T2D has not been widely investigated, but in Antwi et al.'s [18] study, neither pre- nor postdiagnostic statin use had an association with the OS of HCC patients.

As the previous results on this topic have been variable and mostly lacked information on the drug dose and consumption time, this study aimed to evaluate whether the prediagnostic use of metformin, other antidiabetic medications (ADMs), or statins are associated with better overall and cause-specific survival in HCC patients with T2D by using a robust study design and data from multiple high-quality Finnish national registers.

2. Materials and Methods

2.1. Data Sources

In this study, we complied with the Strengthening the Reporting of Observational Studies in Epidemiology guidelines [19]. The data source comprising persons diagnosed with diabetes was the "Diabetes in Finland" (FinDM) database, which was originally generated to make the nationwide epidemiological monitoring of diabetes in Finland possible [20]. Data from numerous registers are included: the Special Reimbursement Register and the Prescription Register from the Social Insurance Institution of Finland, the Care Register for Health and the Hospital Discharge Register from the Finnish Institute for Health and Welfare, and the cause of death statistics from Statistics Finland (Table S1). The Prescription Register provides systematic records of the drugs purchased since 1994, as it incorporates data about the medications prescribed by doctors and reimbursed by the Social Insurance Institution of Finland. In the FinDM database, the onset of diabetes is defined as the first entry regarding diabetes in the aforementioned registers. Individuals with diabetes were classified into type 1 and type 2 based on information on their diagnoses, medication, and age in the first year following the recorded onset of diabetes. The database shows good coverage against a local register in Southern Finland, according to data reliability studies [21].

Data on HCC cases were acquired from the Finnish Cancer Registry, which is linked to the FinDM database. The Finnish Cancer Registry incorporates information on the cancer cases diagnosed since 1953 in Finland, including the date of diagnosis, morphology, histology, and stage [22]. Follow-up data, including causes of death and dates, were obtained from the cause of death statistics, from which the coding experts of the Finnish Cancer Registry further determined the cancer specificity by examining the cause of death records together with other data on the cancer in question.

2.2. Study Population

The cohort formation process is presented in the flowchart below (Figure 1). We identified 2402 people with T2D and HCC. The individuals with T2D who were diagnosed before their 40th birthday were excluded. Furthermore, we excluded the individuals with HCC who were diagnosed before 1998, those with other previous cancer diagnoses (except nonmelanoma skin cancer), and the HCC cases that were diagnosed at autopsy. In addition, those individuals with T2D who were diagnosed less than 365 days before their HCC diagnosis were excluded to avoid reverse causality and immortal time bias as well as to enable the collection of sufficient medication data from before the HCC diagnosis. Follow-up began on the date of the HCC diagnosis. The final cohort consisted of 1383 people who had both type 2 diabetes and HCC diagnosed between 1998 and 2017.

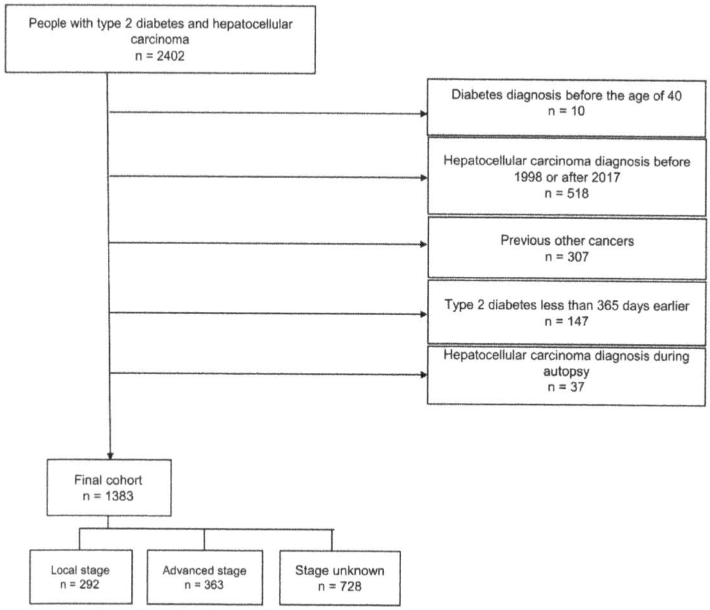

Figure 1. Flowchart of the cohort selection process.

The education levels of the study participants were divided into three categories (basic, intermediate, and higher) based on the most advanced grade or degree achieved by an individual. Basic education refers to a person who has graduated only from obligatory comprehensive schooling, which compromises nine grades. Intermediate education refers to a person who has graduated from upper secondary education, which includes three years of study in a general upper secondary school or in vocational education. Higher education refers to a person who has graduated from a university or a university of applied sciences.

The presence of hepatitis or cirrhosis were identified based on register data which were coded using the *International Classification of Diseases* versions 8, 9, and 10 (Table S2).

2.3. Classification of Medication

ADM use in the cohort was categorized into (1) metformin users and nonusers, (2) insulin users and nonusers, and (3) other ADM users and nonusers. The cohort was also categorized into statin users and nonusers, regardless of the ADM type used. The criterion for statin, metformin, insulin, and other ADM use was the purchase of the medication for a minimum of 180 days within three years before the HCC diagnosis, which guarantees a continuous use of medication. A nonuser was defined as making a statin or an ADM purchase less than 180 days prior to their diagnosis, or not all. A person using multiple medications could be categorized into more than one medication user group. Cumulative medication use was considered by determining the defined daily doses (DDDs) for three years prior to the HCC diagnosis. HCC was defined using the diagnosis code C22.0 of the *International Statistical Classification of Diseases and Related Health Problems* (10th revision) and the *International Classification of Diseases for Oncology* (third edition), as well as the morphology code M8170/3 (HCC, not otherwise specified).

2.4. Staging

The HCC stage was defined based on the Finnish Cancer Registry classification. The stage of HCC at diagnosis is categorized in the Finnish Cancer Registry as follows: (0) unknown; (1) localized; (2) nonlocalized, only regional lymph node metastases; (3) metastasized or an invasion of adjacent tissues; (4) nonlocalized, no information on extent; (5) locally advanced, an invasion of adjacent tissues; and (6) nonlocalized, also distant lymph node metastases. Based on these data, we categorized the stages in our study as local (1), advanced (2–6), and unknown (0).

2.5. Statistical Methods

The follow-up started on the date of the HCC diagnosis and ended on the date of death, emigration, or closure of the follow-up on 31 December 2017. The cumulative mortality from HCC and from other causes of death in the prediagnostic ADM and statin groups was calculated using the Aalen–Johansen estimator of the cumulative incidence function for competing risks. Cause-specific mortality rates were analyzed using Cox proportional hazard models to obtain estimated hazard ratios (HRs) with 95% confidence intervals (CIs), adjusting for the confounding effects of the patients' age, year of diagnosis, duration of diabetes, and HCC stage. A possible nonlinear dose-dependent effect of the medications was assessed by replacing the medication group indicators in the Cox models with cubic spline terms for the average amount of DDDs per day in different medication groups. These models were fitted for patients with all stages of HCC as well as for patients with localized HCC.

The data obtained from the registers were prepared and analyzed using SAS (version 9.4) and R (version 4.0.5). All of the statistical analyses were performed in the R environment. The functions in the "survival" package of R functions were used to compute the Aalen–Johansen estimators of cumulative mortality by cause to fit the Cox models and to diagnose possible deviations from the assumptions of the underlying model. The Schoenfield residuals against the transformed time as well as the cloglog figures were visually inspected to verify that the proportionality assumptions of the Cox regression model were met. Missing data were encountered only concerning the HCC stage, and we labeled these cases as "unknown".

3. Results

3.1. Analysis of the Whole Cohort

A total of 1383 HCC cases were collected, with a median follow-up time of 0.4 years and an interquartile range of 0.08 to 1.3 years (Table 1). Most of the HCC cases were diagnosed when patients were between the ages of 65 and 74 years, with a median age of 72 years (Table S3). The majority of the study population was male (n = 1109, 80%). Two hundred and ninety-two patients (21%) were recorded as local and three hundred and sixty-three (26%) as advanced. In the remaining 728 patients (53%), the stage was unknown.

When comparing the 885 metformin users to the 498 nonusers, the former had a longer diabetes duration at HCC diagnosis, with a median of 9.9 years compared to 9.0 years in the nonusers (Table 1). The most commonly used other ADMs were sulfonylureas (71%) and dipeptidyl peptidase-4 inhibitors (29%) (Table S4). Within the metformin user group, 35% of patients also used insulin; in the metformin nonuser group, 44% used insulin. Similarly, within the metformin user group, 44% used statins, and among metformin nonusers, 27% used statins.

The 529 statin users in the study cohort had a longer median diabetes duration (11.4 years) than statin nonusers (8.6 years) (Table 1). The most commonly used statins were simvastatin (72%) and atorvastatin (23%) (Table S4).

During follow-up, 1210 deaths occurred in the cohort, with 1025 deaths due to HCC. Through the analysis of all the stages, evidence was found for an association with decreased overall mortality among prediagnostic metformin users (HR 0.84, 95% CI 0.74–0.94) compared to metformin nonusers. Similarly, slightly decreased HCC mortality (HR 0.86, 95% CI 0.75–0.99) and other-cause mortality (HR 0.71 95% CI 0.53–0.97) were observed among metformin users. For both overall mortality and HCC mortality, the results were inconclusive for insulin use and other ADM use (Table 2). The estimation results were adjusted for the patients' sex, level of education, duration of diabetes, and presence of hepatitis and cirrhosis, as well as for the year of and age at the HCC diagnosis and the HCC stage (Table S5).

Table 1. Patient characteristics of the whole cohort according to antidiabetic medication and statin use.

	Metformin		Insulin		Other ADM		Statin		
	Yes (%)	No (%)	Yes (%)	No (%)	Yes (%)	No (%)	Yes (%)	No (%)	Total (%)
Total	885 (100)	498 (100)	533 (100)	850 (100)	749 (100)	634 (100)	529 (100)	854 (100)	1383 (100)
Sex									
Male	733 (83)	376 (76)	426 (80)	683 (80)	598 (80)	511 (81)	435 (82)	674 (79)	1109 (80)
Female	152 (17)	122 (24)	107 (20)	167 (20)	151 (20)	123 (19)	94 (18)	180 (21)	274 (20)
Education									
Basic	275 (31)	149 (30)	178 (33)	246 (29)	235 (31)	189 (30)	168 (32)	256 (30)	424 (31)
Intermediate	338 (38)	207 (42)	206 (39)	339 (40)	281 (38)	264 (42)	213 (40)	332 (39)	545 (39)
Higher	272 (31)	142 (29)	149 (28)	265 (31)	233 (31)	181 (29)	148 (28)	266 (31)	414 (30)
Follow-up time (years)									
Median	0.5	0.3	0.4	0.4	0.4	0.4	0.5	0.3	0.4
Interquartile range	0.1–1.5	0.04–1.0	0.07–1.2	0.09–1.3	0.08–1.3	0.09–1.2	0.1–1.4	0.06–1.2	0.08–1.3
Duration of diabetes (years)									
Median	9.9	9.0	13.7	7.7	10.4	8.5	11.4	8.6	9.6
Interquartile range	6.1–14.9	5.1–15.9	9.1–18.1	4.4–11.7	6.9–15.2	4.3–15.2	7.2–16.7	5.0–13.5	5.6–15.2
Hepatitis									
Yes	55 (6)	48 (10)	47 (9)	56 (7)	50 (7)	53 (8)	34 (6)	69 (8)	103 (7)
No	830 (94)	450 (90)	486 (91)	794 (93)	699 (93)	581 (92)	495 (94)	785 (92)	1280 (93)
Cirrhosis									
Yes	190 (21)	144 (29)	152 (29)	182 (21)	170 (23)	164 (26)	91 (17)	243 (28)	334 (24)
No	695 (79)	354 (71)	381 (71)	668 (79)	579 (77)	470 (74)	438 (83)	611 (72)	1049 (76)
Age at HCC diagnosis (years)									
Median	71	72	71	72	72	71	72	71	72
Interquartile range	66–78	65–80	65–77	66–79	66–79	65–78	67–78	65–78	66–78
Stage of HCC									
Local	173 (20)	119 (24)	105 (20)	187 (22)	167 (22)	125 (20)	97 (18)	195 (23)	292 (21)
Advanced	228 (26)	135 (27)	153 (29)	210 (25)	204 (27)	159 (25)	122 (23)	241 (28)	363 (26)
Unknown	484 (55)	244 (49)	275 (52)	453 (53)	378 (50)	350 (55)	310 (59)	418 (49)	728 (53)

ADM = antidiabetic medication, HCC = hepatocellular carcinoma.

Table 2. Estimation results from Cox proportional hazard models of mortality from all causes, HCC, and other causes in the whole cohort, adjusted for sex, education, duration of diabetes, and the presence of hepatitis and cirrhosis, as well as year of and age at HCC diagnosis and HCC stage.

	Overall Mortality			HCC Mortality			Other-Cause Mortality		
	HR	95% CI	*n*	HR	95% CI	*n*	HR	95% CI	*n*
Prediagnostic metformin use									
Yes	0.84	(0.74–0.94)	762	0.86	(0.75–0.99)	660	0.71	(0.53–0.97)	102
No	1.00	Ref.	448	1.00	Ref.	365	1.00	Ref.	83
Prediagnostic other ADM use									
Yes	0.99	(0.88–1.11)	664	0.97	(0.85–1.11)	558	1.04	(0.76–1.42)	106
No	1.00	Ref.	546	1.00	Ref.	467	1.00	Ref.	79
Prediagnostic insulin use									
Yes	1.00	(0.88–1.14)	468	0.99	(0.86–1.14)	397	1.09	(0.78–1.52)	71
No	1.00	Ref.	742	1.00	Ref.	628	1.00	Ref.	114
Prediagnostic statin use									
Yes	0.91	(0.80–1.04)	444	0.91	(0.80–1.05)	384	0.88	(0.62–1.23)	60
No	1.00	Ref.	766	1.00	Ref.	641	1.00	Ref.	125

ADM = antidiabetic medication, HCC = hepatocellular carcinoma, HR = hazard ratio, CI = confidence interval.

The five-year cumulative overall mortality was 93% in metformin users and 95% in nonusers (Figure 2A). Regarding HCC-specific mortality, these proportions were 81% and 77% in metformin users and nonusers, respectively (Figure 2B). The five-year cumulative mortality from other causes was 12% for metformin users and 18% for nonusers (Figure 2C).

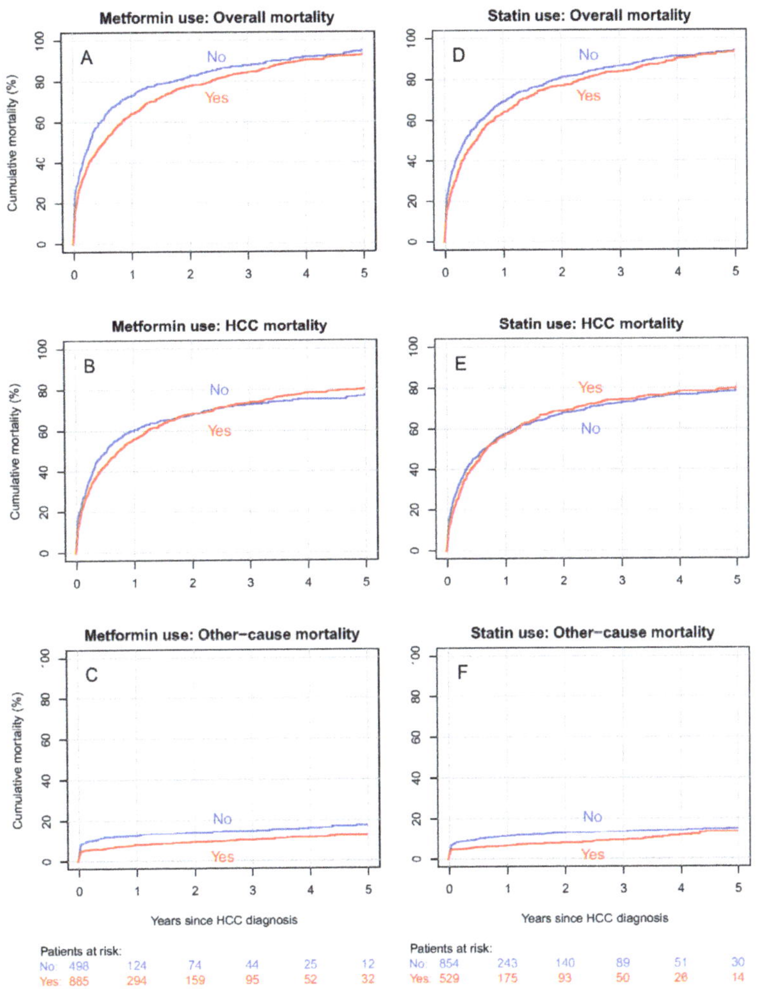

Figure 2. Cumulative overall, hepatocellular carcinoma (HCC) and other-cause mortality curves for the whole cohort according to metformin (**A–C**) and statin (**D–F**) use. Curves (**A**,**D**) represent overall mortality, curves (**B**) and E HCC mortality, and curves (**C**,**F**) other-cause mortality.

No discernible contrast between statin users and nonusers was found in either overall mortality (HR 0.91, 95% CI 0.80–1.04) nor HCC mortality (HR 0.91, 95% CI 0.80–1.05) (Table 2).

The five-year cumulative overall mortality was 94% in the statin user group as well as in the nonuser group (Figure 2D). Furthermore, no significant differences were found in cumulative HCC mortality or mortality from other causes (Figure 2E,F). The DDD analysis indicated no association between the cumulative amount of any medication used and overall (Figure S1) nor HCC mortality.

3.2. Analysis of the Patients with Localized HCC

In the subgroup of patients with localized HCC ($n = 292$) the median follow-up time was 0.7 years, and the interquartile range was 0.1 to 2.7 years (Table 3). Most of the local HCC cases were diagnosed when patients were between the ages of 65 and 74 years, with a median age of 71 years (Table S6).

Table 3. Characteristics of patients with localized tumors according to antidiabetic medication and statin use.

	Metformin		Insulin		Other ADM		Statin		
	Yes (%)	**No (%)**	**Yes (%)**	**No (%)**	**Yes (%)**	**No (%)**	**Yes (%)**	**No (%)**	**Total (%)**
Total	173 (100)	119 (100)	105 (100)	187 (100)	167 (100)	125 (100)	97 (100)	195 (100)	292 (100)
Sex									
Male	143 (83)	92 (77)	79 (75)	156 (83)	139 (83)	96 (77)	78 (80)	157 (81)	235 (80)
Female	30 (17)	27 (23)	26 (25)	31 (17)	28 (17)	29 (23)	19 (20)	38 (19)	57 (20)
Education									
Basic	56 (32)	28 (24)	34 (32)	50 (27)	51 (31)	33 (26)	26 (27)	58 (30)	84 (29)
Intermediate	62 (36)	49 (41)	39 (37)	72 (39)	65 (39)	46 (37)	48 (49)	63 (32)	111 (38)
Higher	55 (32)	42 (35)	32 (30)	65 (35)	51 (31)	46 (37)	23 (24)	74 (38)	97 (33)
Follow-up time (years)									
Median	0.8	0.6	0.6	0.8	0.8	0.7	0.6	0.7	0.7
Interquartile range	0.1–2.9	0.08–2.4	0.06–2.5	0.2–2.7	0.2–2.9	0.08–2.0	0.1–2.5	0.1–2.8	0.1–2.7
Duration of diabetes (years)									
Median	9.6	9.5	12.3	7.8	9.8	8.1	10.2	9.3	9.6
Interquartile range	5.3–13.9	6.0–16.0	8.2–16.9	4.6–12.3	6.8–13.9	3.7–15.8	5.9–15.7	5.3–14.2	5.3–14.9
Hepatitis									
Yes	12 (7)	7 (6)	9 (9)	10 (5)	8 (5)	11 (9)	8 (8)	11 (6)	19 (7)
No	161 (93)	112 (94)	96 (91)	177 (95)	159 (95)	114 (91)	89 (92)	184 (94)	273 (93)
Cirrhosis									
Yes	41 (24)	31 (26)	29 (28)	43 (23)	43 (26)	29 (23)	22 (23)	50 (26)	72 (25)
No	132 (76)	88 (74)	76 (72)	144 (77)	124 (74)	96 (77)	75 (77)	145 (74)	220 (75)
Age at HCC diagnosis (years)									
Median	71	72	70	72	72	70	73	70	71
Interquartile range	65–77	64–80	63–77	65–79	66–79	63–77	66–79	63–78	65–78

ADM = antidiabetic medication, HCC = hepatocellular carcinoma.

There were 173 metformin users in the local HCC group, with a median diabetes duration of 9.6 years. Metformin users had a median follow-up time of 0.8 years. When comparing the metformin users with the nonusers, metformin nonusers had a shorter follow-up time of 0.6 years, but between the two groups there were no remarkable differences in diabetes duration (Table 3).

Statin users with localized HCC (n = 97) had a median diabetes duration of 10.2 years and a median follow-up time of 0.6 years. In the 195 statin nonusers, the median diabetes duration was 9.3 years and the median follow-up time 0.7 years (Table 3).

During the follow-up of patients with localized HCC, 269 deaths occurred, with 207 deaths due to HCC. In this subgroup, the results were inconclusive due to the small number of cases between metformin use and overall mortality (HR 0.96, 95% CI 0.74–1.24), as well as metformin use and HCC mortality (HR 1.03, 95% CI 0.77–1.39) (Table 4). The estimation results were adjusted for the patients' sex, level of education, duration of diabetes, and presence of hepatitis and cirrhosis, as well as the year of and age at the HCC diagnosis and the HCC stage (Table S7).

In the local subgroup, the five-year cumulative overall mortality was 89% in metformin users and 91% in nonusers (Figure 3A). The cumulative HCC mortality was 70% in metformin users and 68% in nonusers (Figure 3B), and the cumulative mortality from other causes was 19% in metformin users and 23% in nonusers (Figure 3C).

The results were inconclusive in terms of statin use and both overall mortality (HR 0.92, 95% CI 0.69–1.23) and HCC mortality (HR 0.87, 95% CI 0.62–1.20) in the local subgroup (Table 4). The estimation results were adjusted for the patients' sex, level of education, duration of diabetes, and presence of hepatitis and cirrhosis, as well as the year of and age at the HCC diagnosis and the HCC stage (Table S6).

In statin users with localized stage HCC, the five-year cumulative overall mortality was 92%, and 89% in nonusers (Figure 3D). The cumulative HCC mortality was 68% in statin users and 70% in nonusers (Figure 3E). Cumulative mortality from other causes was 24% in statin users and 19% in nonusers (Figure 3F). The DDD analysis indicated no association between the cumulative amount of any medication used and the prognosis of localized HCC (Figure S2).

Table 4. Estimation results from Cox proportional hazard models of mortality from all causes, HCC, and other causes in the local subgroup adjusted for sex, education, duration of diabetes and the presence of hepatitis and cirrhosis, as well as year of and age at HCC diagnosis and HCC stage.

	Overall Mortality			HCC Mortality			Other-Cause Mortality		
	HR	95% CI	*n*	HR	95% CI	*n*	HR	95% CI	*n*
Prediagnostic metformin use									
Yes	0.96	(0.74–1.24)	159	1.03	(0.77–1.39)	125	0.78	(0.46–1.31)	34
No	1.00	Ref.	110	1.00	Ref.	82	1.00	Ref.	28
Prediagnostic other ADM use									
Yes	0.84	(0.63–1.11)	157	0.75	(0.55–1.04)	115	1.16	(0.63–2.12)	42
No	1.00	Ref.	112	1.00	Ref.	92	1.00	Ref.	20
Prediagnostic insulin use									
Yes	0.92	(0.69–1.23)	95	0.85	(0.61–1.18)	72	1.19	(0.66–2.16)	23
No	1.00	Ref.	174	1.00	Ref.	135	1.00	Ref.	39
Prediagnostic statin use									
Yes	0.92	(0.69–1.23)	88	0.87	(0.62–1.20)	65	1.03	(0.57–1.85)	23
No	1.00	Ref.	181	1.00	Ref.	142	1.00	Ref.	39

ADM = antidiabetic medication, HCC = hepatocellular carcinoma, HR = hazard ratio, CI = confidence interval.

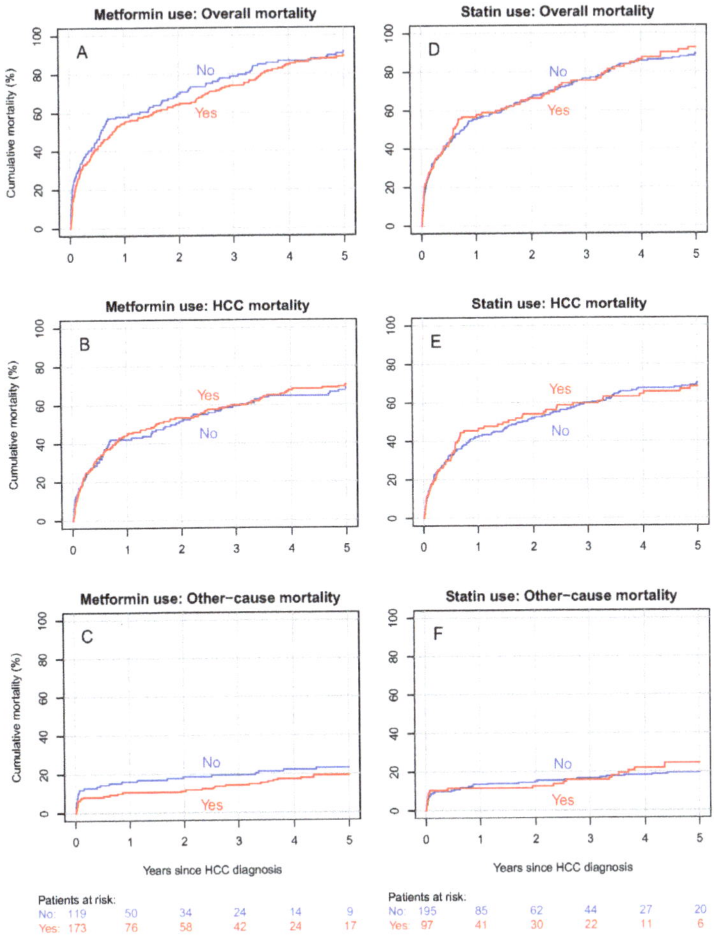

Figure 3. Cumulative overall, HCC, and other-cause mortality curves for the subgroup of patients with local HCC according to metformin (**A–C**) and statin (**D–F**) use. Curves (**A**,**D**) represent overall mortality, curves (**B**) and E HCC mortality, and curves (**C**,**F**) other-cause mortality.

4. Discussion

In this study, prediagnostic metformin use seemed to have an association with decreased overall mortality in patients with HCC and T2D. However, in a subgroup of patients with localized HCC, the results were inconclusive between metformin use and both overall and HCC mortality. In terms of prediagnostic statin use, no discernible contrast between users and nonusers was found in either group in terms of overall mortality nor HCC mortality.

The mechanisms underlying the possible antitumor effects of metformin are of great interest. Through direct activation of adenosine monophosphate-activated protein kinase, metformin can activate p53 and thus stop the cell cycle (Figure 4). In addition, the indirect activation of this protein kinase also decreases the activity of mTOR, which has an influence on protein synthesis and cell growth [23]. In HCC, metformin has been reported to inhibit invasion and growth and activate apoptosis and autophagy [24].

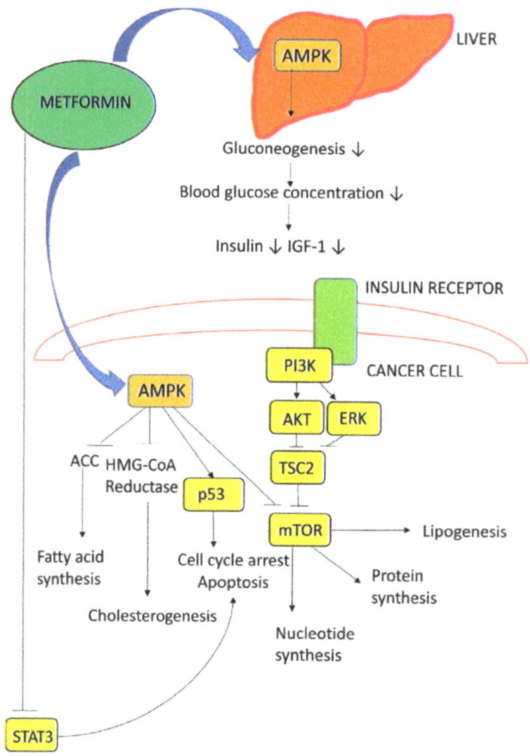

Figure 4. Metformin has both direct and indirect effects on cancer cells. It activates AMP-activated protein kinase (AMPK), leading to the inhibition of the mammalian target of rapamycin (mTOR). It also sensitizes tissues to insulin, reduces hepatic gluconeogenesis, and decreases circulating insulin levels. This leads indirectly to reduced phosphatidylinositol-3-kinase (PI3K) signaling. IGF-1 = insulin-like growth factor 1, ACC = acetyl-CoA carboxylase, HMG-CoA = 3-hydroxy-3-methyl-glutarylcoenzyme A, p53 = tumor protein p53, AKT = serine/threonine-specific protein kinase, and STAT3 = signal transducer and activator of transcription 3, ↓ decreasing effect, ⊥ inhibitory effect [25,26].

According to our analysis of the whole cohort and all of the HCC stages, metformin use seemed to be associated with decreased overall mortality and thus prolonged OS. This finding is in line with a previous meta-analysis in which, with limited knowledge of the HCC stage, metformin use was associated with decreased all-cause mortality and recurrence-free survival in patients with HCC [11]. However, the analysis did not consist of study populations of patients with diabetes only, and there was limited information on the metformin dose and consumption time. According to another meta-analysis of eight retrospective cohort studies, the survival of noncuratively treated advanced-stage HCC patients with T2D was not more strongly associated with metformin use compared to the use of other ADMs [12].

In our study, in a subgroup of patients with localized HCC, the results were inconclusive between metformin use and both overall and HCC mortality. However, in a meta-analysis, Zhou et al. [12] found that after curative treatment of HCC, metformin use had an association with longer OS and recurrence-free survival compared to the use of other ADMs. However, this meta-analysis did not comprise study populations of patients with diabetes alone. Another retrospective cohort study also found that metformin use was associated with decreased HCC-specific mortality after curative HCC treatment in patients with T2D [27]. In addition, in a systematic review, metformin use was associated with prolonged OS and a decreased HCC recurrence rate in patients with T2D after curative HCC therapy [28].

Regarding statin use, an experimental study in a HCC model reported that statins might prolong the survival of animals with HCC [29]. The underlying mechanisms may be linked to statins activating G1/S cell cycle arrest and inducing apoptosis [30], as well as inhibiting the P13K-AKT-mTOR pathway, which is commonly activated in HCC [31] (Figure 5).

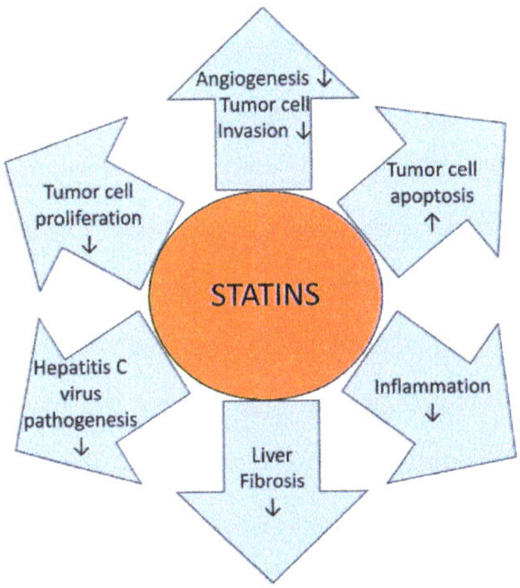

Figure 5. Statins may have multiple antitumoral mechanisms in hepatocellular carcinoma. Statins seems to increase tumor cell apoptosis as well as decrease both tumor cell invasion and proliferation. Additionally, statins decrease angiogenesis, inflammation, liver fibrosis, and hepatitis C virus pathogenesis. ↓ decreasing effect, ↑ increasing effect [32].

In terms of prediagnostic statin use, no discernible contrast between users and nonusers was found in the overall mortality nor HCC mortality in patients with T2D. Therefore, this finding is in line with a previous study that found no association between pre- and postdiagnostic statin use and the OS of elderly HCC patients with T2D [18]. According to our knowledge, the association between statin use and HCC survival in people with T2D has not been widely investigated. In a recent meta-analysis of HCC patients in which diabetes was not taken into account, statin use was associated with decreases in all-cause mortality in HCC patients, HCC-related mortality, and in addition, HCC recurrence after curative treatments [15]. Another recent meta-analysis of HCC patients in general demonstrated an association between statin use and decreased all-cause mortality, but not HCC-related mortality [16].

In our study, the DDD analysis indicated no association with the HCC prognosis. A previous retrospective cohort study found an association between the prediagnostic use of metformin with a dose $\leq$ 1500 mg/day and a decreased risk of death [18]. A null association with OS was found for prediagnostic metformin use with a dose > 1500 mg/day and for postdiagnostic metformin use. However, the study was based only on the data of patients aged 65 years and older [18].

The strengths of our study are the high-quality registers used and the study design, which has a minimal risk of biases. The data in the Finnish registers, such as the Hospital Discharge Register and the Finnish Cancer Registry, are reliable, and the registers are comprehensive [33–35]. Furthermore, the coverage in the Prescription Register of reimbursed medications prescribed by physicians is virtually complete for the study period [36]. We also had detailed data on medication use since our criterion required at least six months of medication use for ADMs in the three years prior to the HCC diagnosis. Data on DDDs were available, and adjustments for the patients' age, sex, level of education, diabetes duration, follow-up time, and the presence of cirrhosis and hepatitis were performed. The study cohort considered virtually all cases of HCC and individuals with T2D in Finland during the study period.

The main weakness of this study is that we only had register information available, with no comprehensive information about the HCC treatments. The registers used did not take lifestyle parameters into account. Furthermore, the degrees of hypercholesterinemia, atherosclerosis, hypertension, and left ventricular function are not available in the register data. Also, the duration of cardiovascular diseases is not available. The laboratory values and severity of diabetes are not known, but insulin use and the duration of diabetes are considered to be surrogate markers for the stage of diabetes. In addition, in a high proportion of HCC cases the stage was recorded as unknown (over 50%). Although the clinical staging of HCC might be challenging, it is highly likely that most unknown cases were advanced. In addition, the median follow-up time in both analyses might seem short, but the five-year survival of the subgroup complied with the general survival time of patients with HCC. The short follow-up time was affected by many patients dying during the first month of the follow-up. In the first two weeks, 165 patients died from HCC. Furthermore, within the first two weeks, 74 patients died from causes other than HCC; the majority of these patients died from cardiovascular related causes (42%) or gastrointestinal incidents (38%), including hepatic cirrhosis.

Challenges of confounding by indication are present in observational studies which contain endpoints that have not yet been studied in randomized controlled trials [37]. As various types of medication are initiated to treat conditions other than the one in the focus of an observational study, differences in participants can have an impact on the results. For example, patients with T2D have worse HCC prognoses compared to patients without T2D [38], but hypercholesterolemia seems not to decrease the survival of HCC patients [39]. Much has been discussed about either metformin or statin use association with healthy user bias, as, for example, statin use is linked to healthy lifestyles, adherence to treatments, better tolerance of side-effects, and the absence of contraindications [40]. However, statin users appear more likely to be elderly and have more coincident severe cardiovascular comorbidities than nonusers of statins [41]. In our study, metformin users had only slightly more insulin, other oral ADM, and statin use compared to metformin nonusers. The prognostic effect of metformin on overall mortality can be partly caused by the reduction of cardiovascular risk factors. However, the prediagnostic metformin use was associated with slightly decreased HCC-specific mortality, which is likely explained by metformin's cardiovascular effects.

In conclusion, prediagnostic metformin use was associated with decreased overall mortality, as well as slightly decreased HCC mortality and other-cause mortality in patients with T2D. In terms of localized HCC, results were inconclusive between prediagnostic metformin use and mortality in patients with HCC. Similarly, no discernible contrast between prediagnostic statin users and nonusers was found in overall mortality nor HCC mortality in either the whole cohort or the local subgroup.

Supplementary Materials: The following supporting information can be downloaded at: https://www.mdpi.com/article/10.3390/biomedicines12081654/s1, Table S1. The FinDM database combines several Finnish national registers which identify all persons who have been diagnosed for diabetes and collect their follow-up data. Table S2: The *International Classification of Diseases* (ICD) versions 8, 9, and 10 code for cirrhosis and hepatitis. Table S3: Patient characteristics of the whole cohort according to antidiabetic medication (ADM) and statin use; Table S4: Distribution of statin and other antidiabetic medication use; Table S5: Estimation results from Cox proportional hazard models of mortality from all causes, HCC, and other causes in the whole cohort; Table S6: Patient characteristics of those with only localized tumors according to antidiabetic medication (ADM) and statin use; Table S7: Estimation results from Cox proportional hazard models of mortality from all causes, HCC, and other causes in the local subgroup, Figure S1: Estimated HRs (with 95% CIs) of overall survival in relation to cumulative use of medications in the whole cohort. Fitted curves are cubic splines estimated from a mutually adjusted Cox regression model. DDD = defined daily doses. Figure S2: Estimated HRs (with 95% CIs) of overall survival in relation to cumulative use of medications in patients with localized HCC. Fitted curves are cubic splines estimated from a mutually adjusted Cox regression model. DDD = defined daily doses.

Author Contributions: All authors were responsible for the conceptualization, review, and editing of the manuscript. Methodology: A.H., H.H., M.A. and R.S.; formal analysis: A.H.; data curation/resources: M.A.; writing of the original draft preparation: I.T. and E.U.; visualization: A.H.; project administration and funding acquisition: P.K., U.P., A.J. and E.U. All authors have read and agreed to the published version of the manuscript.

Funding: This research was funded by the Jane and Aatos Erkko Foundation, the Jenni Piirainen Foundation, and the Finnish government research funds granted to Oulu University Hospital.

Institutional Review Board Statement: This study was conducted in accordance with the Declaration of Helsinki and has received ethical approval from the Ethics Committee of the National Institute for Health and Welfare (May 2018, proceeding §791).

Informed Consent Statement: According to Finnish legislation, no separate informed consent is needed because we utilized only administrative registers.

Data Availability Statement: The data that support the findings of this study are available from the corresponding author upon reasonable request.

Acknowledgments: The authors thank Juha Saarnio for their assistance with the categorization of the HCC stages.

Conflicts of Interest: The authors declare no conflicts of interest.

Abbreviations

ACC	Acetyl-CoA carboxylase
ADM	Antidiabetic medication
AMPK	AMPactivated protein kinase
AKT	Serine/threonine-specific protein kinase
CI	Confidence interval
DDD	Defined daily dose
FinDM	Diabetes in Finland
HCC	Hepatocellular carcinoma
HMG-CoA	3-hydroxy-3-methyl-glutarylcoenzyme A
HR	Hazard ratio
IGF-1	Insulin-like growth factor 1
mTOR	Mammalian target of rapamycin
OS	Overall survival

PI3K	Phosphatidylinositol-3-kinase
p53	Tumor protein p53
STAT3	Signal transducer and activator of transcription 3
T2D	Type 2 diabetes mellitus

References

1. Bray, F.; Laversanne, M.; Sung, H.; Ferlay, J.; Siegel, R.L.; Soerjomataram, I.; Jemal, A. Global cancer statistics 2022: GLOBOCAN estimates of incidence and mortality worldwide for 36 cancers in 185 countries. *CA Cancer J. Clin.* **2024**, *74*, 229–263. [CrossRef] [PubMed]
2. Finnish Cancer Registry. Cancer Statistics. New C22 Cancer Cases of the Latest Year (2022). Updated 29 April 2024. Available online: https://cancerregistry.fi/statistics/cancer-statistics/ (accessed on 23 May 2024).
3. Forner, A.; Hessheimer, A.J.; Isabel Real, M.; Bruix, J. Treatment of hepatocellular carcinoma. *Crit. Rev. Oncol. Hematol.* **2006**, *60*, 89–98. [CrossRef] [PubMed]
4. McGlynn, K.A.; Petrick, J.L.; El-Serag, H.B. Epidemiology of hepatocellular carcinoma. *Hepatology* **2021**, *73*, 4–13. [CrossRef] [PubMed]
5. El-Serag, H.B. Epidemiology of viral hepatitis and hepatocellular carcinoma. *Gastroenterology* **2012**, *142*, 1264–1273.e1. [CrossRef]
6. Foerster, F.; Gairing, S.J.; Müller, L.; Galle, P.R. NAFLD-driven HCC: Safety and efficacy of current and emerging treatment options. *J. Hepatol.* **2022**, *76*, 446–457. [CrossRef]
7. Yang, W.S.; Va, P.; Bray, F.; Gao, S.; Gao, J.; Li, H.L.; Xiang, Y.B. The role of pre-existing diabetes mellitus on hepatocellular carcinoma occurrence and prognosis: A meta-analysis of prospective cohort studies. *PLoS ONE* **2011**, *6*, e27326. [CrossRef] [PubMed]
8. Wang, C.; Wang, X.; Gong, G.; Ben, Q.; Qiu, W.; Chen, Y.I.; Li, G.; Wang, L. Increased risk of hepatocellular carcinoma in patients with diabetes mellitus: A systematic review and meta-analysis of cohort studies. *Int. J. Cancer* **2012**, *130*, 1639–1648. [CrossRef]
9. Wang, Y.G.; Wang, P.; Wang, B.; Fu, Z.J.; Zhao, W.J.; Yan, S.L. Diabetes mellitus and poorer prognosis in hepatocellular carcinoma: A systematic review and meta-analysis. *PLoS ONE* **2014**, *9*, e95485. [CrossRef]
10. Bragg, F.; Holmes, M.V.; Iona, A.; Guo, Y.; Du, H.; Chen, Y.; Bian, Z.; Yang, L.; Herrington, W.; Bennett, D.; et al. Association between diabetes and cause-specific mortality in rural and urban areas of China. *JAMA* **2017**, *317*, 280–289. [CrossRef]
11. Li, Q.; Xu, H.; Sui, C.; Zhang, H. Impact of metformin use on risk and mortality of hepatocellular carcinoma in diabetes mellitus. *Clin. Res. Hepatol. Gastroenterol.* **2022**, *46*, 101781. [CrossRef] [PubMed]
12. Zhou, J.; Ke, Y.; Lei, X.; Wu, T.; Li, Y.; Bao, T.; Tang, H.; Zhang, C.; Wu, X.; Wang, G.; et al. Meta-analysis: The efficacy of metformin and other anti-hyperglycemic agents in prolonging the survival of hepatocellular carcinoma patients with type 2 diabetes. *Ann. Hepatol.* **2020**, *19*, 320–328. [CrossRef]
13. Newman, J.D.; Schwartzbard, A.Z.; Weintraub, H.S.; Goldberg, I.J.; Berger, J.S. Primary prevention of cardiovascular disease in diabetes mellitus. *J. Am. Coll. Cardiol.* **2017**, *70*, 883–893. [CrossRef] [PubMed]
14. Vehko, T.; Sund, R.; Arffman, M.; Manderbacka, K.; Ilanne-Parikka, P.; Keskimäki, I. Monitoring the use of lipid-lowering medication among persons with newly diagnosed diabetes: A nationwide register-based study. *BMJ Open* **2013**, *3*, e003414. [CrossRef]
15. Li, X.; Liu, L.; Hu, Y. Statin use and the prognosis of patients with hepatocellular carcinoma: A meta-analysis. *Biosci. Rep.* **2020**, *40*, BSR20200232. [CrossRef] [PubMed]
16. Wang, J.; Li, X. Impact of statin use on the risk and prognosis of hepatocellular carcinoma: A meta-analysis. *Eur. J. Gastroenterol. Hepatol.* **2021**, *33*, 1603–1609. [CrossRef] [PubMed]
17. Kim, G.; Jang, S.; Han, E.; Lee, Y.; Park, S.; Nam, C.M.; Kang, E.S. Effect of statin on hepatocellular carcinoma in patients with type 2 diabetes: A nationwide nested case-control study. *Int. J. Cancer* **2017**, *140*, 798–806. [CrossRef] [PubMed]
18. Antwi, S.O.; Li, Z.; Mody, K.; Roberts, L.R.; Patel, T. Independent and joint use of statins and metformin by elderly patients with diabetes and overall survival following HCC diagnosis. *J. Clin. Gastroenterol.* **2020**, *54*, 468–476. [CrossRef] [PubMed]
19. Vandenbroucke, J.P.; Elm, E.V.; Altman, D.G.; Gøtzsche, P.C.; Mulrow, C.D.; Pocock, S.J.; Poole, C.; Schlesselman, J.J.; Egger, M. Strengthening the reporting of observational studies in epidemiology (STROBE): Explanation and elaboration. *Int. J. Surg.* **2014**, *12*, 1500–1524. [CrossRef] [PubMed]
20. Arffman, M.; Ilanne-Parikka, P.; Keskimäki, I.; Kurkela, O.; Lindström, J.; Sund, R.; Winel, K. *FinDM Database on Diabetes in Finland*; Discussion Paper 19/2020; Finnish Institute for Health and Welfare: Helsinki, Finland, 2020.
21. Sund, R.; Harno, K.; Ranta, S.; Tolppanen, E. Evaluation of case inclusion in two population-based diabetes registers. *FinJeHeW* **2010**, *2*, 136–146.
22. Leinonen, M.K.; Miettinen, J.; Heikkinen, S.; Pitkäniemi, J.; Malila, N. Quality measures of the population-based Finnish Cancer Registry indicate sound data quality for solid malignant tumours. *Eur. J. Cancer* **2017**, *77*, 31–39. [CrossRef]
23. Saraei, P.; Asadi, I.; Kakar, M.A.; Moradi-Kor, N. The beneficial effects of metformin on cancer prevention and therapy: A comprehensive review of recent advances. *Cancer Manag. Res.* **2019**, *11*, 3295–3313. [CrossRef]
24. Sun, R.; Zhai, R.; Ma, C.; Miao, W. Combination of aloin and metformin enhances the antitumor effect by inhibiting the growth and invasion and inducing apoptosis and autophagy in hepatocellular carcinoma through PI3K/AKT/mTOR pathway. *Cancer Med.* **2020**, *9*, 1141–1151. [CrossRef]

25. Dowling, R.J.; Goodwin, P.J.; Stambolic, V. Understanding the benefit of metformin use in cancer treatment. *BMC Med.* **2011**, *9*, 3–33. [CrossRef] [PubMed]
26. Sosnicki, S.; Kapral, M.; Weglarz, L. Molecular targets of metformin antitumor action. *Pharmacol. Rep.* **2016**, *68*, 918–925. [CrossRef] [PubMed]
27. Seo, Y.S.; Kim, Y.J.; Kim, M.S.; Suh, K.S.; Kim, S.B.; Han, C.J.; Kim, Y.J.; Jang, W.I.; Kang, S.H.; Tchoe, H.J.; et al. Association of metformin use with cancer-specific mortality in hepatocellular carcinoma after curative resection: A nationwide population-based study. *Medicine* **2016**, *95*, e3527. [CrossRef]
28. Yuan, B.; Ma, J.; Wang, J.; Hao, J. The effect of metformin usage on survival outcomes for hepatocellular carcinoma patients with type 2 diabetes mellitus after curative therapy. *Front. Endocrinol.* **2022**, *13*, 1060768. [CrossRef]
29. Taras, D.; Blanc, J.F.; Rullier, A.; Dugot-Senant, N.; Laurendeau, I.; Vidaud, M.; Rosenbaum, J. Pravastatin reduces lung metastasis of rat hepatocellular carcinoma via a coordinated decrease of MMP expression and activity. *J. Hepatol.* **2007**, *46*, 69–76. [CrossRef]
30. Sassano, A.; Platanias, L.C. Statins in tumor suppression. *Cancer Lett.* **2008**, *260*, 11–19. [CrossRef] [PubMed]
31. Gronich, N.; Rennert, G. Beyond aspirin-cancer prevention with statins, metformin and bisphosphonates. *Nat. Rev. Clin. Oncol.* **2013**, *10*, 625–642. [CrossRef]
32. Alipour Talesh, G.; Trézéguet, V.; Merched, A. Hepatocellular Carcinoma and Statins. *Biochemistry* **2020**, *59*, 3393–3400. [CrossRef] [PubMed]
33. Pukkala, E.; Engholm, G.; Højsgaard Schmidt, L.K.; Storm, H.; Khan, S.; Lambe, M.; Pettersson, D.; Ólafsdóttir, E.; Tryggvadóttir, L.; Hakanen, T.; et al. Nordic cancer registries—An overview of their procedures and data comparability. *Acta Oncol.* **2018**, *57*, 440–455. [CrossRef] [PubMed]
34. Mikkelsen, L.; Phillips, D.E.; AbouZahr, C.; Setel, P.W.; De Savigny, D.; Lozano, R.; Lopez, A.D. A global assessment of civil registration and vital statistics systems: Monitoring data quality and progress. *Lancet* **2015**, *386*, 1395–1406. [CrossRef] [PubMed]
35. Sund, R. Quality of the Finnish Hospital Discharge Register: A systematic review. *Scand. J. Public Health* **2012**, *40*, 505–515. [CrossRef] [PubMed]
36. Sund, R.; Gissler, M.; Hakulinen, T.; Rosén, M. Use of health registers. In *Handbook of Epidemiology*; Ahrens, W., Pigeot, I., Eds.; Springer: New York, NY, USA, 2014; pp. 707–730.
37. Jorgensen, N.W.; Sibley, C.T.; McClelland, R.L. Using imputed pre-treatment cholesterol in a propensity score model to reduce confounding by indication: Results from the multi-ethnic study of atherosclerosis. *BMC Med. Res. Methodol.* **2013**, *13*, 81. [CrossRef]
38. Nakatsuka, T.; Tateishi, R. Development and prognosis of hepatocellular carcinoma in patients with diabetes. *Clin. Mol. Hepatol.* **2023**, *29*, 51–64. [CrossRef] [PubMed]
39. Morisco, F.; Guarino, M.; Valvano, M.R.; Auriemma, F.; Farinati, F.; Giannini, E.G.; Ciccarese, F.; Tovoli, F.; Rapaccini, G.L.; Di Marco, M.; et al. Metabolic disorders across hepatocellular carcinoma in Italy. *Liver Int.* **2018**, *38*, 2028–2039. [CrossRef] [PubMed]
40. Beattie, W.S.; Wijeysundera, D.N. Statins and the "healthy user bias" in cardiac surgery. *Anesth. Analg.* **2010**, *111*, 261–263. [CrossRef] [PubMed]
41. Yang, C.C.; Jick, S.S.; Testa, M.A. Who receives lipid-lowering drugs: The effects of comorbidities and patient characteristics on treatment initiation. *Br. J. Clin. Pharmacol.* **2003**, *55*, 288–298. [CrossRef] [PubMed]

biomedicines

MDPI

Article

Atorvastatin Treatment Significantly Increased the Concentration of Bone Marrow-Derived Mononuclear Cells and Transcutaneous Oxygen Pressure and Lowered the Pain Scale after Bone Marrow Cells Treatment in Patients with "No-Option" Critical Limb Ischaemia

Jan Kyselovic [1,2], Adriana Adamičková [1], Andrea Gažová [3,*], Simona Valášková [4], Nikola Chomaničová [4], Zdenko Červenák [1] and Juraj Madaric [5]

1 5th Department of Internal Medicine, Faculty of Medicine, Comenius University Bratislava, Špitálska 24, 81372 Bratislava, Slovakia; kyselovic@uniba.sk (J.K.)
2 Department of Pharmacology and Toxicology, University of Veterinary Medicine and Pharmacy, 04181 Košice, Slovakia
3 Institute of Pharmacology and Clinical Pharmacology, Faculty of Medicine, Comenius University Bratislava, Špitálska 24, 81372 Bratislava, Slovakia
4 International Laser Center, Slovak Centre of Scientific and Technical Information, Lamačská cesta 7315/8A, 84104 Bratislava, Slovakia
5 Department of Angiology, Faculty of Medicine, Comenius University and National Institute of Cardiovascular Disease, Pod Krásnou Hôrkou 1, 83101 Bratislava, Slovakia; madaricjuraj@gmail.com
* Correspondence: andrea.gazova@fmed.uniba.sk

Abstract: Background: The present study investigated the outcomes and possible predictive factors of autologous bone marrow cells (BMCs) therapy in patients with "no-option" critical limb ischaemia (CLI). It was focused on exploring the clinical background and prior statin and renin-angiotensin system (RAS)-acting agents pharmacotherapy related to the therapeutic efficacy of BMCs treatment. Methods: In the present study, we reviewed thirty-three patients (mean age 64.9 ± 10 years; 31 males) with advanced CLI after failed or impossible revascularisation, who were treated with 40 mL of autologous BMCs by local intramuscular application. Patients with limb salvage and wound healing (N = 22) were considered as responders to BMCs therapy, and patients with limb salvage and complete ischemic wound healing (N = 13) were defined as super-responders. Logistic regression models were used to screen and identify the prognostic factors, and a receiver operating characteristics (ROC) curve, a linear regression, and a survival curve were drawn to determine the predictive accuracy, the correlation between the candidate predictors, and the risk of major amputation. Results: Based on the univariate regression analysis, baseline C-reactive protein (CRP) and transcutaneous oxygen pressure ($TcPO_2$) values were identified as prognostic factors of the responders, while CRP value, ankle-brachial index (ABI), and bone marrow-derived mononuclear cells (BM-MNCs) concentration were identified as prognostic factors of the super-responders. An area under the ROC curve of 0.768 indicated good discrimination for CRP > 8.1 mg/L before transplantation as a predictive factor for negative clinical response. Linear regression analysis revealed a significant dependence between the levels of baseline CRP and the concentration of BM-MNCs in transplanted bone marrow. Patients taking atorvastatin before BMCs treatment (N = 22) had significantly improved $TcPO_2$ and reduced pain scale after BMCs transplant, compared to the non-atorvastatin group. Statin treatment was associated with reduced risk for major amputation. However, the difference was not statistically significant. Statin use was also associated with a significantly higher concentration of BM-MNCs in the transplanted bone marrow compared to patients without statin treatment. Patients treated with RAS-acting agents (N = 20) had significantly reduced pain scale after BMCs transplant, compared to the non-RAS-acting agents group. Similar results, reduced pain scale and improved $TcPO_2$, were achieved in patients treated with atorvastatin and RAS-acting agents (N = 17) before BMCs treatment.

Results of the Spearman correlation showed a significant positive correlation between CLI regression, responders, and previous therapy before BMCs transplant with RAS-acting agents alone or with atorvastatin. Conclusions: CRP and $TcPO_2$ were prognostic factors of the responders, while CRP value, ABI, and BM-MNCs concentration were identified as predictive factors of the super-responders. Atorvastatin treatment was associated with a significantly increased concentration of BM-MNCs in bone marrow concentrate and higher $TcPO_2$ and lower pain scale after BMCs treatment in CLI patients. Similarly, reduced pain scales and improved TcPO2 were achieved in patients treated with atorvastatin and RAS-acting agents before BMCs treatment. Positive correlations between responders and previous treatment before BMCs transplant with RAS-acting agents alone or with atorvastatin were significant.

Keywords: critical limb ischaemia, bone marrow cell therapy, mesenchymal stem cells; atorvastatin; RAS-acting agents; predictive analysis; spearman correlation

1. Introduction

As a terminal stage of peripheral arterial disease (PAD), critical limb ischaemia (CLI), which is characterized by chronic ischemic rest pain, ischemic ulcerations, or gangrene, is associated with a significant risk of amputation of the affected limb [1,2]. Revascularisations by percutaneous transluminal angioplasty or bypass graft surgery are essential rescue methods for wound healing and limb salvage. However, up to 30% of patients with CLI are unsuitable for or have failed previous endovascular or surgical revascularisation treatments [3]. Therefore, in these high-risk patients, limb amputation is the only therapeutic option to relieve pain and stop the spread of wound infection. These patients are called "no-option" CLI patients, with an annual mortality of 10% to 40% [4,5].

Several pre-clinical studies of CLI treatment were conducted in recent years, using novel approaches with bone marrow cells (BMCs). The most used stem cells include bone marrow-derived mononuclear cells (BM-MNCs), $CD34^+$ bone marrow cells, or bone marrow-derived mesenchymal stem cells. The implanted stem cells can improve blood circulation and increase blood flow to the transplantation site in patients by promoting ischemic angiogenesis and neovascularisation [6,7]. Notably, several clinical trials have demonstrated the positive therapeutic efficacy of stem cell transplantation and validated its safety and feasibility [8–10]. At the same time, other studies have shown an insignificant moderate prognosis following stem cell therapy, comparable to the placebo group or conservative treatment [11,12]. The heterogeneity of studied populations and differences in specific features of transplants might cause these controversial observations. Another shortcoming of the cells used in therapy is their poor survival and retention of transplants in vivo, caused by the specific properties of individual cell lines and the hostile microenvironment in the ischemic region. For these reasons, attention has been focused on improving stem cell tolerance to the implantation site, which could increase therapeutic efficacy [13].

In addition, it is necessary to consider previous long-term treatment of CLI patients, which could modify the response to the cell therapy. Recommended therapy in all patients with PAD includes statins, widely used as a cholesterol-lowering agent to prevent cardiovascular disease with a favourable safety profile [14,15]. It has been shown that statins can act through various signalling pathways, particularly PI3K/Akt, thus influencing the fate and properties of transplanted bone marrow cells or affecting the implantation site of stem cells [16]. RAS-acting agents (angiotensin-converting enzyme inhibitors (ACEIs) and angiotensin receptor blockers (ARBs)) should be considered as first-line therapy in patients with PAD and hypertension [14]. A study on 31,245 patients recently concluded that statin therapy positively decreased CRP levels and reduced atherosclerotic risk [17].

While previous research has proposed these theoretical frameworks, their efficacy in real-world clinical settings remains unestablished. Existing therapies for cardiovascular diseases provide a readily available platform for clinically verifying these hypotheses through a simplified clinical design. This study investigates the baseline clinical characteristics and prior medication regimens by "no-option" chronic limb ischemia (CLI) patients treated with bone marrow cell therapy. We aim to identify factors associated with treatment response by comparing responders and non-responders. This analysis will contribute to developing and refining selection criteria and prognostic factors for predicting positive clinical outcomes.

2. Materials and Methods

2.1. Patients

Between May 2016 and November 2018, 33 patients (age 65 ± 10 years, 31 males) with advanced CLI (Rutherford category 5 or 6) after failed or impossible revascularisation were treated with 40 mL of bone marrow nucleated cells via the local intramuscular route. The aetiology of arterial obliteration was atherosclerosis in 30 patients and thromboangiitis obliterans (Buerger disease) in three patients. The patients included in this study met the following criteria: (1) at least 18 years of age with ischemic skin lesions (ulcers or gangrene) with a CLI Rutherford category of 4, 5 or 6 according to the Transatlantic Inter-Society Consensus (TASC) classification (minor or major tissue loss), defined as necrosis or gangrene extending proximal to the metatarsal line or as extensive deep heel gangrene [2]; (2) CLI defined by ankle-brachial index (ABI) ≤ 0.4 or ankle systolic pressure < 50 mmHg, or toe systolic pressure < 30 mmHg, and transcutaneous oxygen pressure ($TcPO_2$) < 30 mmHg; (3) no option for endovascular or surgical revascularisation as judged by vascular surgeon and interventionist; (4) failed revascularisation, defined as no change of clinical status with the best standard care four weeks after endovascular or surgical revascularisation. Patients who, at the start of the cell therapy, met any of the following criteria: (1) life expectancy of fewer than six months; (2) presence of malignancy during the last five years; (3) critical coronary artery disease or unstable angina pectoris; (4) patients with end-stage kidney disease and patient on dialysis; (5) bone marrow disease (e.g., severe anaemia, leucopaenia, thrombocytopaenia, myelodysplastic syndrome) were excluded from the study. The local ethical committee of the National Institute of Cardiovascular Diseases, Bratislava, approved the study design. This study was carried out according to the Code of Ethics of the World Medical Association, Declaration of Helsinki (WMA Declaration of Helsinki, 2013).

2.2. Bone Marrow Cell Isolation and Administration

On the day of the transplantation, bone marrow was aspirated from both anterior superior iliac crests under analgosedation with propofol. A total volume of 240 mL of bone marrow was harvested using a standard disposable needle for aspiration. Bone Marrow Aspirate Concentrate System (Harvest, Plymouth, MA, USA), which uses gradient density centrifugation and provides 40 mL of bone marrow-rich product for all blood elements within 15 min, was used to process obtained bone marrow aspirate. After the harvesting and centrifugation of stem cells, 40 mL of bone marrow cells (BMCs) were administered by intramuscular methods using deep injections with a 23-G needle into the muscles of the affected limb along the crural arteries, with each injection being approximately 1 mL. The duration of this procedure was 1 h. A bone marrow cell sample was immediately analyzed using a MACS Quant analyzer (Miltenyi Biotec, Bergisch Gladbach, Germany). The BM-MNCs concentration, MSCs concentration, and viability of cells were determined using an MSC Enumerating kit and propidium iodide solution (Miltenyi Biotec, Bergisch Gladbach, Germany), according to manufacturer's instructions.

2.3. Pre-Procedure Assessment and Follow-Up

All patients were examined before the administration of BMCs, as well as 90 days and six months after the delivery, along with a peripheral blood test to determine basal serological parameters (including C-reactive protein, CRP). Resting ABI was measured according to the validated standards [18]. It was performed by measuring the systolic blood pressure from both brachial arteries and dorsalis pedis and posterior tibial arteries after the patient had rested in the supine position for 10 min (normal values, 0.95–1.2). $TcPO_2$

of the affected limb was assessed using a TCM400 Mk2 monitor (Radiometer Medical ApS, Copenhagen, Denmark). It was measured at the forefoot in the supine position with an electrode temperature of 44 °C. Wound healing was assessed by two independent physicians and documented by digital photography. A visual analogue scale (VAS) was used to measure pain on a scale graded from 0 to 10.

2.4. Endpoints

Primary endpoints were limb salvage and improvement in wound healing without major limb amputation at the six-month of follow-up. Patients who achieved CLI remission were considered responders to BMCs therapy. Patients requiring major limb amputation or patients without signs of wound healing were regarded as non-responders. A group of patients with limb salvage and complete ischemic wound healing were defined as super-responders to BMCs therapy. Patients who underwent major limb amputation were considered as super-non-responders. In addition, patients treated with atorvastatin for a long time (at least six months before BMCs therapy) were included in the atorvastatin group. The other patients were regarded as a non-atorvastatin group. Similarly, patients treated with RAS-acting agents were included in the RAS group, while patients without RAS treatment were considered in the non-RAS-acting agents group. Patients treated with atorvastatin or RAS-acting agents were included in the ATV and RAS group; patients without such therapy were regarded as non-ATV and non-RAS group. The secondary endpoints included changes in $TcPO_2$, ABI, pain scale, and Rutherford category after BMCs transplantation. The local ethical committee of the National Institute of Cardiovascular Diseases, Bratislava, approved the study design. All patients in the study were informed about the nature of the study and gave their written informed consent.

2.5. Statistical Analysis

The baseline characteristics of the responders and non-responders were compared first. Continuous variables were presented as the mean ± standard deviation (SD). Categorical variables were presented as numbers with percentages, and Fisher's exact test was used to analyze the significance of the differences. Gaussian distribution of data was tested by the Shapiro-Wilk test. The independent Student *t*-test or Mann-Whitney test was used to analyze the significance of the differences between responders and non-responders. The paired *t*-test or Wilcoxon signed-rank test was used to analyze the longitudinal changes from baseline to 6 months post-transplantation. The candidate prognostic factors of the responders and super-responders were screened through a univariate binary logistic regression analysis. The correlations between the candidate predictors or the variables at different time points were analyzed with linear regression or Spearman nonparametric correlation. Receiver operating characteristics analysis was used to study predictors of clinical response after bone marrow transplantation. The Kaplan–Meier method estimated the survival curve and was compared using the log-rank test. We considered p values < 0.05 to be statistically significant. All statistical analyses were performed using Microsoft Office Excel (2007), XLSTAT statistical and data analysis solution (Addinsoft 2021, New York, NY, USA) or GraphPad Prism version 9.0 (GraphPad Software, San Diego, CA, USA).

3. Results

3.1. Baseline Information and Endpoints

The mean age of 33 patients included and analyzed in the study was 64.9 ± 10 years, and the male ratio was 94%. There were 32 lower limbs and one upper limb involved in the study. The baseline Rutherford class was 5 in 32 patients (97%) and 6 in one patient (3%) (Table 1). The six-month major amputation-free survival rate was 81.8% (27/33), wherein six patients underwent major amputations due to CLI progression. The combined primary endpoint of limb salvage and wound healing was met in 22 of the 33 patients (66.7%) at the six-month follow-up and were regarded as responders to the BMCs therapy. A total of

13 patients (39.4%) achieved limb salvage and complete wound healing at six months and were regarded as super-responders to the BM-MNCs transplantation (Figure 1).

Table 1. Characteristics of patients before stem cell treatment.

	All Patients (N = 33)	Responders (N = 22)	Non-Responders (N = 11)	*p* Value
Age (years)	64.9 ± 10	67.4 ± 9.3	59.8 ± 10.7	0.014 *
Sex (males)	31 (94%)	21 (95%)	10 (91%)	1.000
Rutherford class (1–6)	5.0 ± 0.30	5.0	4.9 ± 0.54	0.208
Body mass index (kg/m^2)	27 ± 4.1	27.2 ± 3.8	27.6 ± 4.9	0.756
		Risk factors of limb ischaemia		
Diabetes mellitus	11 (33%)	7 (32%)	4 (36%)	1.000
Arterial hypertension	27 (82%)	18 (82%)	9 (82%)	1.000
Hyperlipidaemia	23 (70%)	15 (68%)	8 (73%)	1.000
Smoker	10 (30%)	6 (27%)	4 (36%)	0.696
		Blood examination		
CRP (mg/L)	13.3 ± 21.3	8.1 ± 12.3	23.3 ± 30.5	0.013 *
Creatinine (μmol/L)	95.9 ± 34.6	95.4 ± 35.7	96.7 ± 34.2	0.946
		Treatment history		
Statins	22 (67%)	16 (73%) (NNT 5.5)	6 (55%)	0.255
Antiplatelet drugs	24 (73%)	17 (77%)	7 (64%)	0.438
Aspirin	16 (48%)	11 (50%)	5 (45%)	0.4074
Clopidogrel	17 (52%)	10 (45%)	7 (64%)	0.1711
RAS-acting agents	20 (61%)	16 (73%) (NNT 2.75)	4 (36%)	0.065
Statins and RAS-acting agents	17 (52%)	13 (59%) (NNT4.4)	4 (36%)	0.282
Naftidrofuryl	28 (85%)	18 (82%)	10 (91%)	0.643
Post-MI	31 (94%)	22 (100%)	9 (82%)	0.104
		Parameters of limb ischaemia		
$TcPO_2$ < 10 mmHg	19 (58%)	11 (50%)	8 (73%)	0.278
ABI	0.51 ± 0.38	0.57 ± 0.35	0.37 ± 0.43	0.183
Pain scale (0–10)	5.75 ± 1.6	5.62 ± 1.75	6.14 ± 1.07	0.366

Where appropriate, data are presented as mean ± standard deviation or numbers and percentages. CRP, C-reaction protein; RAS, renin-angiotensin system; MI, myocardial infarct; $TcPO_2$, transcutaneous oxygen pressure; ABI, ankle-brachial index; NNT, number needed to treat. Statistical analysis was performed by the Mann-Whitney test and by Student's *t*-test (depending on data distribution determined by the Shapiro-Wilk test) or Fisher's exact test; *p*-value = responders vs. non-responders. * The difference between six months and baseline in responders was statistically significant.

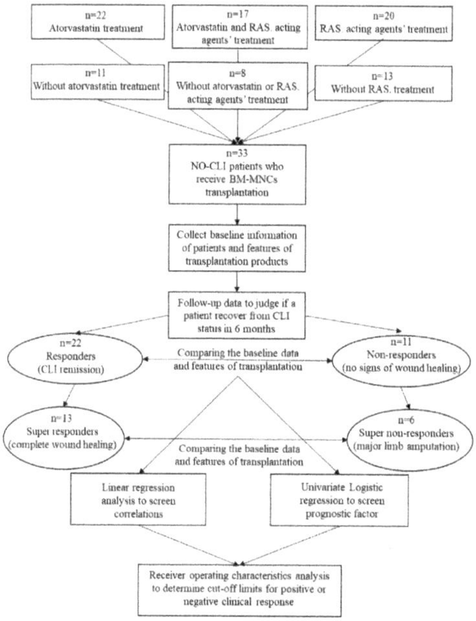

Figure 1. Study flow diagram. NO-CLI, "no-option" critical limb ischaemia.

3.2. Characteristics of Responders and Non-Responders

The baseline information of patients before the BMCs therapy is presented in Table 1. The mean age of the responders was higher than that of the non-responders; the difference was significant (67.4 ± 9.3 vs. 59.8 ± 10.7, p = 0.014). No significant variations regarding limb ischaemia risk factors were observed between the responders and non-responders. When the baseline blood parameters were evaluated, the responders had significantly lower CRP levels than the patients in the non-responders category (p = 0.013).

Regarding the treated limbs, the responders were characterized by fewer patients with baseline $TcPO_2$ < 10 mmHg than the non-responders (p = 0.278). Based on the available complete longitudinal data (N = 28), the mean $TcPO_2$ of the responders increased from 12.5 ± 14.0 mmHg at baseline to 22.7 ± 15.2 mmHg at six months post-transplantation (p = 0.008). At the same time, that of the non-responders did not improve significantly, from 2.4 ± 0.63 mmHg at baseline to 3.18 ± 8.4 mmHg at six months post-transplantation (p = 0.573) (Table 2, Figure 2A). $TcPO_2$ at baseline correlated significantly with that at six months (R^2 = 0.371, p = 0.001) (Figure 2B).

Table 2. Outcomes of BMCs treatment after six months in responders and non-responders.

Parameters of Limb Ischaemia	Responders			Non-Responders		
	Baseline (N = 22)	Six Months (N = 17)	p Value	Baseline (N = 11)	Six Months (N = 11)	p Value
Rutherford class (1–6)	5.0 ± 0.30	4.2 ± 1.0	0.008 *	4.9 ± 0.54	5.55 ± 0.52	0.059
$TcPO_2$ (mmHg)	12.5 ± 14.0	22.7 ± 15.2	0.008 *	2.4 ± 1.77	3.18 ± 8.4	0.573
ABI	0.57 ± 0.35	0.60 ± 0.34	0.480	0.37 ± 0.43	0.029 ± 0.08	0.043 *
Pain scale (0–10)	5.62 ± 1.75	1.78 ± 1.22	<0.001 *	6.14 ± 1.07	6.86 ± 3.76	0.445

Data are presented as mean ± standard deviation. ABI, ankle-brachial index; $TcPO_2$, transcutaneous oxygen pressure. Statistical analysis was performed by the Wilcoxon matched-pair test and Student's t-test (depending on data distribution determined by the Shapiro-Wilk test). p = six months vs. baseline.* The difference between six months and baseline in responders was statistically significant.

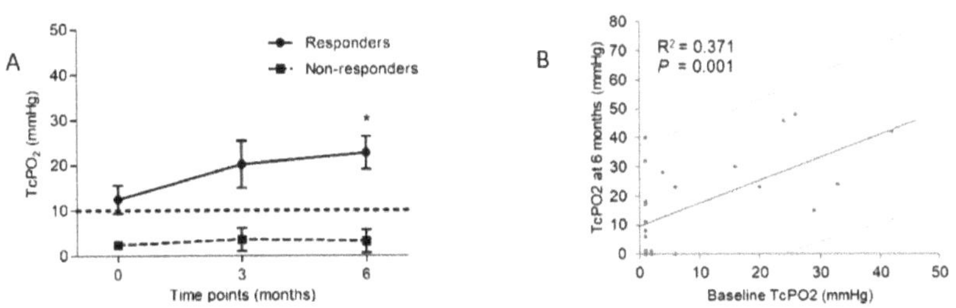

Figure 2. Comparison of longitudinal $TcPO_2$ changes (mean with SEM) in the ischemic limbs of the responders and non-responders (**A**) and linear regression between $TcPO_2$ at baseline and at six months post-transplantation, depicted with a solid fitting line, dotted 95% confidence interval bars and lined 95% prediction intervals (**B**). * The difference between six months and baseline in responders was statistically significant (p = 0.008). $TcPO_2$, transcutaneous oxygen pressure.

No differences were observed between the responders and the non-responders in baseline ABI (p = 0.183), and there was no significant improvement during the six-month follow-up. Despite this, a significant ABI decrease was observed in the non-responder group (p = 0.043). Moreover, we did not find a significant variation in the pain scale between groups at the baseline (p = 0.366). Still, a significant pain reduction was observed in the responder group during the six-month follow-up (p < 0.001). We did not see any significant changes in the non-responder group regarding the pain scale (p = 0.445). In addition, no difference was revealed between groups in terms of the Rutherford class at the baseline (p = 0.208). Still, significant improvement was observed at the six-month follow-up in the responder group (p = 0.008), with no difference in the non-responder group (p = 0.059) (Table 2).

3.3. Characteristics of Super-Responders and Super-Non-Responders

Table 3 presents baseline information of patients before BMCs therapy. The mean age of super-responders tended to be lower than that of the super-non-responders, though the difference was not significant (64.8 ± 10.4 vs. 66.8 ± 4.0, $p = 0.690$). Comparing blood parameters at baseline demonstrated lower CRP levels in the super-responder group than patients in the super non-responder group ($p < 0.001$).

Table 3. Characteristics of super-responders and super-non-responders before stem cell treatment.

	All Patients (N = 33)	Super-Responders (N = 13)	Super-Non-Responders (N = 6)	*p* Value
Age (years) (mean ± SD)	64.9 ± 10	64.8 ± 10.4	66.8 ± 4.0	0.690
Sex (males)	31 (94%)	12 (92%)	6 (100%)	1.000
Rutherford class (1–6)	5.0 ± 0.30	5.0	4.83 ± 0.75	0.175
Body mass index (kg/m^2)	27 ± 4.1	27.1 ± 4.04	25.6 ± 3.76	0.450
Risk factors of limb ischaemia				
Diabetes mellitus (N, %)	11 (33%)	5 (38%)	3 (50%)	1.000
Arterial hypertension	27 (82%)	11 (85%)	6 (100%)	1.000
Hyperlipidaemia	23 (70%)	10 (77%)	5 (83%)	1.000
Smoker	10 (30%)	3 (23%)	2 (33%)	1.000
Blood examination				
CRP (mg/L)	13.3 ± 21.3	5.2 ± 3.45	36.6 ± 37.01	<0.001 *
Creatinine (μmol/L)	95.9 ± 34.6	98.7 ± 41.02	102.5 ± 39.78	0.914
Treatment history				
Statins (N, %)	22 (67%)	11 (85%)	3 (50%)	0.262
Antiplatelet drugs	24 (72%)	12 (92%)	3 (50%)	0.071
Aspirin	16 (48%)	8 (62%)	2 (33%)	0.1463
Clopidogrel	17 (52%)	8 (62%)	3 (50%)	0.3361
RAS-acting agents	20 (61%)	9 (69%)	3 (50%)	0.617
Statins and RAS-acting agents	17 (52%)	9 (69%)	2 (33%)	0.319
Naftidrofuryl	28 (85%)	12 (92%)	6 (100%)	1.000
Post-MI	31 (94%)	12 (92%)	5 (83%)	1.000
Parameters of limb ischaemia				
$TcPO_2$ < 10 mmHg	19 (58%)	6 (46%)	4 (67%)	0.629
ABI	0.51 ± 0.38	0.57 ± 0.37	0.18 ±0.36	0.101
Pain scale (0–10)	5.75 ± 1.6	5.61 ± 1.71	6.33 ± 0.58	0.907

Where appropriate, data are presented as mean ± standard deviation or numbers and percentages. CRP, C-reaction protein; RAS, renin-angiotensin system; MI, myocardial infarct; $TcPO_2$, transcutaneous oxygen pressure; ABI, ankle-brachial index. Statistical analysis was performed by the Mann-Whitney test and by Student's *t*-test (depending on data distribution determined by the Shapiro-Wilk test) or Fisher's exact test; *p*-value = responders vs. non-responders. * The difference between six months and baseline in responders was statistically significant.

The super-responders were characterized by higher baseline $TcPO_2$ (14.17 ± 14.69 mmHg) and ABI (0.57 ± 0.37) than the super-non-responders ($TcPO_2$ 3.0 ± 2.65 mmHg, $p = 0.536$, ABI 0.18 ± 0.36, $p = 0.101$); however, these differences were not statistically significant (Table 3). Based on the available complete longitudinal data, the mean $TcPO_2$ of the super-responders increased from 14.17 ± 14.69 mmHg at baseline to 25.92 ± 14.92 mmHg at six months post-transplantation ($p = 0.012$). In contrast, that of the super-non-responders did not improve because of the deteriorating health and amputation of the affected limb. There was no significant improvement in the case of ABI of the super-responders (0.57 ± 0.37 at baseline, 0.57 ± 0.29 at six months, $p = 0.983$), while significant improvement of pain scale was demonstrated in the super-responders group (5.61 ± 1.71 at baseline, 1.46 ± 1.2 at six months post-transplantation, $p < 0.0001$), compared to the worsened pain scale in the super-non-responder group (6.33 ± 0.58 at baseline, 9.0 at six months, $p = 0.102$). Regarding the Rutherford scale, the super-responder group had significantly improved from 5.0 at baseline to 3.92 ± 1.04 at six months post-transplantation ($p = 0.008$). In comparison, the Rutherford scale decreased from 4.83 ± 0.75 at baseline to 6.0 ($p = 0.038$) at six months post-transplantation.

3.4. Characteristics of Transplanted Bone Marrow Cells

According to the characteristics of BMCs transplant, several variables differed between groups (Table 4). The concentration of BM-MNCs appeared to be higher in the responders ($3.53 \pm 1.5 \times 10^9$) than in the non-responders ($2.86 \pm 1.13 \times 10^9$), although the difference was not statistically significant ($p = 0.213$). However, in the case of subgroup analysis of super-responders and super-non-responders, we found a significantly higher number of BM-MNCs in the super-responders compared to super-non-responders ($3.68 \pm 1.51 \times 10^9$ vs. $2.26 \pm 0.74 \times 10^9$, $p = 0.049$).

Table 4. Characteristics of transplanted BMCs.

Group Analysis	Responders (N = 22)	Non-Responders (N = 11)	*p* Value
BM-MNCs (109 cells/mL)	3.53 ± 1.5	2.86 ± 1.13	0.213
Viability of BM-MNCs (%)	99.70 ± 0.3	99.27 ± 0.86	0.464
MSCs (104 cells/mL)	0.79 ± 0.61	1.46 ± 1.56	0.123
Subgroup analysis	super-responders (limb salvage and complete ischemic wound healing, N = 13)	super-non-responders (major limb amputation, N = 6)	*p* value
BM-MNCs (109 cells/mL)	3.68 ± 1.51	2.26 ± 0.74	0.049 *
Viability of BM-MNCs (%)	99.71 ± 0.32	99.05 ± 0.94	0.263
MSCs (104 cells/mL)	0.83 ± 0.52	1.68 ± 2.14	0.639

Data are presented as mean ± standard deviation. BMCs, bone marrow cells; BM-MNCs, bone marrow mononuclear cells; MSCs, mesenchymal stem cells. Statistical analysis was performed by the Mann-Whitney test and Student's *t*-test (depending on data distribution determined by the Shapiro-Wilk test). *p* = responders vs. non-responders; super-responders vs. super-non-responders. * The difference between six months and baseline in responders was statistically significant.

3.5. Prognostic Factors and Predictors of BMCs Treatment Outcomes

According to the results of the univariate logistic regression, two variables were screened out for responders: CRP [OR 0.955, 95% CI 0.901–1.012, $p = 0.044$] and $TcPO_2$ [OR 1.149, 95% CI 0.949–1.392, $p = 0.021$] (Table 5). The results of univariate logistic regression for super-responders showed that CRP [OR 0.544, 95% CI 0.221–1.341, $p < 0.0001$], ABI [OR 56.140, 95% CI 0.531–5932.9, $p = 0.035$] and BM-MNCs concentration [OR 1.0, 95% CI 0.999–1.0, $p = 0.035$] were screened out for super-responders (Table 5).

Table 5. Univariate logistic regression analysis of prognostic factors.

Candidate Variable	Responder		Super-Responder	
	OR (95% CI)	*p* Value	OR (95% CI)	*p* Value
Age ≥ 50 years	1.097 (0.993–1.212)	0.056	0.972 (0.844–1.095)	0.689
Rutherford class	2.803 (0.221–35.552)	0.411	3.026 (0.222–41.289)	0.389
Body mass index (kg/m^2)	0.977 (0.819–1.166)	0.800	1.118 (0.847–1.476)	0.412
Smoker	0.808 (0.169–3.858)	0.653	0.500 (0.050–4.978)	0.712
CRP (mg/L)	0.958 (0.905–1.014)	0.044 *	0.563 (0.242–1.312)	<0.0001 *
Creatinine (µmol/L)	0.990 (0.965–1.017)	0.919	0.984 (0.950–1.020)	0.843
$TcPO_2$ (mmHg)	1.134 (0.933–1.380)	0.021 *	1.104 (0.926–1.317)	0.071
ABI	5.084 (0.347–126.09)	0.199	46.635 (0.393–5533.96)	0.035
BM-MNCs (109 cells/mL)	1.560 (0.896–3.138)	0.189	1.0 (0.999–1.0)	0.035

OR, odds ratio; CI, confidential interval; CRP, C-reaction protein; ABI, ankle-brachial index; $TcPO_2$, transcutaneous oxygen pressure. * The difference between six months and baseline in responders was statistically significant.

The receiver operating characteristics (ROC) analysis (Figure 3) was performed based on the univariate logistic regression results for the responder. An ROC curve was generated to address the sensitivity and specificity of CRP. The area under the ROC curve for CRP was 0.768 (95% CI 0.572–0.96, $p = 0.014$), indicating good discrimination for non-responders. Analysis showed that a cut-off limit of baseline CRP > 8.1 mg/L before transplantation was predictive for negative clinical response, with 81% specificity and 82% sensitivity

(Figure 3A). Analysis of linear regression showed a significant dependence between the levels of baseline CRP and the concentration of BM-MNCs in transplanted bone marrow ($R^2 = 0.162$, $p = 0.03$) (Figure 3B).

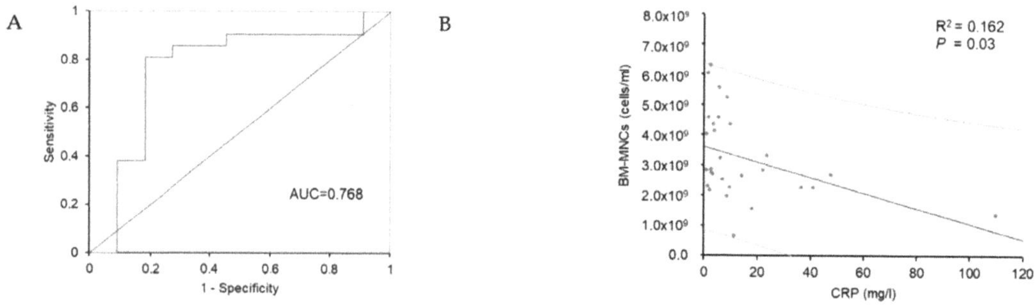

Figure 3. Receiver operating characteristics of CRP levels for predicting the BMCs therapeutic response. Area under the receiver operating characteristic (ROC) curve: CRP = 0.768 (CI 0.572–0.96, $p = 0.014$) (**A**) and linear regression between CRP and BM-MNCs, with lined 95% confidence interval bars and lined 95% prediction intervals (**B**). CRP, C-reaction protein; BMCs, bone marrow cells; BM-MNCs, bone marrow-derived mononuclear cells.

3.6. Effect of Atorvastatin Therapy before BMCs Treatment on the Outcomes of Stem Cell Treatment

The patients' baseline characteristics before BMCs therapy are presented in Table 6. No significant differences were observed between the atorvastatin and non-atorvastatin groups regarding the basic characteristics, previous blood examination, or parameters of limb ischaemia at baseline (Table 6).

Table 6. Characteristics of patients before stem cell treatment.

	All Patients (N = 33)	ATV Group (N = 22)	Non-ATV Group (N = 11)	*p* Value
Age (years) (mean ± SD)	64.9 ± 10	64.3 ± 11	65.9 ± 9.2	0.983
Sex (males)	31 (94%)	21 (95%)	10 (91%)	1.000
Rutherford class (1–6)	5 ± 0.30	5 ± 0.21	5 ± 0.45	0.829
Body mass index (kg/m^2)	27 ± 4.1	27.5 ± 3.8	26.9 ± 4.9	0.080
		Risk factors of limb ischaemia		
Diabetes mellitus (N, %)	11 (33%)	8 (22%)	3 (27%)	0.709
Arterial hypertension	27 (82%)	19 (86%)	8 (73%)	0.375
Hyperlipidaemia	23 (70%)	17 (77%)	6 (55%)	0.240
Smoker	10 (30%)	5 (23%)	5 (45%)	0.240
		Blood examination		
CRP (mg/L)	13.3 ± 21.3	12.8 ± 24.6	14.2 ± 14	0.341
Creatinine (µmol/L)	95.9 ± 34.6	97 ± 37.6	94 ± 29.7	0.977
		Parameters of limb ischaemia		
$TcPO_2 < 10$ mmHg	19 (58%)	11 (50%)	8 (73%)	0.278
ABI	0.51 ± 0.38	0.51 ± 0.36	0.52 ± 0.47	0.951
Pain scale (0–10)	5.75 ± 1.6	5.74 ± 1.52	5.78 ± 1.86	0.951

Data are presented as mean ± standard deviation or numbers and percentages, where appropriate. CRP, C-reaction protein; $TcPO_2$, transcutaneous oxygen pressure; ABI, ankle-brachial index. Statistical analysis was performed by the Mann-Whitney test and by Student's *t*-test (depending on data distribution determined by the Shapiro-Wilk test) or Fisher's exact test. p = ATV vs. non-ATV group.

3.7. Parameters of Limb Ischaemia after BMCs Delivery in Atorvastatin or Non-Atorvastatin Group

Based on the functional outcomes after BMCs treatment, significant improvement of $TcPO_2$ was observed in the atorvastatin group ($p = 0.015$), compared to nonsignificant improvement in the non-atorvastatin group (p = 0.611) (Table 7). Reduction in pain scoring was statistically significant in the atorvastatin group (p = 0.004), while no difference was observed in the non-atorvastatin group (p = 0.202). Amputation-free survival was achieved in 18 patients (82%) in the ATV group, while in the non-ATV group was achieved in 8 patients (73%, p = 0.661). The risk of major amputation was decreased in those prescribed statins (Hazard ratio (HR) 0.44, 95% CI 0.08–2.5, p = 0.36) but did not differ significantly (Figure 4C).

Table 7. Outcomes of BMCs treatment after three and six months in all patients with or without atorvastatin treatment prior to BMCs transplant.

	ATV Group (N = 22)				Non-ATV Group (N = 11)			
	before BMCs	Three Months	Six Months	p Value	before BMCs	Three Months	Six Months	p Value
Rutherford category	4.95 ± 0.21	4.95 ± 0.60	4.55 ± 1.1	0.092	5.0 ± 0.45	5.0 ± 0.78	5.0 ± 0.93	0.655
$TcPO_2$ (mmHg)	10.72 ± 13.01	14.4 ± 19.9	17.3 ± 16.5	0.015 *	7.5 ± 12.46	10.7 ± 14.9	10.2 ± 14.7	0.611
ABI	0.51 ± 0.36	0.44 ± 0.41	0.42 ± 0.34	0.532	0.52 ± 0.47	0.47 ± 0.47	0.38 ± 0.51	0.655
Pain scale (0–10)	5.74 ± 1.52	4.45 ± 2.7	3.6 ± 3.35	0.004 *	5.78 ± 1.86	5.2 ± 3.42	4.8 ± 4.07	0.202

Data are presented as mean ± standard deviation. ABI, ankle-brachial index; BMCs, bone marrow cells; $tcPO_2$, transcutaneous oxygen pressure. Statistical analysis was performed by the Wilcoxon matched-pair test and by Student's t-test (depending on data distribution determined by the Shapiro-Wilk test). p = six months vs. baseline. * The difference between six months and baseline in responders was statistically significant.

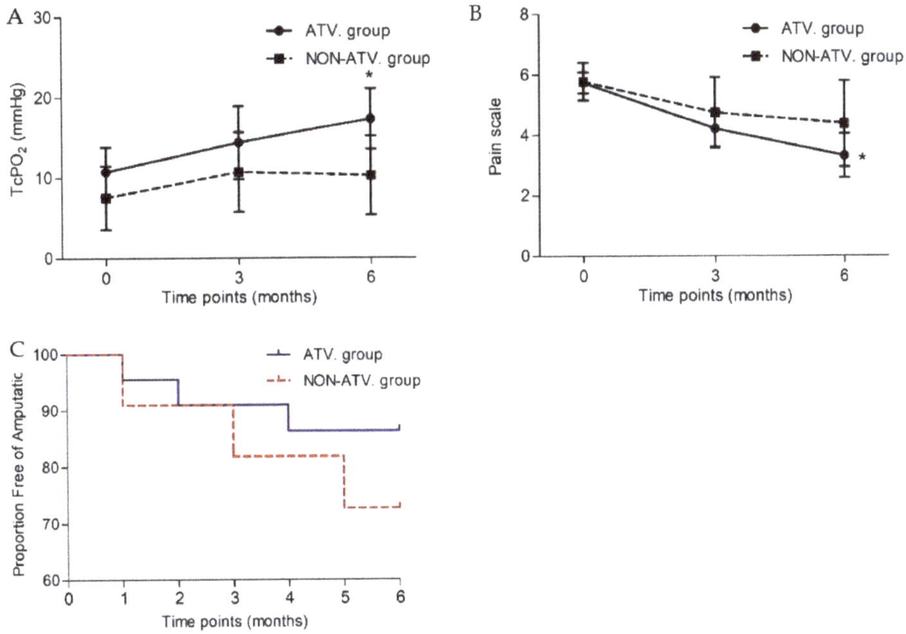

Figure 4. Comparison of longitudinal $TcPO_2$ changes (mean with SEM) in the ischemic limbs of patients treated with or without atorvastatin prior to BMCs treatment (**A**); comparison of longitudinal pain scale changes (mean with SEM) in the ischemic limbs of patients treated with or without atorvastatin prior to BMCs treatment (**B**); Kaplan-Meier curve to six months post-transplantation showing the proportion free of amputation (**C**). $TcPO_2$, transcutaneous oxygen pressure. * The difference between six months and baseline in responders was statistically significant.

3.8. Characteristics of Transplanted Bone Marrow Cells in ATV and Non-ATV Group

Table 8 compares the characteristics of BMCs transplants administered to the affected limb. The concentration of BM-MNCs was significantly higher in the atorvastatin group ($3.64 \pm 1.53 \times 10^9$) than in the non-atorvastatin group ($2.58 \pm 0.73 \times 10^9$, $p = 0.038$) (Table 8). No other statistically significant differences were observed between groups in terms of cell viability and count of MSCs in the transplant.

Table 8. Characteristics of transplanted BMCs.

	ATV Group (N = 22)	non-ATV Group (N = 11)	*p* Value
BM-MNCs (10^9 cells/mL)	3.64 ± 1.53	2.58 ± 0.73	0.038
Viability of BM-MNCs (%)	99.5 ± 0.57	99.6 ± 0.67	0.537
MSCs (10^4 cells/mL)	0.79 ± 0.52	1.47 ± 1.62	0.281

Data are presented as mean ± standard deviation. BMCs, bone marrow cells; BM-MNCs, bone marrow mononuclear cells; MSCs, mesenchymal stem cells. The Mann-Whitney test was used to perform statistical analysis. p = ATV vs. non-ATV group.

3.9. Effect of RAS-Acting Agents Therapy Prior to BMCs Treatment on the Outcomes of Stem Cell Treatment

Table 9 presents the baseline characteristics of patients before BMCs therapy. Patients with RAS-acting agents treatment were characterized by higher age ($p = 0.006$) and higher rate of arterial hypertension ($p = 0.025$).

Table 9. Characteristics of patients before stem cell treatment.

	All Patients (N = 33)	RAS Group (N = 20)	Non-RAS Group (N = 13)	*p* Value
Age (years) (mean ± SD)	64.9 ± 10	68.65 ± 8.82	59.0 ± 9.80	0.006 *
Sex (males)	31 (94%)	19 (95%)	12 (92%)	1.000
Rutherford class (1–6)	5 ± 0.30	4.95 ± 0.22	5.0 ± 0.41	0.652
Body mass index (kg/m^2)	27 ± 4.1	26.56 ± 2.85	28.47 ± 5.57	0.385
		Risk factors of limb ischaemia		
Diabetes mellitus (N, %)	11 (33%)	8 (40%)	3 (23%)	0.277
Arterial hypertension	27 (82%)	19 (95%)	8 (62%)	0.025 *
Hyperlipidaemia	23 (70%)	14 (70%)	9 (69%)	1.000
Smoker	10 (30%)	4 (21%)	6 (46%)	0.244
		Blood examination		
CRP (mg/L)	13.3 ± 21.3	16.09 ± 26.1	9.26 ± 10.77	0.367
Creatinine (μmol/L)	95.9 ± 34.6	100.1 ± 37.77	89.69 ± 29.8	0.258
		Parameters of limb ischaemia		
$TcPO_2 < 10$ mmHg	19 (58%)	10 (50%)	9 (69%)	0.310
ABI	0.51 ± 0.38	0.59 ± 0.37	0.38 ± 0.37	0.165
Pain scale (0–10)	5.75 ± 1.6	5.56 ± 1.42	6.10 ± 1.91	0.426

Data are presented as mean ± standard deviation or numbers and percentages, where appropriate. CRP, C-reaction protein; $TcPO_2$, transcutaneous oxygen pressure; ABI, ankle-brachial index. Statistical analysis was performed by the Mann-Whitney test and by Student's t-test (depending on data distribution determined by the Shapiro-Wilk test) or Fisher's exact test. p value = RAS vs. non-RAS group. * The difference between six months and baseline in responders was statistically significant.

3.10. Parameters of Limb Ischaemia after BMCs Delivery in RAS or Non-RAS Group

Based on the functional outcomes after BMCs treatment, significant improvement in pain scale was observed in the RAS group ($p = 0.005$), compared to nonsignificant improvement in the non-RAS group ($p = 0.139$). We have not seen any significant changes in the RAS or non-RAS group comparing Rutherford class, $TcPO_2$, or ABI during the six-month follow-up (Table 10).

Table 10. Outcomes of BMCs treatment after six months in all patients with or without RAS treatment prior to BMCs transplant.

Parameters of Limb Ischaemia	RAS Group			Non-RAS Group		
	Baseline (N = 20)	Six Months (N = 18)	p Value	Baseline (N = 13)	Six Months (N = 10)	p Value
Rutherford class (1–6)	4.95 ± 0.22	4.61 ± 0.41	0.164	5.0 ± 0.41	4.8 ± 1.03	0.276
$TcPO_2$ (mmHg)	11.4 ± 13.5	15.5 ± 14.5	0.077	6.7 ± 11.4	14.3 ± 18.8	0.201
ABI	0.59 ± 0.37	0.53 ± 0.41	0.408	0.38 ± 0.37	0.38 ± 0.26	0.500
Pain scale (0–10)	5.56 ± 1.42	3.33 ± 3.25	0.005 *	6.10 ± 1.91	4.22 ± 3.83	0.139

Data are presented as mean ± standard deviation. ABI, ankle-brachial index; BMCs, bone marrow cells; $TcPO_2$, transcutaneous oxygen pressure. Statistical analysis was performed using the Wilcoxon matched-pair test and Student's t-test (depending on data distribution determined by the Shapiro-Wilk test). p value = six months vs. baseline. * The difference between six months and baseline in responders was statistically significant.

In the RAS group, 16 patients (80%) achieved major amputation-free survival six months post-transplantation, while in the non-RAS group amputation-free survival was achieved in 10 patients (77%, p = 1.0). The risk of major amputation was decreased in those prescribed RAS-acting agents (HR 0.438, 95% CI 0.08–2.4, p = 0.34) but did not differ significantly (Figure 5).

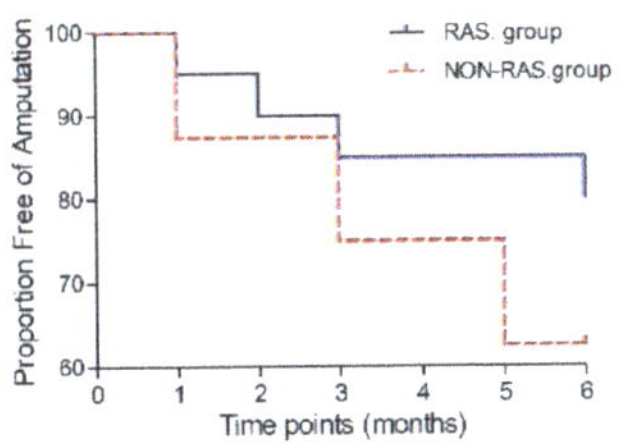

Figure 5. Kaplan-Meier curve to six months post-transplantation showing the proportion free of amputation.

3.11. Characteristics of Transplanted Bone Marrow Cells in RAS or Non-RAS Group

No statistical differences were observed between the RAS and non-RAS groups in terms of characteristics of BMCs transplants administered to the affected limb (Table 11).

Table 11. Characteristics of transplanted BMCs.

	RAS Group (N = 18)	non-RAS Group (N = 12)	p Value
BM-MNCs (10^9 cells/mL)	3.44 ± 1.55	3.05 ± 1.61	0.462
Viability of BM-MNCs (%)	99.6 ± 0.49	99.5 ± 0.75	0.859
MSCs (10^4 cells/mL)	0.86 ± 0.60	1.23 ± 1.50	0.730

Data are presented as mean ± standard deviation. BMCs, bone marrow cells; BM-MNCs, bone marrow mononuclear cells; MSCs, mesenchymal stem cells. The Mann-Whitney test was used to perform statistical analysis. p value = RAS. vs. non-RAS group.

3.12. Effect of Atorvastatin and RAS-Acting Agents Therapy Prior to BMCs Treatment on the Outcomes of Stem Cell Treatment

Of the 33 patients, 17 were treated with atorvastatin together with RAS-acting agents before stem cell treatment, while eight patients were without atorvastatin and RAS-acting agents treatment. The baseline characteristics of these groups were compared first, with only a significant difference in the mean age of patients (p = 0.026) (Table 12).

Table 12. Characteristics of patients before stem cell treatment.

	All Patients (N = 33)	ATV and RAS Group (N = 17)	Non-ATV and Non-RAS Group (N = 8)	*p* Value
Age (years) (mean ± SD)	64.9 ± 10	67.41 ± 9	62.25 ± 7.94	0.026 *
Sex (males)	31 (94%)	16 (94%)	7 (88%)	1.000
Rutherford class (1–6)	5 ± 0.30	4.94 ± 0.24	5 ± 0.54	0.817
Body mass index (kg/m^2)	27 ± 4.1	26.37 ± 2.73	26.87 ± 5.50	0.763
		Risk factors of limb ischaemia		
Diabetes mellitus (N, %)	11 (33%)	7 (41%)	2 (25%)	0.661
Arterial hypertension	27 (82%)	16 (94%)	5 (63%)	0.081
Hyperlipidaemia	23 (70%)	13 (76%)	5 (63%)	0.640
Smoker	10 (30%)	4 (24%)	5 (63%)	0.087
		Blood examination		
CRP (mg/L)	13.3 ± 21.3	16.06 ± 27.51	13.43 ± 12.05	0.653
Creatinine (µmol/L)	95.9 ± 34.6	100.7 ± 41.31	93.06 ± 35.29	0.425
		Parameters of limb ischaemia		
$TcPO_2$ < 10 mmHg	9.6 ± 12.7	8 (47%)	6 (75%)	0.234
ABI	0.51 ± 0.38	0.54 ± 0.33	0.34 ± 0.32	0.540
Pain scale (0–10)	5.75 ± 1.6	5.80 ± 1.42	6.50 ± 1.87	0.063

Data are presented as mean ± standard deviation or numbers and percentages, where appropriate. CRP, C-reaction protein; $TcPO_2$, transcutaneous oxygen pressure; ABI, ankle-brachial index. Statistical analysis was performed using the Mann-Whitney test and Student's *t*-test (depending on data distribution determined by the Shapiro-Wilk test) or Fisher's exact test. *p* = ATV and RAS group vs. non-ATV and non-RAS group. * The difference between six months and baseline in responders was statistically significant.

3.13. Parameters of Limb Ischaemia after BMCs Delivery in ATV and RAS Group or Non-ATV and Non-RAS Group

According to the results of BMCs treatment after six months, several variables were screened out in the ATV and RAS group (Table 13). Based on the available complete longitudinal data, the mean $TcPO_2$ of the RAS and ATV group increased from 11.6 ± 13.5 mmHg at baseline to 16.5 ± 15.0 mmHg at six months post-transplantation (p = 0.033). In contrast, that of the non-ATV and non-RAS groups did not improve significantly (p = 0.344). Regarding the results of improvement in the pain scale, the ATV and RAS group was associated with significant improvement of the pain scale from 5.80 ± 1.42 at baseline to 3.50 ± 3.43 at six months (p = 0.009), while assessment of the pain scale did not change significantly in the non-ATV and non-RAS group (p = 0.279). Amputation-free survival was achieved in 13 patients (76%) in the ATV and RAS group, while in the non-ATV and non-RAS group it was achieved in 5 patients (62.5%, p = 0.344). The risk of major amputation was decreased in those prescribed atorvastatin and RAS-acting agents (HR 0.39, 95% CI 0.07–2.3, p = 0.36) but did not differ significantly (Figure 6).

Table 13. Outcomes of BMCs treatment after six months in all patients with or without ATV-RAS treatment prior to BMCs transplant.

Parameters of Limb Ischaemia	ATV and RAS Group			Non-ATV and Non-RAS Group		
	Baseline (N = 17)	Six Months (N = 15)	*p* Value	Baseline (N = 8)	Six Months (N = 7)	*p* Value
Rutherford class (1–6)	4.94 ± 0.24	4.56 ± 1.15	0.164	5.0 ± 0.54	5.0 ± 1.10	0.655
$TcPO_2$ (mmHg)	11.6 ± 13.5	16.5 ± 15.0	0.033 *	6.3 ± 11.8	10.9 ± 16.4	0.344
ABI	0.54 ± 0.33	0.47 ± 0.36	0.409	0.34 ± 0.32	0.18 ± 0.32	0.650
Pain scale (0–10)	5.80 ± 1.42	3.50 ± 3.43	0.009 *	6.50 ± 1.87	5.17 ± 4.45	0.279

Data are presented as mean ± standard deviation. ABI, ankle-brachial index; BMCs, bone marrow cells; $TcPO_2$, transcutaneous oxygen pressure. Statistical analysis was performed using the Wilcoxon matched-pair test and Student's *t*-test (depending on data distribution determined by the Shapiro-Wilk test). *p* = six months vs. baseline.
* The difference between six months and baseline in responders was statistically significant.

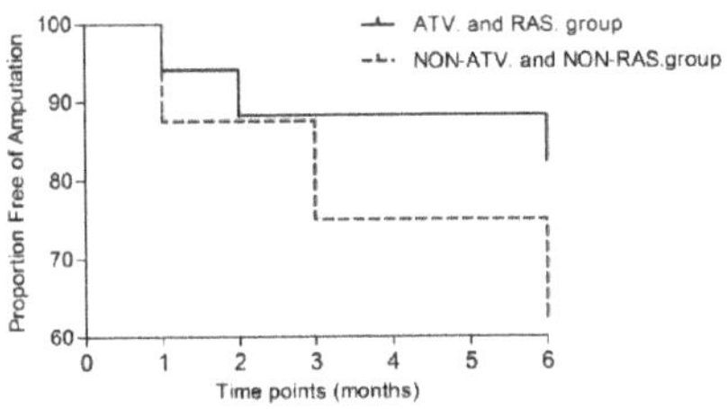

Figure 6. Kaplan-Meier curve to six months post-transplantation showing the proportion free of amputation.

3.14. Characteristics of Transplanted Bone Marrow Cells in ATV and RAS Group or Non-ATV and Non-RAS Group

Regarding the transplants, the transplanted BM-MNCs count appeared to be higher in the ATV and RAS group ($3.56 \pm 1.60 \times 10^9$) than in the non-ATV and non-RAS group ($2.60 \pm 0.81 \times 10^9$). However, the difference was not statistically significant ($p = 0.064$) (Table 14).

Table 14. Characteristics of transplanted BMCs.

	ATV and RAS Group (N = 17)	Non-ATV and Non-RAS Group (N = 8)	*p* Value
BM-MNCs (10^9 cells/mL)	3.56 ± 1.60	2.60 ± 0.81	0.064
Viability of BM-MNCs (%)	99.6 ± 0.51	99.6 ± 0.75	0.642
MSCs (10^4 cells/mL)	0.78 ± 0.56	1.53 ± 1.89	0.549

BMCs, bone marrow cells; BM-MNCs, bone marrow mononuclear cells; MSCs, mesenchymal stem cells. The Mann-Whitney test was used to perform statistical analysis. p = ATV and RAS vs. non-ATV and non-RAS group.

3.15. Results of Spearman Correlation Analysis for the Investigated Treatment Option

The Spearman correlation between investigated treatment options before BMCs transplantation and baseline characteristics is shown in Table 15. Patients with CLI regression, patients considered as responders, showed a significant positive correlation with age ($R = 0.430$, $p = 0.012$) and RAS treatment ($R = 0.351$, $p = 0.045$). Relevantly, there was a negative correlation with CRP ($R = -0.442$, $p = 0.011$). Statin treatment before BMCs administration correlated with RAS treatment ($R = 0.482$, $p = 0.005$). RAS-acting agents treatment was highly correlated with age of patients ($R = 0.566$, $p = 0.0006$). Treatment with both investigated pharmacotherapies, statin and RAS treatment, showed a significant positive correlation with CLI regression, responder status ($R = 0.618$, $p = 0.001$), and age of patients ($R = 0.454$, $p = 0.023$).

Table 15. Results of Spearman correlation analysis (R) for the investigated treatment option and baseline characteristics of patients.

		Responder	Age	CRP	RAS-Acting Agents Treatment
Responder	Spearman's r	-	0.430	−0.442	0.351
	p value	-	0.012	0.011	0.045
Statin treatment	Spearman's r	-	-	-	0.482
	p value	-	-	-	0.005
RAS-acting agents treatment	Spearman's r	0.351	0.566	-	-
	p value	0.045	0.0006	-	-
Statin and RAS-acting agents treatment	Spearman's r	0.618	0.454	-	1
	p value	0.001	0.023	-	<0.0001

4. Discussion

4.1. Summary of the Results

This study investigated the outcomes and possible predictive factors of autologous bone marrow cell transplantation in treating "no-option" CLI patients. It was focused on exploring clinical background and prior statin pharmacotherapy related to the therapeutic efficacy of BMCs treatment. Our results revealed that CRP and $TcPO_2$ values positively correlated with the probability of being a responder. In contrast, CRP value, ABI, and BM-MNCs concentration were identified as prognostic factors of the super-responders. Based on the results of univariate logistic regression for responders, ROC analysis of CRP revealed that a cut-off limit of CRP > 8.1 mg/L before transplantation was predictive for negative clinical response after BMCs transplantation. Linear regression analysis demonstrated a significant dependence between the levels of baseline CRP and the concentration of BM-MNCs in transplanted bone marrow.

Atorvastatin treatment prior to BMCs transplant revealed significant improvement of $TcpO_2$ and reduction of pain scale after BMCs transplant compared to nonsignificant changes in the non-atorvastatin group. Our results showed that atorvastatin use was associated with decreased risk for major amputation. However, the difference was not statistically significant. Furthermore, our findings showed a significantly higher concentration of BM-MNCs in the transplanted bone marrow cells of patients in the atorvastatin group than in the non-atorvastatin group, which might contribute to the beneficial effect of cell therapy.

Patients treated with RAS-acting agents before BMCs transplant had significantly reduced pain scale after six months, compared to the non-RAS group. Similar results, reduced pain scale as well as improved $TcPO_2$, were achieved in a group of patients treated with atorvastatin and RAS-acting agents before BMCs treatment. Results of Spearman correlation showed a significant positive correlation between CLI regression, patients considered as responders, and previous treatment before BMCs transplant with RAS-acting agents alone or together with atorvastatin.

4.2. Prognostic Factors of the Therapeutic Responses to Autologous BMCs Treatment

As the terminal stage of peripheral arterial disease, CLI is characterized by an extremely high risk of amputation and other vascular issues, causing severe morbidity and mortality in affected patients. Therapeutic angiogenesis with cell-based therapies aims to increase blood flow to ischemic regions. One of the most encouraging cells used as an alternative for the surgical treatment of CLI is mesenchymal stem cells appearing in the bone marrow-derived mononuclear stem cells population [19]. Although stem cell therapies are studied clinically for their benefit in the treatment of cardiac repair or patients with CLI, their effects are still controversial and considered experimental [13,20,21]. The published data show that treatment with bone marrow stem cells is associated with limb salvage, increased $TcPO_2$, ABI, or blood flow perfusion [22]. The results of our study present the beneficial effects of autologous BMCs transplantation in $TcPO_2$, pain scoring, and Rutherford category, but not ABI. ABI did not change after six months, similar to the results of other authors [23,24], but it was inconsistent with the report of Gupta et al. 2013 and Benoit et al. 2013 [25,26]. The prevalence of amputation-free survival at 82% was similar to the results of Zafarhandi et al. 2010, who also reported the effects of cell therapy after six months [27].

$TcPO_2$ represents the tension of oxygen disseminated from subcutaneous microcirculation and can reflect the distal peripheral perfusion [28]. $TcPO_2$ measurement is a metabolic test and is considered a helpful predictor for chronic ischemic ulcer healing, with a threshold value of 20–40 mmHg [29]. On the contrary, the unfavourable value for spontaneous healing is less than 10 mmHg [30,31]. In our study, the evaluation of the baseline characteristics showed that responders had higher baseline $TcPO_2$ than non-responders, but the difference was not statistically significant. The univariate regression analysis showed that the baseline $TcPO_2$ value was a prognostic factor for being a responder to BMCs treatment.

Moreover, according to the longitudinal data, we found significant improvement of $TcPO_2$ at six months post-transplantation in the responder group, whereas little improvement was found in the non-responders group. Moreover, the $TcPO_2$ at baseline correlated significantly with values at six months post-transplantation. Based on these data, we assume that baseline $TcPO_2$ represents an important criterion for the patients undergoing transplantation of bone marrow stem cells, consistent with several previous studies [29,32,33]. These results suggest that the restoration of peripheral perfusion after BMCs therapy is characterized by a favourable baseline condition of local microcirculation, which might explain the predictive role of baseline $TcPO_2$.

Inflammatory markers such as C-reactive protein (CRP), fibrinogen, and serum amyloid A are associated with an increased risk of cardiovascular events. They are considered critical risk factors for the development and progression of PAD [34,35]. Our study demonstrates that responders to BMCs therapy are characterized by significantly lower baseline CRP levels than non-responders. The univariate regression analysis showed that the baseline CRP value was a prognostic factor for being a responder to BMCs treatment. CRP belongs to acute-phase reactant protein and is produced during inflammation, which negatively modulates the local inflammatory reaction in the transplantation site and, thus, the entire process of therapeutic angiogenesis after BM-MNCs transplantation [36]. Moreover, CRP influences the systemic inflammatory reaction and can negatively regulate bone marrow cells' characteristics. Indeed, we found that depressed numbers of BM-MNCs in the bone marrow transplant were associated with elevated levels of CRP in patients with critical limb ischaemia. We found that these two characteristics are significantly dependent upon each other. The receiver operating characteristics analysis showed a cut-off limit of baseline CRP > 8.1 mg/L before transplantation was predictive for negative clinical response after BMCs transplantation.

In addition to the patient's clinical background, the characteristic of the bone marrow transplant plays a critical role in the healing prognosis. An important predictor of the therapeutic response is the number of administered nucleated cells, bone marrow-derived mononuclear cells, which strongly relate to clinical benefit in the PROVASA trial and are considered an independent predictor of improved ulcer healing [12]. On the other hand, in the study of Yusoff et al. 2020, the authors found that the difference in the number of BM-MNCs derived from bone marrow did not alter the major amputation-free survival rate or mortality rate in atherosclerotic PAD patients with CLI [37]. Our results demonstrate a significant difference in the concentration of BM-MNCs, however, in the subgroup analysis of super-responders, patients with limb salvage and complete ischemic wound healing, compared to super-non-responders, patients with major limb amputation. Specifically, a significantly higher number of BM-MNCs was present in the BMCs transplant of the super-responder group compared to the super-non-responder group.

Moreover, the univariate regression analysis showed that the concentration of BM-MNCs was a prognostic factor for being a super-responder to BMCs treatment. Accordingly, we believe that the concentration of BM-MNCs in transplant might be feasible for NO-CLI patients. A longer-term follow-up study will be needed to compare the outcomes and advantages of transplantation types.

4.3. Subgroup Analysis of Treatment Approach before BMCs Transplant

Many studies demonstrated the poor survival and retention of transplanted bone marrow cells in vivo, caused by stem cells' properties, the extremely hostile microenvironment of implantation, or a combination of both [13]. For these reasons, the effort has been focused on improving the tolerance of transplanted stem cells to the microenvironment. This would lead to developing a clinical approach with enhanced stem cell survival and angiogenesis in the implantation site. Recent pre-clinical and clinical studies describe the use of statin drugs to augment the function of MSCs or endothelial progenitor cells (EPC) for regenerative cell-based therapy. Promising results have been reported in treating AMI in animal models but have yet to be reported in human studies. Pre-clinical and clinical studies reported a beneficial effect of statin therapy that improves MSCs or EPC function and their numbers. However, statin use in enhancing cell-based vascular repair warrants further study [38–40]. Systematic review and meta-analysis of nineteen studies with 26,985 patients with CLI showed that statin use was associated with decreased risk of major amputation, mortality, and more remarkable amputation-free survival and overall patency rates [16].

In this study, we examined the efficacy of atorvastatin treatment before BMCs transplant on outcomes of cell-based therapy. Our data confirmed a significant improvement of $TcPO_2$ and a reduction of pain scoring in the atorvastatin group, compared to a nonsignificant improvement in the non-atorvastatin group. Our results showed that statin use was associated with a decreased risk of major amputation. However, the difference was not statistically significant. Furthermore, our findings showed a significantly higher concentration of BM-MNCs in transplanted bone marrow cells in patients with prior atorvastatin treatment compared to the non-atorvastatin group. We suggest that these beneficial effects of atorvastatin contribute to the valuable effect of cell therapy in CLI patients and are related to the clinical benefit of stem cell treatment.

Moreover, we focused on the effects of RAS-acting agents treatment before BMCs transplant on the outcomes of cell-based therapy. RAS-acting agents (angiotensin-converting enzyme inhibitors (ACEIs) and angiotensin receptor blockers (ARBs)) should be considered as first-line therapy in patients with PAD and hypertension [14]. Bodewes et al. 2018 revealed the long-term mortality benefit of RAS inhibitors in chronic limb-threatening ischaemia patients, whereas limb events were unaffected [41]. Our study has demonstrated that patients treated with RAS-acting agents before BMCs transplant had significantly reduced pain scale after six months, compared to the non-RAS group. Similar results, reduced pain scale and improved $TcPO_2$, were achieved in patients treated with atorvastatin and RAS-acting agents before BMCs treatment.

Results of the Spearman correlation showed a significant positive correlation between CLI regression, responders, and previous treatment before BMCs transplant with RAS-acting agents alone or with atorvastatin.

5. Limitations

There were several limitations to this study. First, no parallel placebo control group is present due to ethical concerns and one single centre. Additionally, the sample size was insufficient to evaluate more specific variables. Moreover, our study focused on short-term responders (six months) to BMCs therapy rather than long-term remission from CLI, which is also the target of therapeutic angiogenesis. Therefore, a prolonged cohort follow-up with larger numbers of patients is needed in the future.

6. Conclusions

Our data suggest the potential benefits of carefully managing patients with CLI before BMCs transplantation, as this approach appears to enhance the effectiveness of cell therapy.

CRP and $TcPO_2$ values were positively associated with a positive response to BMCs transplantation. Additionally, our analyzed factors (CRP value, ABI, and BM-MNCs concentration) may help predict responders and super-responders to cell therapy. A baseline CRP level above 8.1 mg/L could indicate a reduced positive clinical response after BMCs transplantation. In line with recommended guidelines for treating CLI patients, long-term atorvastatin use appears to improve outcomes after BMCs therapy, potentially through increased BM-MNCs in the transplant. The long-term treatment of CLI patients with RAS-acting agents significantly reduced pain scale after BMCs transplant. The combination of atorvastatin and RAS-acting agents shows promise for reducing pain and improving TcPO2 values in CLI patients after BMCs therapy.

While these findings are encouraging, further research is needed to confirm them in larger studies, to explore the exact mechanisms by which statins and RAS-acting agents might improve BMCs therapy outcomes, and to determine the optimal timing and combination of these therapies with BMCs transplantation.

Author Contributions: Resources, A.A., S.V., N.C. and Z.Č.; Writing—review & editing, A.A. and A.G.; Supervision, J.K. and J.M. All authors have read and agreed to the published version of the manuscript.

Funding: This research was funded by a grant from the Ministry of the Health of the Slovak Republic 2016/13-FAUK-1.

Institutional Review Board Statement: The local ethical committee of the National Institute of Cardiovascular Diseases, Bratislava, approved the study design. This study was carried out by the Code of Ethics of the World Medical Association, Declaration of Helsinki (WMA Declaration of Helsinki, 2013).

Informed Consent Statement: All patients in the study were informed about the nature of the study and gave their written informed consent.

Data Availability Statement: The data that support the findings of this study are available upon request.

Conflicts of Interest: The authors declare no conflicts of interest.

Abbreviations

ABI	ankle-brachial index
ACEIs	angiotensin-converting enzyme inhibitors
ARBs	angiotensin receptor blockers
ATV	atorvastatin
AUC	area under the ROC curve
BMCs	bone marrow cells
BM-MNCs	bone marrow-derived mononuclear cells
CI	confidence interval
CLI	critical limb ischaemia
CRP	C-reactive protein
EPC	endothelial progenitor cells
HR	hazard ratio
MI	myocardial infarct
MSCs	mesenchymal stem cells
NO-CLI	"no-option" critical limb ischaemia
non-RAS	non-renin-angiotensin system
OR	odds ratio
PAD	peripheral arterial disease
RAS	renin-angiotensin system
ROC	receiver operating characteristics
SD	standard deviation
SEM	standard error
TASC	Transatlantic Inter-Society Consensus
$TcPO_2$	transcutaneous oxygen pressure
VAS	Visual analogue scale

References

1. Paola, L.D.; Cimaglia, P.; Carone, A.; Scavone, G.; Boscarino, G.; Bernucci, D.; Sbarzaglia, P.; Censi, S.; Ferrari, R.; Campo, G. Limb salvage in diabetic patients with no-option critical limb ischemia: Outcomes of a specialized center experience. *Diabet. Foot Ankle* **2019**, *10*, 1696012. [CrossRef]
2. Norgren, L.; Hiatt, W.R.; Dormandy, J.A.; Nehler, M.R.; Harris, K.A.; Fowkes, F.G.R. Inter-Society Consensus for the Management of Peripheral Arterial Disease (TASC II). *J. Vasc. Surg.* **2007**, *45*, S5–S67. [CrossRef]
3. Wahid, S.F.A.; Ismail, N.A.; Jamaludin, W.F.W.; Muhamad, N.A.; Hamid, M.K.A.A.; Harunarashid, H.; Lai, N.M. Autologous cells derived from different sources and administered using different regimens for "no-option" critical lower limb ischaemia patients. *Cochrane Database Syst. Rev.* **2018**, *2018*, CD010747. [CrossRef]

4. Hassanshahi, M.; Khabbazi, S.; Peymanfar, Y.; Hassanshahi, A.; Hosseini-Khah, Z.; Su, Y.W.; Xian, C.J. Critical limb ischemia: Current and novel therapeutic strategies. *J. Cell. Physiol.* **2019**, *234*, 14445–14459. [CrossRef]
5. Uccioli, L.; Meloni, M.; Izzo, V.; Giurato, L.; Merolla, S.; Gandini, R. Critical limb ischemia: Current challenges and future prospects. *Vasc. Heal. Risk Manag.* **2018**, *14*, 63–74. [CrossRef]
6. Fang, G.; Jiang, X.; Fang, Y.; Pan, T.; Liu, H.; Ren, B.; Wei, Z.; Gu, S.; Chen, B.; Jiang, J.; et al. Autologous peripheral blood-derived stem cells transplantation for treatment of no-option angiitis-induced critical limb ischemia: 10-year management experience. *Stem Cell Res. Ther.* **2020**, *11*, 458. [CrossRef]
7. Lu, D.; Jiang, Y.; Deng, W.; Zhang, Y.; Liang, Z.; Wu, Q.; Jiang, X.; Zhang, L.; Gao, F.; Cao, Y.; et al. Long-Term Outcomes of BMMSC Compared with BMMNC for Treatment of Critical Limb Ischemia and Foot Ulcer in Patients with Diabetes. *Cell Transplant.* **2019**, *28*, 645–652. [CrossRef] [PubMed]
8. Procházka, V.; Gumulec, J.; Jalůvka, F.; Šalounová, D.; Jonszta, T.; Czerný, D.; Krajča, J.; Urbanec, R.; Klement, P.; Martinek, J.; et al. Cell Therapy, a New Standard in Management of Chronic Critical Limb Ischemia and Foot Ulcer. *Cell Transplant.* **2010**, *19*, 1413–1424. [CrossRef] [PubMed]
9. Szabó, G.V.; Kövesd, Z.; Cserepes, J.; Daróczy, J.; Belkin, M.; Acsády, G. Peripheral blood-derived autologous stem cell therapy for the treatment of patients with late-stage peripheral artery disease—Results of the short- and long-term follow-up. *Cytotherapy* **2013**, *15*, 1245–1252. [CrossRef]
10. Ozturk, A.; Kucukardali, Y.; Tangi, F.; Erikci, A.; Uzun, G.; Bashekim, C.; Sen, H.; Terekeci, H.; Narin, Y.; Ozyurt, M.; et al. Therapeutical potential of autologous peripheral blood mononuclear cell transplantation in patients with type 2 diabetic critical limb ischemia. *J. Diabetes Complicat.* **2012**, *26*, 29–33. [CrossRef]
11. Teraa, M.; Sprengers, R.W.; Schutgens, R.E.; Slaper-Cortenbach, I.C.; Van Der Graaf, Y.; Algra, A.; Van Der Tweel, I.; Doevendans, P.A.; Mali, W.P.; Moll, F.L.; et al. Effect of Repetitive Intra-Arterial Infusion of Bone Marrow Mononuclear Cells in Patients with No-Option Limb Ischaemia: The Randomized, Double-Blind, Placebo-Controlled Rejuvenating Endothelial Progenitor Cells via Transcutaneous Intra-arterial Supplementation (JUVENTAS) Trial. *Circulation* **2015**, *131*, 851–860. [CrossRef] [PubMed]
12. Walter, D.H.; Krankenberg, H.; Balzer, J.O.; Kalka, C.; Baumgartner, I.; Schlüter, M.; Tonn, T.; Seeger, F.; Dimmeler, S.; Lindhoff-Last, E.; et al. Intraarterial Administration of Bone Marrow Mononuclear Cells in Patients with Critical Limb Ischemia. *Circ. Cardiovasc. Interv.* **2011**, *4*, 26–37. [CrossRef] [PubMed]
13. Dai, G.; Xu, Q.; Luo, R.; Gao, J.; Chen, H.; Deng, Y.; Li, Y.; Wang, Y.; Yuan, W.; Wu, X. Atorvastatin treatment improves effects of implanted mesenchymal stem cells: Meta-analysis of animal models with acute myocardial infarction. *BMC Cardiovasc. Disord.* **2015**, *15*, 170. [CrossRef] [PubMed]
14. Aboyans, V.; Ricco, J.-B.; Bartelink, M.-L.E.L.; Björck, M.; Brodmann, M.; Cohnert, T.; Collet, J.-P.; Czerny, M.; De Carlo, M.; Debus, S.; et al. 2017 ESC Guidelines on the Diagnosis and Treatment of Peripheral Arterial Diseases, in collaboration with the European Society for Vascular Surgery (ESVS). *Eur. Heart J.* **2018**, *39*, 763–816. [CrossRef] [PubMed]
15. Kokkinidis, D.G.; Arfaras-Melainis, A.; Giannopoulos, S.; Katsaros, I.; Jawaid, O.; Jonnalagadda, A.K.; Parikh, S.A.; Secemsky, E.A.; Giri, J.; Kumbhani, D.J.; et al. Statin therapy for reduction of cardiovascular and limb-related events in critical limb ischemia: A systematic review and meta-analysis. *Vasc. Med.* **2020**, *25*, 106–117. [CrossRef] [PubMed]
16. Samakova, A.; Gazova, A.; Sabova, N.; Valaskova, S.; Jurikova, M.; Kyselovic, J. The pi3k/Akt Pathway Is Associated With Angiogenesis, Oxidative Stress and Survival of Mesenchymal Stem Cells in Pathophysiologic Condition in Ischaemia 2019;68:8. *Physiol. Res.* **2019**, *68*, 8.
17. Ridker, P.M.; Bhatt, D.L.; Pradhan, A.D.; Glynn, R.J.; MacFadyen, J.G.; Nissen, S.E. Inflammation and cholesterol as predictors of cardiovascular events among patients receiving statin therapy: A collaborative analysis of three randomised trials. *Lancet* **2023**, *401*, 1293–1301. [CrossRef]
18. Rutherford, R.B.; Baker, J.; Ernst, C.; Johnston, K.; Porter, J.M.; Ahn, S.; Jones, D.N. Recommended standards for reports dealing with lower extremity ischemia: Revised version. *J. Vasc. Surg.* **1997**, *26*, 517–538. [CrossRef] [PubMed]
19. Shirbaghaee, Z.; Hassani, M.; Heidari Keshel, S.; Soleimani, M. Emerging roles of mesenchymal stem cell therapy in patients with critical limb ischemia. *Stem Cell Res. Ther.* **2022**, *13*, 462. [CrossRef]
20. Weem, S.P.; Teraa, M.; de Borst, G.; Verhaar, M.; Moll, F. Bone Marrow derived Cell Therapy in Critical Limb Ischemia: A Meta-analysis of Randomized Placebo Controlled Trials. *Eur. J. Vasc. Endovasc. Surg.* **2015**, *50*, 775–783. [CrossRef]
21. Jaluvka, F.; Ihnat, P.; Madaric, J.; Vrtkova, A.; Janosek, J.; Prochazka, V. Current Status of Cell-Based Therapy in Patients with Critical Limb Ischemia. *Int. J. Mol. Sci.* **2020**, *21*, 8999. [CrossRef] [PubMed]
22. Compagna, R.; Amato, B.; Massa, S.; Amato, M.; Grande, R.; Butrico, L.; de Franciscis, S.; Serra, R. Cell Therapy in Patients with Critical Limb Ischemia. *Stem Cells Int.* **2015**, *2015*, 931420. [CrossRef] [PubMed]
23. Klepanec, A.; Mistrik, M.; Altaner, C.; Valachovicova, M.; Olejarova, I.; Slysko, R.; Balazs, T.; Urlandova, T.; Hladikova, D.; Liska, B.; et al. No Difference in Intra-Arterial and Intramuscular Delivery of Autologous Bone Marrow Cells in Patients with Advanced Critical Limb Ischemia. *Cell Transplant.* **2012**, *21*, 1909–1918. [CrossRef] [PubMed]
24. Matoba, S.; Tatsumi, T.; Murohara, T.; Imaizumi, T.; Katsuda, Y.; Ito, M.; Saito, Y.; Uemura, S.; Suzuki, H.; Fukumoto, S.; et al. Long-term clinical outcome after intramuscular implantation of bone marrow mononuclear cells (Therapeutic Angiogenesis by Cell Transplantation [TACT] trial) in patients with chronic limb ischemia. *Am. Hear. J.* **2008**, *156*, 1010–1018. [CrossRef] [PubMed]
25. Benoit, E.; O'Donnell, T.F.; Patel, A.N.; O'Donnell, J.T.F. Safety and Efficacy of Autologous Cell Therapy in Critical Limb Ischemia: A Systematic Review. *Cell Transplant.* **2013**, *22*, 545–562. [CrossRef] [PubMed]

26. Gupta, P.K.; Chullikana, A.; Parakh, R.; Desai, S.; Das, A.; Gottipamula, S.; Krishnamurthy, S.; Anthony, N.; Pherwani, A.; Majumdar, A.S. A double blind randomized placebo controlled phase I/II study assessing the safety and efficacy of allogeneic bone marrow-derived mesenchymal stem cell in critical limb ischaemia. *J. Transl. Med.* **2013**, *11*, 143. [CrossRef]
27. Zafarghandi, M.R.; Ravari, H.; Aghdami, N.; Namiri, M.; Moazzami, K.; Taghiabadi, E.; Fazel, A.; Pournasr, B.; Farrokhi, A.; Sharifian, R.A.; et al. Safety and efficacy of granulocyte–colony-stimulating factor administration following autologous intramuscular implantation of bone marrow mononuclear cells: A randomized controlled trial in patients with advanced lower limb ischemia. *Cytotherapy* **2010**, *12*, 783–791. [CrossRef]
28. Leenstra, B.; Wijnand, J.; Verhoeven, B.; Koning, O.; Teraa, M.; Verhaar, M.C.; de Borst, G.J. Applicability of Transcutaneous Oxygen Tension Measurement in the Assessment of Chronic Limb-Threatening Ischemia. *Angiology* **2019**, *71*, 208–216. [CrossRef]
29. Pan, T.; Liu, H.; Fang, Y.; Wei, Z.; Gu, S.; Fang, G.; Liu, Y.; Luo, Y.; Guo, D.; Xu, X.; et al. Predictors of responders to mononuclear stem cell-based therapeutic angiogenesis for no-option critical limb ischemia. *Stem Cell Res. Ther.* **2019**, *10*, 15. [CrossRef]
30. Got, I. Transcutaneous oxygen pressure (TcPO2): Advantages and limitations. *Diabetes Metab.* **1998**, *24*, 379–384.
31. Yang, C.; Weng, H.; Chen, L.; Yang, H.; Luo, G.; Mai, L.; Jin, G.; Yan, L. Transcutaneous oxygen pressure measurement in diabetic foot ulcers: Mean values and cut-point for wound healing. *J. Wound Ostomy Cont. Nurs. Publ. Wound Ostomy Cont. Nurses Soc.* **2013**, *40*, 585–589. [CrossRef]
32. Madaric, J.; Klepanec, A.; Valachovicova, M.; Mistrik, M.; Bucova, M.; Olejarova, I.; Necpal, R.; Madaricova, T.; Paulis, L.; Vulev, I. Characteristics of responders to autologous bone marrow cell therapy for no-option critical limb ischemia. *Stem Cell Res. Ther.* **2016**, *7*, 116. [CrossRef] [PubMed]
33. Aoyama, N.; Nishinari, M.; Ohtani, S.; Kanai, A.; Noda, C.; Hirata, M.; Miyamoto, A.; Watanabe, M.; Minamino, T.; Izumi, T.; et al. Clinical features and predictors of patients with critical limb ischemia who responded to autologous mononuclear cell transplantation for therapeutic angiogenesis. *Hear. Vessel.* **2017**, *32*, 1099–1108. [CrossRef] [PubMed]
34. Hazarika, S.; Annex, B.H. Biomarkers and Genetics in Peripheral Artery Disease. *Clin. Chem.* **2017**, *63*, 236–244. [CrossRef] [PubMed]
35. Owens, C.D.; Ridker, P.M.; Belkin, M.; Hamdan, A.D.; Pomposelli, F.; Logerfo, F.; Creager, M.A.; Conte, M.S. Elevated C-reactive protein levels are associated with postoperative events in patients undergoing lower extremity vein bypass surgery. *J. Vasc. Surg.* **2007**, *45*, 2–9. [CrossRef] [PubMed]
36. Verma, S.; Kuliszewski, M.A.; Li, S.-H.; Szmitko, P.E.; Zucco, L.; Wang, C.-H.; Badiwala, M.V.; Mickle, D.A.; Weisel, R.D.; Fedak, P.W.; et al. C-Reactive Protein Attenuates Endothelial Progenitor Cell Survival, Differentiation, and Function: Further Evidence of a Mechanistic Link Between C-Reactive Protein and Cardiovascular Disease. *Circulation* **2004**, *109*, 2058–2067. [CrossRef] [PubMed]
37. Yusoff, F.M.; Kajikawa, M.; Takaeko, Y.; Kishimoto, S.; Hashimoto, H.; Maruhashi, T.; Nakashima, A.; Wahid, S.F.S.A.; Higashi, Y. Relationship between cell number and clinical outcomes of autologous bone-marrow mononuclear cell implantation in critical limb ischemia. *Sci. Rep.* **2020**, *10*, 19891. [CrossRef] [PubMed]
38. Park, A.; Barrera-Ramirez, J.; Ranasinghe, I.; Pilon, S.; Sy, R.; Fergusson, D.; Allan, D.S. Use of Statins to Augment Progenitor Cell Function in Preclinical and Clinical Studies of Regenerative Therapy: A Systematic Review. *Stem Cell Rev. Rep.* **2016**, *12*, 327–339. [CrossRef] [PubMed]
39. Jia, W.; Zhao, Y.; Yang, J.; Wang, W.; Wang, X.; Ling, L.; Ge, L. Simvastatin Promotes Dental Pulp Stem Cell–induced Coronal Pulp Regeneration in Pulpotomized Teeth. *J. Endod.* **2016**, *42*, 1049–1054. [CrossRef]
40. Tahamtan, S.; Shirban, F.; Bagherniya, M.; Johnston, T.P.; Sahebkar, A. The effects of statins on dental and oral health: A review of preclinical and clinical studies. *J. Transl. Med.* **2020**, *18*, 155. [CrossRef]
41. Bodewes, T.C.; Darling, J.D.; O'Donnell, T.F.; Deery, S.E.; Shean, K.E.; Mittleman, M.A.; Moll, F.L.; Schermerhorn, M.L. Long-term mortality benefit of renin-angiotensin system inhibitors in patients with chronic limb-threatening ischemia undergoing vascular intervention. *J. Vasc. Surg.* **2018**, *67*, 800–808. [CrossRef] [PubMed]

biomedicines

MDPI

Article

Sacubitril/Valsartan Alleviates Cardiac Remodeling and Dysfunction in L-NAME-Induced Hypertension and Hypertensive Heart Disease

Peter Stanko [1,2,†], Kristina Repova [1,†], Tomas Baka [1], Kristina Krajcirovicova [1], Silvia Aziriova [1], Andrej Barta [3], Stefan Zorad [4], Michaela Adamcova [5] and Fedor Simko [1,4,6,*]

1 Institute of Pathophysiology, Faculty of Medicine, Comenius University, 81108 Bratislava, Slovakia; pete.stanko@gmail.com (P.S.); kristina.repova@fmed.uniba.sk (K.R.); tomasko.baka@gmail.com (T.B.); krikratina@gmail.com (K.K.); silvia.aziriova@gmail.com (S.A.)

2 Department of Pneumology, Phthisiology and Functional Diagnostics, Slovak Medical University and Bratislava University Hospital, 82606 Bratislava, Slovakia

3 Institute of Normal and Pathological Physiology, Centre of Experimental Medicine, Slovak Academy of Sciences, 81371 Bratislava, Slovakia; andrej.barta@savba.sk

4 Institute of Experimental Endocrinology, Biomedical Research Center, Slovak Academy of Sciences, 84505 Bratislava, Slovakia; stefan.zorad@savba.sk

5 Department of Physiology, Faculty of Medicine in Hradec Kralove, Charles University, 50003 Hradec Kralove, Czech Republic; adamcova@lfhk.cuni.cz

6 3rd Department of Internal Medicine, Faculty of Medicine, Comenius University, 83305 Bratislava, Slovakia

* Correspondence: fedor.simko@fmed.uniba.sk

† These authors contributed equally to this work.

Abstract: There is ample evidence on the benefit of angiotensin receptor-neprilysin inhibitors (ARNIs) in heart failure, yet data regarding the potential protective action of ARNIs in hypertensive heart disease are sparse. The aim of this study was to show whether an ARNI exerts a protective effect in a model of Nω-nitro-L-arginine methyl ester (L-NAME)-induced hypertension with a hypertensive heart and to compare this potential benefit with an angiotensin-converting enzyme inhibitor, captopril. Five groups of adult male *Wistar rats* were studied (14 per group) for four weeks: untreated controls; ARNI (68 mg/kg/day); L-NAME (40 mg/kg/day); L-NAME treated with ARNI; and L-NAME treated with captopril (100 mg/kg/day). L-NAME administration induced hypertension, accompanied by increased left ventricular (LV) weight and fibrotic rebuilding of the LV in terms of increased concentration and content of hydroxyproline in insoluble collagen and in total collagen and with a histological finding of fibrosis. These alterations were associated with a compromised systolic and diastolic LV function. Treatment with either an ARNI or captopril reduced systolic blood pressure (SBP), alleviated LV hypertrophy and fibrosis, and prevented the development of both systolic and diastolic LV dysfunction. Moreover, the serum levels of prolactin and prolactin receptor were reduced significantly by ARNI and slightly by captopril. In conclusion, in L-NAME-induced hypertension, the dual inhibition of neprilysin and AT1 receptors by ARNI reduced SBP and prevented the development of LV hypertrophy, fibrosis, and systolic and diastolic dysfunction. These data suggest that ARNI could provide protection against LV structural remodeling and functional disorders in hypertensive heart disease.

Keywords: sacubitril/valsartan; L-NAME; hypertensive heart disease; hypertrophy; fibrosis; prolactin

1. Introduction

Arterial hypertension is the principal risk factor for cardiovascular diseases [1] resulting in target organ damage, including heart, kidney, and brain damage. Hypertensive heart disease, due to chronic pressure overload, is characterized by structural remodeling of the LV in terms of hypertrophic growth and fibrosis, which are associated with a worsening of diastolic and systolic function, alterations in energetic metabolism, and electrical abnormalities [2]. Although initial mass enlargement aims to normalize LV wall stress under conditions of higher hemodynamic load while maintaining adequate performance, thus representing a compensatory reaction, maladaptive growth of the hypertensive heart in later periods is associated with worse prognosis and frequently results in the development of overt heart failure (HF). Thus, LV hypertrophy has been a target of therapeutic interventions aimed at mitigating or even reversing pathological heart growth, and novel means of treatment are continuously being searched for [3].

In the population with HF, the inhibition of neurohumoral activation by angiotensin inhibitors, beta-blockers, and aldosterone receptor blockers is an effective means of reducing mortality. Besides the inhibition of excessive activation of heart performance and vasoconstriction, the promotion of hormones with vasodilative and antiproliferative action is considered for HF treatment. Natriuretic peptides (NPs), which are released during atrial and ventricular dilation due to pressure or volume overload [4], have been shown to exert desirable protective effects [5,6]. In the PARADIGM-HF trial, a significant reduction of cardiovascular events and mortality in patients with systolic HF was achieved by increasing plasma NP levels via inhibition of the endopeptidase neprilysin by sacubitril in combination with the angiotensin II receptor blocker valsartan [7]. However, the PARAGON-HF (Prospective Comparison of ARNI (angiotensin receptor-neprilysin inhibitor) with ARB (angiotensin-receptor blockers) Global Outcomes in HF with Preserved Ejection Fraction) trial has not shown any benefit of sacubitril–valsartan in patients who had HF with preserved ejection fraction [8]. According to the latest ACC/AHA/HFSA Guideline for the Management of Heart Failure, ARNI is recommended to reduce mortality and morbidity in patients with HF with reduced ejection fraction (HFrEF) and NYHA class II to III [9].

In contrast to the accepted evidence of the mortality-reducing benefit of ARNI in HF, there is a shortage of data regarding the potential protective action of ARNI on the hypertensive heart in patients with increased blood pressure [10,11]. Considering that hypertensive heart disease is a relatively common pathology, the possible protective effect of ARNI in this indication could bring considerable benefits to the population. The aim of our study was to detect the potential cardioprotective effects of ARNI in a model of L-NAME-induced hypertension with a hypertensive heart and to compare it with an angiotensin-converting enzyme inhibitor, captopril.

2. Materials and Methods

2.1. Animals and Treatment

Adult (12-week-old) male *Wistar rats* (Department of Toxicology and Laboratory Animals Breeding, Slovak Academy of Sciences, Dobra Voda, Slovakia) were randomly divided into five groups (14 per group) with the following treatment lasting for four weeks: no treatment (C); treated with ARNI (68 mg/kg/day; Novartis, Basel, Switzerland) (ARNI); treated with L-NAME (40 mg/kg/day; Cayman Chemical Company, Ann Arbor, MI, USA) (LN); LN treated with ARNI (LN + ARNI); and LN treated with captopril (100 mg/kg/day; Cayman Chemical Company, Ann Arbor, MI, USA) (LN + CAP). The medications were dissolved in drinking water and aligned with daily water consumption. The rats were kept in separate cages and were given an unlimited supply of a regular pellet diet. They were kept in standard laboratory conditions, including a 12 h light and dark cycle, a temperature of 22 ± 2 °C, and humidity of 55 ± 10%. The study was conducted in compliance with the Guide for the Care and Use of Laboratory Animals published by the US National Institutes of Health (NIH publication no. 85-23, revised 1996). The Ethics Committee of the Institute of Pathophysiology, Faculty of Medicine, Comenius University, Bratislava, Slovakia approved the protocol (approval number: 809/19-221/3; approval date: 23 April 2019).

2.2. Blood Pressure Measurement, Collection and Processing of Samples

During treatment, the SBP was measured once a week using a non-invasive tail-cuff plethysmography (Hugo Sachs Elektronik, Freiburg, Germany). Following the four-week treatment period, the rats were humanely euthanized by isoflurane inhalation. Body weight (BW), tibia length (TL), left ventricular weight (LVW), right ventricular weight (RVW), and lungs and liver weights were measured. Afterward, the left ventricular weight to body weight (LVW/BW), left ventricular weight to tibia length (LVW/TL), right ventricular weight to body weight (RVW/BW), and right ventricular weight to tibia length (RVW/TL) ratios were calculated. LV tissue samples were frozen at −80 °C and subsequently analyzed for hydroxyproline concentrations.

2.3. Echocardiography

All animals underwent transthoracic echocardiography after four weeks of treatment using a 14 MHz matrix probe (M12L) and the GE Medical Vivid 7 Dimension System (GE Medical Systems CZ Ltd., Prague, Czech Republic) [12]. The animals were anesthetized throughout the procedure with isoflurane (2.5% inspiratory concentration at a flow rate of 2 L/min) while breathing spontaneously. In this study, the thoracic wall of the rats was shaved while they were placed in a supine position on a warming pad at a temperature of 38 °C. Continuous monitoring of the rats' heart rate (HR) and body temperature was carried out during the procedure.

Using the parasternal long-axis images, the end-diastolic (IVSd) and end-systolic thickness of the interventricular septum (IVSs) were measured. The LV end-diastolic (LVIDd) and end-systolic (LVIDs) internal diameters, the LV end-diastolic (PWd) and end-systolic (PWs) posterior wall thickness, and end-diastolic (EDV) and end-systolic volumes (ESV) were measured using anatomical M-mode in a parasternal long-axis view.

The systolic function of the LV was evaluated by calculating the LV fractional shortening (LVFS) and ejection fraction (LVEF) using the Teichholz formula. The diastolic function of the LV was evaluated by measuring the diastolic transmitral peak early (E) and late (A) filling velocities from the two-dimensionally guided Doppler spectra of mitral inflow in the apical four-chamber view. The E/A ratio and deceleration time (DecT) were then calculated to evaluate the LV diastolic function.

From the pulsed-wave Doppler flow in the apical five-chamber view, the LV inflow (mitral inflow) and outflow (aortic flow velocity) signals were recorded, and the isovolumic relaxation time (IVRT), the time between the closing of the aortic valve and the opening of the mitral valve, was calculated.

An experienced echocardiographer blinded to the group identity performed all echocardiography measurements, which were averaged over three consecutive cardiac cycles.

2.4. Hydroxyproline in the Left Ventricle

To isolate collagenous proteins in the LV, LV samples were treated with different buffers [13]. Soluble collagenous proteins were extracted using CH3COOH-pepsin buffer (pH 1.4, 24 h at 4 °C), and the remaining insoluble collagenous proteins were extracted using NaOH (1.1 mol/L, 45 min at 105 °C). Subsequently, the hydrolyzed samples were oxidized using chloramine T and acetate-citrate buffer at pH 6.0. After incubation (20 min at room temperature), the reaction was stopped by adding Ehrlich's reagent, followed by incubation at 65 °C for 15 min. Spectrophotometry at 550 nm was used to measure the LV hydroxyproline concentration, a marker of LV fibrosis, in both collagenous fractions. The hydroxyproline content in the LV was then calculated and expressed as mg per total weight of the LV.

2.5. Quantitative Analysis of the Left Ventricular Fibrosis

The LV samples from 6 subjects per treatment group, preserved in a solution of 4% formaldehyde, underwent embedding in paraffin and were subsequently sectioned into slices measuring 5 μm in thickness. Following this, sample sections underwent a process of deparaffinization, rehydration, and staining with picrosirius red (PSR) for a quantitative assessment of LV fibrosis. Photomicrographs were captured utilizing a NIKON Eclipse

Ti C2+ microscope (NIKON, Tokyo, Japan) equipped with polarized light, and thereafter subjected to analysis using NIKON NIS-Elements Analysis software (v 4.50.00, NIKON, Tokyo, Japan) and ImageJ software (1.54f, National Institutes of Health, Bethesda, MD, USA) [14].

To achieve a quantitative assessment of LV fibrosis, sections stained with PSR were subjected to analysis at a magnification of 10× using polarized light microscopy in conjunction with ImageJ software (1.54f). PSR enhances the birefringence of collagen fibers in a manner dependent on their type, thereby facilitating the visualization of thick type I collagen (Col I, 1.6–2.4 μm in diameter) appearing in red–orange hues and thin type III collagen (Col III, <0.8 μm in diameter) appearing in green–yellow hues. By appropriately configuring the hue, brightness, and saturation thresholds of the color spectrum, the areas exhibiting red–orange and green–yellow shades were quantified as percentages of the total area of interest (AOI) through ImageJ processing. Upon ascertaining the volume of Col I and Col III, we proceeded to compute the sum of Col I and Col III (Col I + III), as well as the ratio of Col I to Col III (Col I/III).

2.6. Serum Concentration of Prolactin and Prolactin Receptor

Rat enzyme-linked immunosorbent assay (ELISA) kits designed for the quantification of prolactin and prolactin receptor (prolactin R) were employed to determine their respective serum concentrations in 6 subjects per treatment group (RayBiotech Life, Inc., 3607 Parkway Ln, Suite 200, Peachtree Corners, GA, USA).

2.7. Statistical Analysis

The results are presented as the means and standard error of the mean (SEM). To analyze the data statistically, we used a one-way, repeated-measures analysis of variance (ANOVA) followed by multiple comparisons with a Bonferroni post hoc test. We considered differences to be significant if the p-value was less than 0.05. All statistical analyses were conducted using GraphPad Prism 9 for Windows (GraphPad Software, La Jolla, CA, USA).

3. Results

3.1. Cardiovascular Parameters

3.1.1. Systolic Blood Pressure Was Reduced by ARNI and Captopril in L-NAME-Induced Hypertension

After four weeks of treatment, the SBP was 131.7 ± 3.02 mmHg in the controls, while ARNI administration did not change it (Figure 1A). The chronic L-NAME treatment significantly increased the SBP to 183.4 ± 2.52 mmHg (by 39%, $p < 0.05$), while both ARNI (by 29%, $p < 0.05$) and captopril (by 30%, $p < 0.05$) significantly reduced it.

3.1.2. ARNI and Captopril Reduced LVW in L-NAME-Induced Hypertension

Following a period of 4 weeks of treatment, discernible alterations in body weight were not observed across the respective groups (Table 1). The absolute LV weight in the control group was 499 ± 21.81 mg, while ARNI treatment did not change it (Figure 1B). The L-NAME administration increased LV weight to 582 ± 25 mg (by 17%, $p < 0.05$), while both ARNI (by 24%, $p < 0.05$) and captopril (by 18%, $p < 0.05$) reduced it significantly. In the control group, the LVW/BW and LVW/TL ratio after four weeks was 1.28 ± 0.05 mg/g and 135.1 ± 5 mg/cm, respectively, while ARNI administration did not change it (Figure 1C,D). The L-NAME treatment increased the LVW/BW and LVW/TL ratio significantly to 1.49 ± 0.06 mg/g (by 16%, $p < 0.05$) and 140.12 ± 5.3 mg/cm (15%, $p < 0.05$), respectively, and ARNI (by 17% and 16%, respectively, $p < 0.05$) and captopril (by 30% and 31%, respectively, $p < 0.05$) reduced it significantly. The BW, LVW, RVW, RVW/BW, and RVW/TL ratios are described in Table 1.

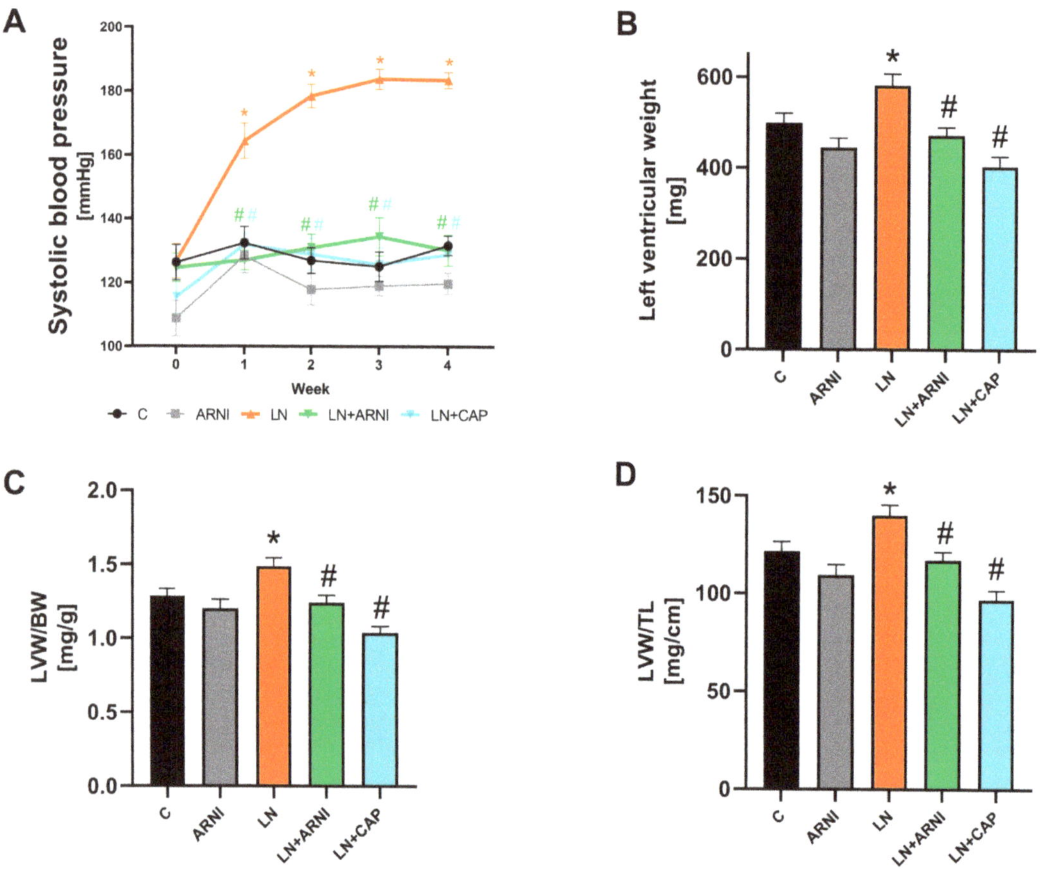

Figure 1. Effect of ARNI and captopril on systolic blood pressure (**A**), left ventricular weight (**B**), left ventricular weight to body weight (LVW/BW) (**C**), and to tibia length ratio (LVW/TL) (**D**) in L-NAME-induced hypertension and hypertensive heart disease after four weeks of treatment. C, controls; LN, L-NAME; ARNI, sacubitril/valsartan; CAP, captopril. * $p < 0.05$ vs. C; # $p < 0.05$ vs. LN.

Table 1. Body weight (BW), tibia length (TL), right ventricular weight (RVW), RVW to body weight (BW) ratio (RVW/BW), RVW to TL ratio (RVW/TL), lungs weight, and liver weight in L-NAME-induced hypertension and hypertensive heart disease after four weeks of treatment. Values are mean ± SEM. C, controls; LN, L-NAME; ARNI, sacubitril/valsartan; CAP, captopril.

	C	ARNI	LN	LN + ARNI	LN + CAP
BW [mg]	388 ± 5.5	370 ± 5.6	391 ± 7.94	380 ± 9.23	388 ± 11.43
TL [cm]	4.09 ± 0.04	4.06 ± 0.04	4.14 ± 0.03	4.02 ± 0.07	4.14 ± 0.05
RVW [mg]	172.6 ± 6.90	175.3 ± 5.49	176.00 ± 11.28	167.90 ± 13.29	158.30 ± 7.99
RVW/BW [mg/g]	0.45 ± 0.02	0.47 ± 0.01	0.45 ± 0.03	0.44 ± 0.03	0.41 ± 0.01
RVW/TL [mg/cm]	42.41 ± 2.01	43.57 ± 1.59	42.43 ± 2.59	42.39 ± 3.13	37.62 ± 1.69
Lungs [mg]	1.61 ± 0.05	1.58 ± 0.04	1.53 ± 0.03	1.51 ± 0.03	1.57 ± 0.03
Liver [mg]	11.64 ± 0.27	10.99 ± 0.27	11.89 ± 0.31	11.33 ± 0.4	11.69 ± 0.38

3.1.3. ARNI and Captopril Improved LV Function in L-NAME-Induced Hypertension

After four weeks, the echocardiographic parameters of the control group did not change with ARNI treatment. However, administration of L-NAME decreased LVEF by 17% ($p < 0.05$) and LVFS by 27% ($p < 0.05$) (Figure 2A,B). On the other hand, both ARNI and captopril significantly increased these parameters in the L-NAME-administered group. In the hypertensive

L-NAME group, ARNI increased LVEF by 14% ($p < 0.05$) and LVFS by 21% ($p < 0.05$), while captopril increased LVEF by 15% ($p < 0.05$) and LVFS by 24% ($p < 0.05$).

In contrast, LV diastolic function parameters, such as the E/A ratio (by 51%, $p < 0.05$), DecT (by 52%, $p < 0.05$), and IVRT (by 52%, $p < 0.05$), increased after L-NAME administration (Figure 2C–E). Both ARNI and captopril effectively reduced these parameters in the L-NAME group, as follows: ARNI reduced the E/A ratio by 22% ($p < 0.05$), DecT by 36% ($p < 0.05$), and IVRT by 46% ($p < 0.05$), while captopril reduced the E/A ratio by 29% ($p < 0.05$), DecT by 36% ($p < 0.05$) and IVRT by 50% ($p < 0.05$).

The HR, IVSd, IVSs, LVIDd, LVIDs, PWd, PWs, EDV, and ESV are described in Table 2.

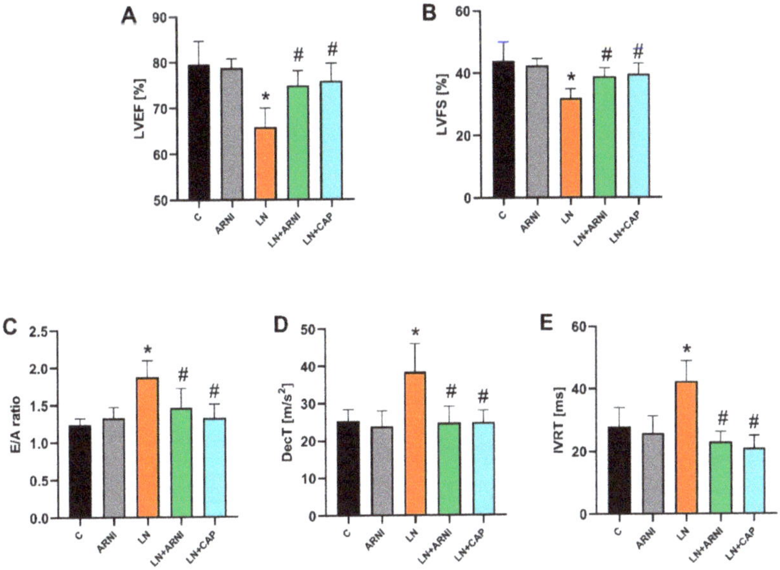

Figure 2. Effect of ARNI and captopril on left ventricular ejection fraction (LVEF) (**A**), left ventricular fractional shortening (LVFS) (**B**), the ratio of the diastolic transmitral peak early and late filling velocities (E/A ratio) (**C**), deceleration time (DecT) (**D**) and isovolumic relaxation time (IVRT) (**E**) in L-NAME-induced hypertension and hypertensive heart disease after four weeks of treatment. C, controls; LN, L-NAME; ARNI, sacubitril/valsartan; CAP, captopril. * $p < 0.05$ vs. C; # $p < 0.05$ vs. LN.

Table 2. Effect of ARNI and captopril on left ventricular echocardiographic functional parameters in L-NAME-induced hypertension and hypertensive heart disease after four weeks of treatment; heart rate (HR), end-diastolic interventricular septum thickness (IVSd), end-systolic interventricular septum thickness (IVSs), end-diastolic LV internal diameter (LVIDd), end-systolic LV internal diameter (LVIDs), end-diastolic posterior wall diameter (PWd), end-systolic posterior wall diameter (PWs), end-diastolic LV volume (EDV), end-systolic LV volume (ESV). C, controls; LN, L-NAME; ARNI, sacubitril/valsartan; CAP, captopril. * $p < 0.05$ vs. C; # $p < 0.05$ vs. LN.

	C	ARNI	LN	LN + ARNI	LN + CAP
HR [min^{-1}]	380.90 ± 0.16	361.43 ± 11.15	343.05 ± 10.17	353.64 ± 11.54	355.55 ± 11.79
IVSd [cm]	0.91 ± 0.02	0.89 ± 0.02	0.94 ± 0.03	0.79 ± 0.02 #	0.73 ± 0.02 #
IVSs [cm]	0.87 ± 0.03	0.85 ± 0.03	0.85 ± 0.03	0.75 ± 0.02 #	0.74 ± 0.03 #
LVIDd [cm]	6.67 ± 0.15	6.55 ± 0.11	6.63 ± 0.16	6.33 ± 0.15	6.20 ± 0.18
LVIDs [cm]	3.77 ± 0.16	3.77 ± 0.08	4.52 ± 0.14 *	3.89 ± 0.12 #	3.75 ± 0.13 #
PWd [cm]	0.98 ± 0.04	0.92 ± 0.02	1.02 ± 0.03	0.83 ± 0.04 #	0.77 ± 0.03 #
PWs [cm]	1.14 ± 0.04	1.05 ± 0.02	1.13 ± 0.03	0.96 ± 0.03 #	0.85 ± 0.03 #
EDV [mL]	0.69 ± 0.04	0.65 ± 0.03	0.68 ± 0.04	0.60 ± 0.04	0.57 ± 0.05
ESV [mL]	0.15 ± 0.01	0.14 ± 0.01	0.24 ± 0.02 *	0.15 ± 0.01 #	0.14 ± 0.01 #

3.2. Hydroxyproline Concentration and Content in Soluble, Insoluble and Total Collagenous Proteins in the Left Ventricle Was Decreased by ARNI and Captopril in L-NAME-Induced Hypertension

After four weeks of treatment, the hydroxyproline concentration in the soluble collagenous protein was 0.202 ± 0.013 mg/g in the controls, and ARNI did not change it (Figure 3A). The L-NAME administration increased the hydroxyproline concentration in the soluble collagenous protein numerically to 0.288 ± 0.019 mg/g (ns), while captopril only significantly reduced it, by 28% ($p < 0.05$). In the controls, the hydroxyproline concentration in the insoluble collagenous fraction was 0.384 ± 0.022 mg/g, while ARNI had no effect. After four weeks of L-NAME treatment, the concentration of hydroxyproline in the insoluble collagenous fraction was 0.786 ± 0.085 mg/g, and both ARNI (by 46%, $p < 0.05$) and captopril (by 42%, $p < 0.05$) reduced it significantly. The total hydroxyproline concentration was 0.585 ± 0.026 mg/g in the controls, while ARNI had no effect. L-NAME administration increased the total hydroxyproline concentration to 1.014 ± 0.087 mg/g ($p < 0.05$), and both ARNI (by 37%, $p < 0.05$) and captopril (by 39%, $p < 0.05$) reduced it significantly.

After four weeks of treatment, the hydroxyproline content in the soluble collagenous proteins was 0.102 ± 0.009 mg/LV in the controls, and ARNI did not change it (Figure 3B). The L-NAME administration increased the content in the soluble collagenous proteins numerically to 0.133 ± 0.014 mg/LV (ns), and both ARNI (by 27%, $p < 0.05$) and captopril (by 50%, $p < 0.05$) reduced it significantly. The hydroxyproline content in the insoluble collagenous fraction was 0.192 ± 0.015 mg/LV in the controls, and ARNI had no effect. After L-NAME treatment, the hydroxyproline content in the insoluble collagenous proteins was 0.453 ± 0.051 mg/LV ($p < 0.05$), and both ARNI (by 56%, $p < 0.05$) and captopril (by 59%, $p < 0.05$) reduced it significantly. The total hydroxyproline content was 0.294 ± 0.021 mg/LV in the controls, while ARNI did not change it. L-NAME administration increased the total hydroxyproline concentration to 0.587 ± 0.054 mg/LV ($p < 0.05$), and both ARNI (by 50%, $p < 0.05$) and captopril (by 57%, $p < 0.05$) reduced it significantly.

3.3. Left Ventricular Fibrosis Was Reduced by ARNI and Captopril in L-NAME-Induced Hypertension

Following a duration of four weeks from the initiation of the experiment, the volume of Col I and Col III in the LV AOI in the control group was 0.47 ± 0.2 and 0.37 ± 0.12, respectively, and were not affected by ARNI (Figure 4P,Q); L-NAME increased ($p < 0.05$) the proportion of Col I (by 59%, $p < 0.05$) and Col III (by 52%, $p < 0.05$). In the L-NAME group, both ARNI and captopril decreased ($p < 0.05$) the proportion of Col I (by 54% and 34%, respectively) and Col III (by 53% and 38%, respectively). The sum of Col I + III in the control group was 0.85 ± 0.22 and ARNI did not influence it (Figure 4R); chronic administration of L-NAME increased the sum of Col I and Col III (by 57%, $p < 0.05$), while both ARNI and captopril significantly reduced it (by 54% and 35%, respectively, $p < 0.05$). The Col I/III ratio was 1.4 ± 0.7 in the control group and no statistically significant differences were observed among the groups (Figure 4S).

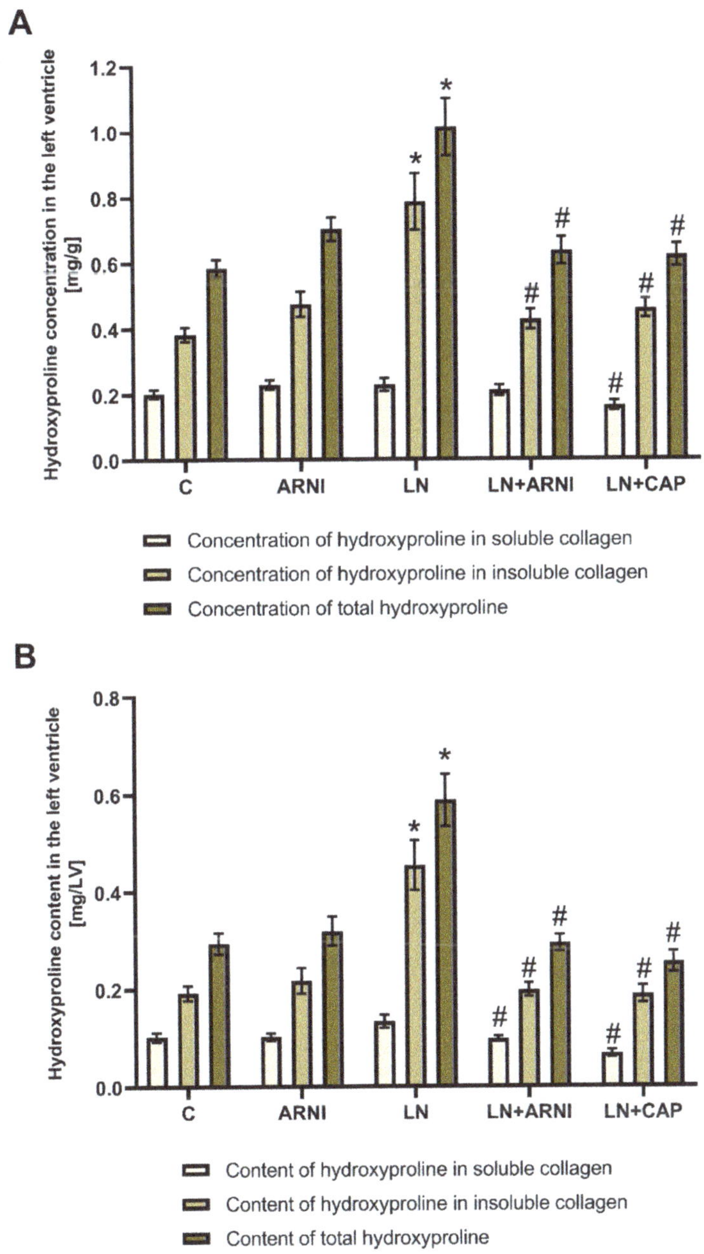

Figure 3. Effect of ARNI and captopril on the concentration (**A**) and content (**B**) of hydroxyproline in soluble and insoluble collagenous proteins and total hydroxyproline in L-NAME-induced hypertension and hypertensive heart disease after four weeks of treatment. C, controls; LN, L-NAME; ARNI, sacubitril/valsartan; CAP, captopril. * $p < 0.05$ vs. C; # $p < 0.05$ vs. LN.

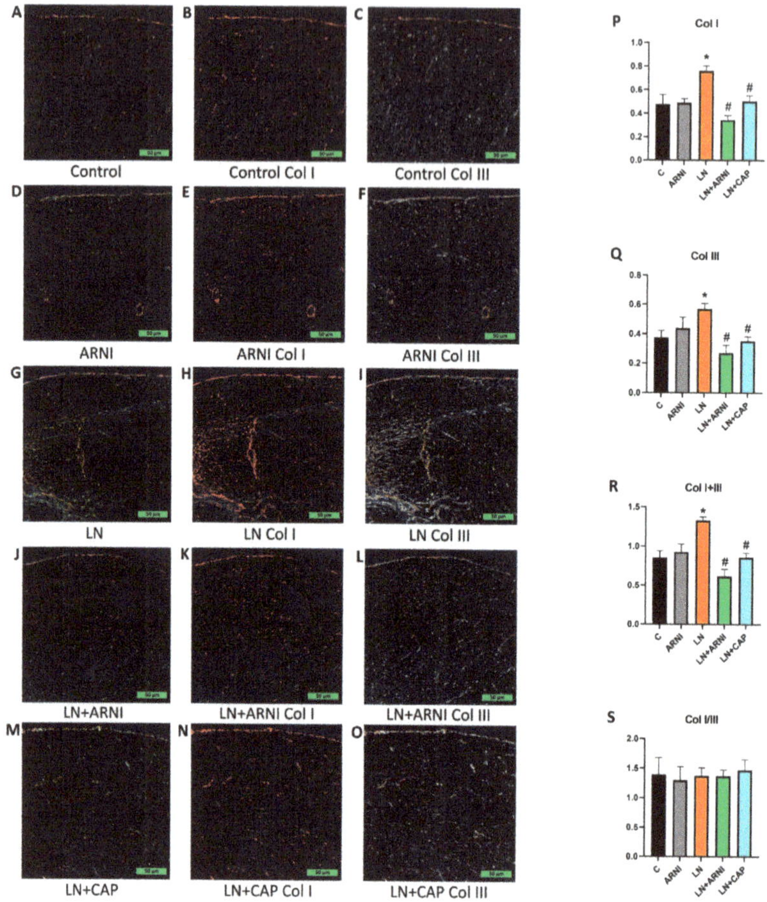

Figure 4. Effect of ARNI and captopril on left ventricular fibrosis in L-NAME-induced hypertension and hypertensive heart disease. PSR-stained sections at 10× magnification using polarized light microscopy showing collagen I in red and collagen III in white (**A–O**), the volume of collagen I (Col I) (**P**), collagen III (Col III) (**Q**), the sum of collagen I and III (Col I + III) (**R**), and the ratio of Col I/Col III (Col I/III) (**S**). C, controls; LN, L-NAME; ARNI, sacubitril/valsartan; CAP, captopril. * $p < 0.05$ vs. C; # $p < 0.05$ vs. LN.

3.4. Serum Levels of Prolactin and Prolactin Receptor Were Reduced by ARNI in L-NAME-Induced Hypertension

After four weeks, the serum level of prolactin and prolactin R in the control group was 1 165.1 ± 139.6 pg/mL and 4 336.7 ± 576.8 pg/mL, respectively, and ARNI did not have an effect on these molecules (Figure 5A,B). L-NAME numerically increased serum levels of prolactin (by 28%, $p < 0.05$) and prolactin R (by 63%, $p < 0.05$), while only ARNI reduced these monitored serum parameters (by 54% and 51%, respectively, $p < 0.05$). Captopril reduced prolactin or prolactin receptor levels only numerically (without statistical significance).

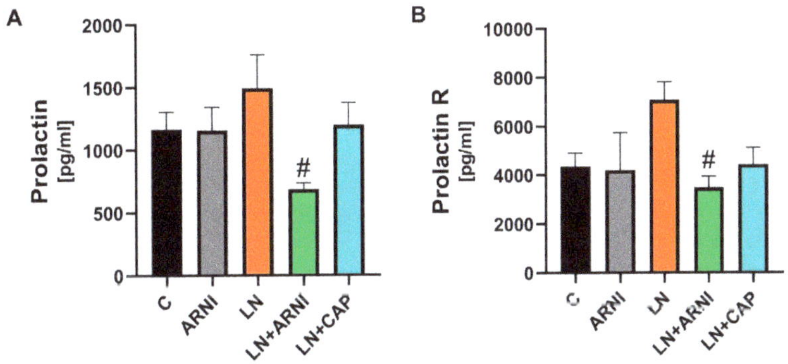

Figure 5. Effect of ARNI and captopril on serum levels of prolactin (**A**) and prolactin receptor (prolactin R) (**B**) in the L-NAME-induced hypertension and hypertensive heart disease. C, controls; LN, L-NAME; ARNI, sacubitril/valsartan; CAP, captopril. # $p < 0.05$ vs. LN.

4. Discussion

In this experiment, four weeks of L-NAME administration resulted in hypertension accompanied by increased LV weight and fibrotic rebuilding of the LV in terms of increased hydroxyproline concentration and content and histological findings of increased fibrosis. These hemodynamic and structural alterations were associated with compromised systolic and diastolic LV function. Treatment with either ARNI or captopril reduced systolic blood pressure, alleviated LV hypertrophy and fibrosis, and prevented the development of LV dysfunction. Additionally, the serum level of prolactin and prolactin receptor, supposedly associated with endothelial dysfunction, pathological remodeling, and compromised cardiovascular health, was significantly reduced by ARNI and slightly by captopril.

L-NAME-induced hypertension is a well-established model of hypertension and target organ damage. L-NAME acts as a false substrate for endothelial nitric oxide synthase (eNOS), thus reducing the formation of nitric oxide (NO), resulting in the development of NO-deficient hypertension [14]. Besides the shortage of vasodilative action of NO itself, reduced NO availability in the renal artery is thought to stimulate renin release, followed by angiotensin II (Ang II)—aldosterone axis activation in the circulation [15] and in tissues such as the heart and aorta [16] or kidney [14,17], thus contributing to hypertension development and end-stage organ damage [15]. Nonetheless, our recent investigation revealed that L-NAME-induced hypertension is linked not to heightened, but rather to the normal or reduced activation of the renin–angiotensin II system (RAS) in both serum and LV tissue [18]. The normal-to-low level of renin–angiotensin system activation has also been previously documented in spontaneously hypertensive rats [19]. Yet, the serum aldosterone level and the ratio of aldosterone to Ang II were increased in L-NAME-hypertension [18,20], which is consistent with the results obtained by other research groups [21,22]. In agreement with our recent results with an L-NAME model of hypertension, aldosterone activation was previously demonstrated in various models of experimental hypertension [23]. Consequently, it is possible that the pivotal factor contributing to LV remodeling in L-NAME-induced hypertension is the activation of aldosterone rather than Ang II [18]. The described pro-proliferative effect of aldosterone receptor stimulation [24] with the enhancement of the collagenous concentration and content and histological signs of fibrosis in myocardial tissue seen in this experiment may underly the deterioration of diastolic and systolic LV function. The rise in the level of insoluble collagen with numerous cross-linking in particular may deteriorate the myocardial elasticity and participate in the LV diastolic dysfunction development [18].

Neprilysin is an endopeptidase cleaving various biologically active peptides. Some of these compounds, such as atrial natriuretic peptide (ANP), brain natriuretic peptide (BNP), and C-type natriuretic peptide (CNP), along with adrenomedullin and bradykinin, support vasodilation, natriuresis, insulin sensitivity, and antifibrotic action [25]. On the other hand, neprilysin also degrades Ang II or endothelin-1 with opposing effects in terms of vasoconstriction, pro-aggregation, and pro-proliferation. Thus, inhibition of neprilysin by sacubitril not only increases the bioavailability of presumably protective substances but also raises the levels of vasoconstrictors and growth promotors, including Ang II. This might partially counterbalance the protective effects of natriuretic peptides [26]. To avoid these adverse effects, neprilysin inhibitor was combined with the Ang II type 1 (AT1) receptor blocker valsartan in one pill (sacubitril/valsartan—ARNI) in order to eliminate the undesirable effect of increased Ang II [27,28].

The neprilysin AT1 blocker ARNI has been shown to be effective in a number of heart failure studies [29] and is recommended for the treatment of HF with reduced ejection fraction [9]. Yet, it is not entirely clear whether ARNI could provide additional benefits in the treatment of hypertension and in the protection of the hypertensive heart [10,11]. The situation with hypertensive heart disease is complex because the nature of essential hypertension and the corresponding target organ damage can be related to various interfering factors, such as endothelial dysfunction, chronic neurohumoral activation, or genetic predisposition. Therefore, testing the effect of a particular drug in different experimental models of hypertension is unavoidable. Although ARNI has been investigated in several models of hypertension and associated cardiac injury, to the best of our knowledge, ARNI has not been used in the L-NAME model of hypertension, which is primarily induced by a deficit of nitric oxide production and is considered to be a NO-deficient model of hypertension [15,30]. The disclosing of the protective effect of ARNI in the L-NAME model in this work may contribute to understanding the pathomechanism of ARNI in hypertensive disease with endothelial dysfunction and limited nitric oxide production and could support the consideration of ARNI in the treatment of essential hypertension, which is currently not the case [10].

In our experiment, both ARNI and the angiotensin-converting enzyme (ACE)-inhibitor captopril reduced SBP and LV hypertrophy, along with improving the systolic and diastolic functional parameters of the LV. These results are in agreement with previous results from our and other laboratories. In L-NAME hypertension, captopril prevented SBP enhancement and the development of LV hypertrophy and fibrosis [30] and reduced DNA and RNA concentration and protein synthesis in the LV, aorta, kidney, and brain [31] without restoring nitric oxide synthase activity and even induced the regression of hypertrophic and fibrotic remodeling, when LV hypertrophy was already developed [32]. Although ARNI was not investigated in L-NAME hypertension, protection was shown in various other models of experimental cardiovascular pathologies. ARNI treatment attenuated structural changes in terms of myocardial hypertrophy and fibrosis after myocardial infarction [33,34] and in salt-induced heart damage in rats [35], and reduced cardiomyocyte hypertrophy in Ang II-induced hypertension [36]. ARNI improved LV function in anthracycline-induced cardiomyopathy [37] in models of myocardial infarction in rats [33] and mice [34], as well as in high-salt diet-induced diastolic dysfunction in rats [35]. In SHR, ARNI improved atrial remodeling and reduced susceptibility to atrial fibrillation [38], and a novel ARNI S086 effectively reduced myocardial cell necrosis and fibrosis development [39]. A meta-analysis of clinical studies spanning the decade from 2010 to 2019 [40] demonstrated the remarkable ability of ARNI to reverse LV remodeling in individuals suffering from HF accompanied by systolic dysfunction [40], and ARNI's antifibrotic potential is to be investigated in the REVERSE-LVH clinical trial in a regression experiment on hypertensive patients with LVH [11].

Various cardiac markers in plasma are under investigation to obtain a general overview of the extent of cardiovascular changes induced by hypertension in clinical or experimental conditions. One of them, prolactin, a polypeptide hormone of lactation, exerts pleiotropic cytokine effects that are associated with hypertension and cardiac remodeling [41]. Elevated serum prolactin has been associated with the development of hypertension through a reduction in endothelial nitric oxide synthase activity in mice [42]. In addition, hyperprolactinemia is associated with endothelial dysfunction and impaired insulin sensitivity [43,44], increased arterial stiffness [45], and the risk of atherosclerosis and cardiovascular events in high-risk patients [44]. In addition, prolactin receptor expression appears to be linked to myocardial hypertrophy [46]. Although prolactin did not reliably reflect cardiometabolic risk in an analysis of 3232 subjects from the Framingham Heart Study [47], a recent study of 10,907 patients with type 2 diabetes showed a positive association of serum prolactin with mortality [48], and a recent meta-analysis of 14 studies involving 23,596 patients confirmed that serum prolactin is an independent predictor of all-cause mortality and cardiovascular mortality [49]. The results of our experiment correlated well with these data from the literature. An increase in prolactin and prolactin receptor levels was revealed in the L-NAME group, which is consistent with the LV remodeling observed in this experiment and the decreased activity of endothelial NO activity in the heart, aorta, kidneys, and brain mentioned in a number of our previous studies [30,31,50,51]. Importantly, ARNI significantly and captopril slightly reduced serum prolactin and prolactin R levels, suggesting slightly better protective potential with ARNI, despite similar hemodynamic and structural effects of the two drugs.

The findings of our current experiment support the hypothesis that the simultaneous inhibition of neprilysin and AT1 receptors could exert protective effects in the hypertensive heart. These benefits include not only mitigating structural remodeling but also averting functional impairments. It has to be recognized, however, that in most animal and clinical experiments, ARNI outperformed the ACE-inhibition or AT1 blockade, whereas in our experiment with an L-NAME-induced hypertensive heart, ARNI and captopril yielded comparable outcomes. The appropriate dose of ARNI and captopril should thus be considered. Both the dual inhibitor and the classical ACE-inhibitor captopril were given in a high pharmacologic dose. A dose of captopril of 100 mg/kg was chosen in relation to a number of our prior experiments, where this dose yielded protection while keeping side effects unnoticeable. The dose of ARNI of 68 mg/kg was in agreement with the highest dose used in experiments from other laboratories. The adequacy of the choice of both doses is supported by the equal SBP reduction by both drugs during the whole experiment. However, one should consider several other issues, which may have potentially influenced the level of protection. First, captopril (unlike enalapril used in the PARADIGH-HF Trial) contains SH groups that are claimed to enhance its antioxidant properties [52]. In the condition of decreased NO production in the L-NAME-induced hypertension, this factor might have improved NO availability and thus enhanced the protection by captopril. Second, L-NAME-induced hypertension was previously shown to be a model with low renin–angiotensin II pathway activation. Under these circumstances, the space for RAS inhibitors might be restricted, thus hiding subtle differences of the drugs tested. Third, in a condition of hypertension with the absence of HF and fluid accumulation, there may be no need for increased natriuretic peptide availability. Furthermore, even the very similar effects of ARNI and captopril on the surrogate endpoint represented by hypertensive heart diseases do not automatically indicate the same effect on morbidity and mortality in subjects with hypertensive heart remodeling, which could only be disclosed in a long-term experiment focused on the hard endpoints. This consideration is supported by the more pronounced attenuation of the serum level of prolactin and prolactin R by ARNI than by captopril.

In conclusion, we have shown that in L-NAME-induced hypertension, the dual inhibition of neprilysin and AT1 receptor by ARNI reduced SBP and prevented the development of LV hypertrophy, fibrosis, and systolic and diastolic dysfunction. The data suggest that in hypertensive individuals with hypertensive heart disease, ARNI could yield protection against LV structural remodeling and functional disorders.

5. Limitations

Investigating natriuretic peptides could help reflect neurohumoral modifications. However, in a number of papers on ARNI from several laboratories, NPs were not presented as standard. This may be due to the following reasons. Since the recent advent of ARNIs, it is necessary to investigate how these two biomarkers should be interpreted in HF or ventricular dysfunction. ARNI use is associated with a decrease in NT-proBNP but an increase in BNP levels [53]. Moreover, due to the large species specificities of NP, it is necessary to use rat-specific kits, while standardization in experimental animals is lacking. Different kits have been used with different results in the literature. For these reasons, it seems that only experienced laboratories are able to adequately interpret complex changes in NPs under specific conditions.

Furthermore, in vitro experiments of the effects of neurohumoral inhibitors on isolated myocardial cells, along with thorough histological investigation, may supply deeper insight into the protective effects of the drug used. However, these investigations were beyond the technical equipment and possibilities of our laboratory.

Author Contributions: Conceptualization, F.S.; methodology, P.S., M.A. and F.S.; validation, P.S., K.R., M.A. and F.S.; formal analysis, P.S., K.R. and M.A.; investigation, P.S., K.R., A.B. and M.A.; resources, K.K., M.A. and F.S.; data curation, P.S., K.R. and M.A.; writing—original draft preparation, P.S., K.R. and F.S.; writing—review and editing, P.S., K.R., T.B., S.A., S.Z., M.A. and F.S.; visualization, P.S., K.R. and M.A.; supervision, F.S.; project administration, K.K. and F.S.; funding acquisition, K.K., S.Z. and F.S. All authors have read and agreed to the published version of the manuscript.

Funding: This work was supported by the research grant VEGA (grant of the Scientific Grant Agency of the Ministry of Education of the Slovak Republic) 1/0048/23 and grant APVV-20-0421.

Institutional Review Board Statement: The study was conducted in conformity with the Guide for the Care and Use of Laboratory Animals published by the US National Institutes of Health (NIH publication no. 85-23, revised 1996). The protocol was approved by the Ethics Committee of the Institute of Pathophysiology, Faculty of Medicine, Comenius University, Bratislava, Slovak Republic (approval number: 809/19-221/3; approval date: 23 April 2019).

Informed Consent Statement: Not applicable.

Data Availability Statement: Data supporting the reported results are available from the corresponding author per request.

Conflicts of Interest: The authors declare no conflict of interest. The funders had no role in the design of the study; in the collection, analyses, or interpretation of data; in the writing of the manuscript, or in the decision to publish the results.

References

1. Al Ghorani, H.; Götzinger, F.; Böhm, M.; Mahfoud, F. Arterial Hypertension—Clinical Trials Update 2021. *Nutr. Metab. Cardiovasc. Dis.* **2022**, *32*, 21–31. [CrossRef] [PubMed]
2. Masenga, S.K.; Kirabo, A. Hypertensive Heart Disease: Risk Factors, Complications and Mechanisms. *Front. Cardiovasc. Med.* **2023**, *10*, 1205475. [CrossRef] [PubMed]
3. Zile, M.R.; Brutsaert, D.L. New Concepts in Diastolic Dysfunction and Diastolic Heart Failure: Part II: Causal Mechanisms and Treatment. *Circulation* **2002**, *105*, 1503–1508. [CrossRef] [PubMed]
4. Kuwahara, K. The Natriuretic Peptide System in Heart Failure: Diagnostic and Therapeutic Implications. *Pharmacol. Ther.* **2021**, *227*, 107863. [CrossRef]
5. Huo, J.-Y.; Jiang, W.-Y.; Chen, C.; Chen, R.; Ge, T.-T.; Chang, Q.; Zhu, L.; Geng, J.; Jiang, Z.-X.; Shan, Q.-J. Effects of Angiotensin Receptor Neprilysin Inhibitors on Inducibility of Ventricular Arrhythmias in Rats with Ischemic Cardiomyopathy. *Int. Heart J.* **2019**, *60*, 1168–1175. [CrossRef] [PubMed]
6. McMurray, J.J.V. Neprilysin Inhibition to Treat Heart Failure: A Tale of Science, Serendipity, and Second Chances. *Eur. J. Heart Fail.* **2015**, *17*, 242–247. [CrossRef]
7. Packer, M.; McMurray, J.J.V.; Desai, A.S.; Gong, J.; Lefkowitz, M.P.; Rizkala, A.R.; Rouleau, J.L.; Shi, V.C.; Solomon, S.D.; Swedberg, K.; et al. Angiotensin Receptor Neprilysin Inhibition Compared with Enalapril on the Risk of Clinical Progression in Surviving Patients with Heart Failure. *Circulation* **2015**, *131*, 54–61. [CrossRef] [PubMed]
8. Solomon, S.D.; McMurray, J.J.V.; Anand, I.S.; Ge, J.; Lam, C.S.P.; Maggioni, A.P.; Martinez, F.; Packer, M.; Pfeffer, M.A.; Pieske, B.; et al. Angiotensin-Neprilysin Inhibition in Heart Failure with Preserved Ejection Fraction. *N. Engl. J. Med.* **2019**, *381*, 1609–1620. [CrossRef] [PubMed]

9. Heidenreich, P.A.; Bozkurt, B.; Aguilar, D.; Allen, L.A.; Byun, J.J.; Colvin, M.M.; Deswal, A.; Drazner, M.H.; Dunlay, S.M.; Evers, L.R.; et al. 2022 AHA/ACC/HFSA Guideline for the Management of Heart Failure: A Report of the American College of Cardiology/American Heart Association Joint Committee on Clinical Practice Guidelines. *J. Am. Coll. Cardiol.* **2022**, *79*, e263–e421. [CrossRef]
10. Ali, A.; Ortega-Legaspi, J.M. Is It Time to Adopt Angiotensin Receptor-Neprilysin Inhibitors (ARNI) Therapy as Standard of Care for the Management of Hypertension? *Ann. Palliat. Med.* **2022**, *11*, 3040–3042. [CrossRef]
11. Lee, V.; Zheng, Q.; Toh, D.-F.; Pua, C.J.; Bryant, J.A.; Lee, C.-H.; Cook, S.A.; Butler, J.; Díez, J.; Richards, A.M.; et al. Sacubitril/Valsartan versus Valsartan in Regressing Myocardial Fibrosis in Hypertension: A Prospective, Randomized, Open-Label, Blinded Endpoint Clinical Trial Protocol. *Front. Cardiovasc. Med.* **2023**, *10*, 1248468. [CrossRef] [PubMed]
12. Liu, J.; Rigel, D.F. Echocardiographic Examination in Rats and Mice. *Methods Mol. Biol.* **2009**, *573*, 139–155. [CrossRef] [PubMed]
13. Reddy, G.K.; Enwemeka, C.S. A Simplified Method for the Analysis of Hydroxyproline in Biological Tissues. *Clin. Biochem.* **1996**, *29*, 225–229. [CrossRef] [PubMed]
14. Stanko, P.; Baka, T.; Repova, K.; Aziriova, S.; Krajcirovicova, K.; Barta, A.; Janega, P.; Adamcova, M.; Paulis, L.; Simko, F. Ivabradine Ameliorates Kidney Fibrosis in L-NAME-Induced Hypertension. *Front. Med.* **2020**, *7*, 325. [CrossRef] [PubMed]
15. Simko, F.; Simko, J. The Potential Role of Nitric Oxide in the Hypertrophic Growth of the Left Ventricle. *Physiol. Res.* **2000**, *49*, 37–46. [PubMed]
16. Takemoto, M.; Egashira, K.; Usui, M.; Numaguchi, K.; Tomita, H.; Tsutsui, H.; Shimokawa, H.; Sueishi, K.; Takeshita, A. Important Role of Tissue Angiotensin-Converting Enzyme Activity in the Pathogenesis of Coronary Vascular and Myocardial Structural Changes Induced by Long-Term Blockade of Nitric Oxide Synthesis in Rats. *J. Clin. Investig.* **1997**, *99*, 278–287. [CrossRef]
17. Corremans, R.; D'Haese, P.C.; Vervaet, B.A.; Verhulst, A. L-NAME Administration Enhances Diabetic Kidney Disease Development in an STZ/NAD Rat Model. *Int. J. Mol. Sci.* **2021**, *22*, 12767. [CrossRef] [PubMed]
18. Simko, F.; Baka, T.; Poglitsch, M.; Repova, K.; Aziriova, S.; Krajcirovicova, K.; Zorad, S.; Adamcova, M.; Paulis, L. Effect of Ivabradine on a Hypertensive Heart and the Renin-Angiotensin-Aldosterone System in L-NAME-Induced Hypertension. *Int. J. Mol. Sci.* **2018**, *19*, 3017. [CrossRef] [PubMed]
19. Simko, F.; Baka, T.; Stanko, P.; Repova, K.; Krajcirovicova, K.; Aziriova, S.; Domenig, O.; Zorad, S.; Adamcova, M.; Paulis, L. Sacubitril/Valsartan and Ivabradine Attenuate Left Ventricular Remodelling and Dysfunction in Spontaneously Hypertensive Rats: Different Interactions with the Renin-Angiotensin-Aldosterone System. *Biomedicines* **2022**, *10*, 1844. [CrossRef]
20. Simko, F.; Baka, T.; Krajcirovicova, K.; Repova, K.; Aziriova, S.; Zorad, S.; Poglitsch, M.; Adamcova, M.; Reiter, R.J.; Paulis, L. Effect of Melatonin on the Renin-Angiotensin-Aldosterone System in l-NAME-Induced Hypertension. *Molecules* **2018**, *23*, 265. [CrossRef]
21. Muldowney, J.A.S.; Davis, S.N.; Vaughan, D.E.; Brown, N.J. NO Synthase Inhibition Increases Aldosterone in Humans. *Hypertension* **2004**, *44*, 739–745. [CrossRef] [PubMed]
22. Suehiro, T.; Tsuruya, K.; Ikeda, H.; Toyonaga, J.; Yamada, S.; Noguchi, H.; Tokumoto, M.; Kitazono, T. Systemic Aldosterone, But Not Angiotensin II, Plays a Pivotal Role in the Pathogenesis of Renal Injury in Chronic Nitric Oxide-Deficient Male Rats. *Endocrinology* **2015**, *156*, 2657–2666. [CrossRef] [PubMed]
23. Klug, D.; Robert, V.; Swynghedauw, B. Role of Mechanical and Hormonal Factors in Cardiac Remodeling and the Biologic Limits of Myocardial Adaptation. *Am. J. Cardiol.* **1993**, *71*, A46–A54. [CrossRef]
24. Tu, W.; Pratt, J.H. Autonomous Aldosterone Production and Left Ventricular Hypertrophy. *Hypertension* **2020**, *75*, 1409–1411. [CrossRef] [PubMed]
25. Clerico, A.; Vittorini, S.; Passino, C. Measurement of the Pro-Hormone of Brain Type Natriuretic Peptide (proBNP): Methodological Considerations and Pathophysiological Relevance. *Clin. Chem. Lab. Med.* **2011**, *49*, 1949–1954. [CrossRef]
26. Docherty, K.F.; Vaduganathan, M.; Solomon, S.D.; McMurray, J.J.V. Sacubitril/Valsartan. *JACC Heart Fail.* **2020**, *8*, 800–810. [CrossRef]
27. Jiang, W.-Y.; Huo, J.-Y.; Chen, C.; Chen, R.; Ge, T.-T.; Chang, Q.; Hu, J.-W.; Geng, J.; Jiang, Z.-X.; Shan, Q.-J. Renal Denervation Ameliorates Post-Infarction Cardiac Remodeling in Rats through Dual Regulation of Oxidative Stress in the Heart and Brain. *Biomed. Pharmacother.* **2019**, *118*, 109243. [CrossRef]
28. Uijl, E.; 't Hart, D.C.; Roksnoer, L.C.W.; Groningen, M.C.C.; van Veghel, R.; Garrelds, I.M.; de Vries, R.; van der Vlag, J.; Zietse, R.; Nijenhuis, T.; et al. Angiotensin-Neprilysin Inhibition Confers Renoprotection in Rats with Diabetes and Hypertension by Limiting Podocyte Injury. *J. Hypertens.* **2020**, *38*, 755–764. [CrossRef]
29. Abdin, A.; Schulz, M.; Riemer, U.; Hadëri, B.; Wachter, R.; Laufs, U.; Bauersachs, J.; Kindermann, I.; Vukadinović, D.; Böhm, M. Sacubitril/Valsartan in Heart Failure: Efficacy and Safety in and Outside Clinical Trials. *ESC Heart Fail.* **2022**, *9*, 3737–3750. [CrossRef]
30. Pecháňová, O.; Bernátová, I.; Pelouch, V.; Simko, F. Protein Remodelling of the Heart in NO-Deficient Hypertension: The Effect of Captopril. *J. Mol. Cell Cardiol.* **1997**, *29*, 3365–3374. [CrossRef]
31. Bernátová, I.; Pecháňová, O.; Simko, F. Effect of Captopril in L-NAME-Induced Hypertension on the Rat Myocardium, Aorta, Brain and Kidney. *Exp. Physiol.* **1999**, *84*, 1095–1105. [PubMed]
32. Bernátová, I.; Pecháňová, O.; Pelouch, V.; Simko, F. Regression of Chronic L -NAME-Treatment-Induced Left Ventricular Hypertrophy: Effect of Captopril. *J. Mol. Cell Cardiol.* **2000**, *32*, 177–185. [CrossRef] [PubMed]

33. von Lueder, T.G.; Wang, B.H.; Kompa, A.R.; Huang, L.; Webb, R.; Jordaan, P.; Atar, D.; Krum, H. Angiotensin Receptor Neprilysin Inhibitor LCZ696 Attenuates Cardiac Remodeling and Dysfunction after Myocardial Infarction by Reducing Cardiac Fibrosis and Hypertrophy. *Circ. Heart Fail.* **2015**, *8*, 71–78. [CrossRef] [PubMed]
34. Liu, J.; Zheng, X.; Zhang, C.; Zhang, C.; Bu, P. Lcz696 Alleviates Myocardial Fibrosis After Myocardial Infarction Through the sFRP-1/Wnt/β-Catenin Signaling Pathway. *Front. Pharmacol.* **2021**, *12*, 724147. [CrossRef] [PubMed]
35. Zhang, W.; Liu, J.; Fu, Y.; Ji, H.; Fang, Z.; Zhou, W.; Fan, H.; Zhang, Y.; Liao, Y.; Yang, T.; et al. Sacubitril/Valsartan Reduces Fibrosis and Alleviates High-Salt Diet-Induced HFpEF in Rats. *Front. Pharmacol.* **2020**, *11*, 600953. [CrossRef] [PubMed]
36. Tashiro, K.; Kuwano, T.; Ideishi, A.; Morita, H.; Idemoto, Y.; Goto, M.; Suematsu, Y.; Miura, S.-I. Sacubitril/Valsartan Inhibits Cardiomyocyte Hypertrophy in Angiotensin II-Induced Hypertensive Mice Independent of a Blood Pressure-Lowering Effect. *Cardiol. Res.* **2020**, *11*, 376–385. [CrossRef] [PubMed]
37. Sobiborowicz-Sadowska, A.M.; Kamińska, K.; Cudnoch-Jędrzejewska, A. Neprilysin Inhibition in the Prevention of Anthracycline-Induced Cardiotoxicity. *Cancers* **2023**, *15*, 312. [CrossRef] [PubMed]
38. Li, Q.; Fang, Y.; Peng, D.-W.; Li, L.-A.; Deng, C.-Y.; Yang, H.; Kuang, S.-J.; Li, Q.-Q.; Zhang, M.-Z.; Zeng, P.; et al. Sacubitril/Valsartan Reduces Susceptibility to Atrial Fibrillation by Improving Atrial Remodeling in Spontaneously Hypertensive Rats. *Eur. J. Pharmacol.* **2023**, *952*, 175754. [CrossRef] [PubMed]
39. Xiao, Y.; Zhou, Z.-Y.; Sun, J.-C.; Xing, W.; Yan, J.; Xu, W.-J.; Lu, Y.-S.; Liu, T.; Jin, Y. Protective Effect of Novel Angiotensin Receptor Neprilysin Inhibitor S086 on Target Organ Injury in Spontaneously Hypertensive Rats. *Biomed. Pharmacother.* **2024**, *170*, 115968. [CrossRef]
40. Wang, Y.; Zhou, R.; Lu, C.; Chen, Q.; Xu, T.; Li, D. Effects of the Angiotensin-Receptor Neprilysin Inhibitor on Cardiac Reverse Remodeling: Meta-Analysis. *J. Am. Heart Assoc.* **2019**, *8*, e012272. [CrossRef]
41. Bole-Feysot, C.; Goffin, V.; Edery, M.; Binart, N.; Kelly, P.A. Prolactin (PRL) and Its Receptor: Actions, Signal Transduction Pathways and Phenotypes Observed in PRL Receptor Knockout Mice. *Endocr. Rev.* **1998**, *19*, 225–268. [CrossRef] [PubMed]
42. Chang, A.S.; Grant, R.; Tomita, H.; Kim, H.-S.; Smithies, O.; Kakoki, M. Prolactin Alters Blood Pressure by Modulating the Activity of Endothelial Nitric Oxide Synthase. *Proc. Natl. Acad. Sci. USA* **2016**, *113*, 12538–12543. [CrossRef] [PubMed]
43. Yavuz, D.; Deyneli, O.; Akpinar, I.; Yildiz, E.; Gözü, H.; Sezgin, O.; Haklar, G.; Akalin, S. Endothelial Function, Insulin Sensitivity and Inflammatory Markers in Hyperprolactinemic Pre-Menopausal Women. *Eur. J. Endocrinol.* **2003**, *149*, 187–193. [CrossRef] [PubMed]
44. Carrero, J.J.; Kyriazis, J.; Sonmez, A.; Tzanakis, I.; Qureshi, A.R.; Stenvinkel, P.; Saglam, M.; Stylianou, K.; Yaman, H.; Taslipinar, A.; et al. Prolactin Levels, Endothelial Dysfunction, and the Risk of Cardiovascular Events and Mortality in Patients with CKD. *Clin. J. Am. Soc. Nephrol.* **2012**, *7*, 207–215. [CrossRef] [PubMed]
45. Georgiopoulos, G.A.; Stamatelopoulos, K.S.; Lambrinoudaki, I.; Lykka, M.; Kyrkou, K.; Rizos, D.; Creatsa, M.; Christodoulakos, G.; Alevizaki, M.; Sfikakis, P.P.; et al. Prolactin and Preclinical Atherosclerosis in Menopausal Women with Cardiovascular Risk Factors. *Hypertension* **2009**, *54*, 98–105. [CrossRef]
46. Aguayo-Cerón, K.A.; Calzada-Mendoza, C.C.; Méndez-Bolaina, E.; Romero-Nava, R.; Ocharan-Hernández, M.E. The Regulatory Effect of Bromocriptine on Cardiac Hypertrophy by Prolactin and D2 Receptor Modulation. *Clin. Exp. Hypertens.* **2020**, *42*, 675–679. [CrossRef]
47. Therkelsen, K.E.; Abraham, T.M.; Pedley, A.; Massaro, J.M.; Sutherland, P.; Hoffmann, U.; Fox, C.S. Association Between Prolactin and Incidence of Cardiovascular Risk Factors in the Framingham Heart Study. *J. Am. Heart Assoc.* **2016**, *5*, e002640. [CrossRef]
48. Shen, Y.; Yang, Q.; Hu, T.; Wang, Y.; Chen, L.; Gao, F.; Zhu, W.; Hu, G.; Zhou, J.; Wang, C.; et al. Association of Prolactin with All-Cause and Cardiovascular Mortality among Patients with Type 2 Diabetes: A Real-World Study. *Eur. J. Prev. Cardiol.* **2023**, *30*, 1439–1447. [CrossRef] [PubMed]
49. Papazoglou, A.S.; Leite, A.R.; Moysidis, D.V.; Anastasiou, V.; Daios, S.; Borges-Canha, M.; Giannopoulos, G.; Neves, J.S.; Ziakas, A.; Giannakoulas, G. Serum Prolactin Levels and Mortality in Adults without Prolactinoma: A Meta-Analysis. *J. Clin. Endocrinol. Metab.* **2024**, dgae087, *ahead of print*. [CrossRef]
50. Simko, F.; Matuskova, J.; Luptak, I.; Krajcirovicova, K.; Kucharska, J.; Gvozdjakova, A.; Babal, P.; Pechanova, O. Effect of Simvastatin on Remodeling of the Left Ventricle and Aorta in L-NAME-Induced Hypertension. *Life Sci.* **2004**, *74*, 1211–1224. [CrossRef]
51. Simko, F.; Luptak, I.; Matuskova, J.; Krajcirovicova, K.; Sumbalova, Z.; Kucharska, J.; Gvozdjakova, A.; Simko, J.; Babal, P.; Pechanova, O.; et al. L-Arginine Fails to Protect against Myocardial Remodelling in L-NAME-Induced Hypertension. *Eur. J. Clin. Investig.* **2005**, *35*, 362–368. [CrossRef]
52. Bartosz, M.; Kedziora, J.; Bartosz, G. Antioxidant and Prooxidant Properties of Captopril and Enalapril. *Free Radic. Biol. Med.* **1997**, *23*, 729–735. [CrossRef] [PubMed]
53. Bettencourt, P.; Fonseca, C.; Franco, F.; Andrade, A.; Brito, D. Interpretation of B-Type Natriuretic Peptides in the Era of Angiotensin Receptor-Neprilysin Inhibitors. *Rev. Port. Cardiol.* **2017**, *36*, 881–884. [CrossRef] [PubMed]

biomedicines

Article

Repurposing of the Cardiovascular Drug Statin for the Treatment of Cancers: Efficacy of Statin–Dipyridamole Combination Treatment in Melanoma Cell Lines

Nanami Irie [1,†], Kana Mizoguchi [1,†], Tomoko Warita [2,*,†], Mirai Nakano [3], Kasuga Sasaki [3], Jiro Tashiro [3], Tomohiro Osaki [4], Takuro Ishikawa [5], Zoltán N. Oltvai [6] and Katsuhiko Warita [3,*]

1 Graduate School of Science and Technology, Kwansei Gakuin University, 1 Gakuen Uegahara, Sanda 669-1330, Japan
2 Department of Biomedical Sciences, School of Biological and Environmental Sciences, Kwansei Gakuin University, 1 Gakuen Uegahara, Sanda 669-1330, Japan
3 Department of Veterinary Anatomy, School of Veterinary Medicine, Tottori University, 4-101 Koyama Minami, Tottori 680-8553, Japan
4 Department of Veterinary Clinical Medicine, School of Veterinary Medicine, Tottori University, 4-101 Koyama Minami, Tottori 680-8553, Japan
5 Department of Anatomy, School of Medicine, Aichi Medical University, 1-1 Yazakokarimata, Nagakute 480-1195, Japan
6 Department of Pathology and Laboratory Medicine, University of Rochester, 601 Elmwood Ave, Rochester, NY 14642, USA; zoltan_oltvai@urmc.rochester.edu
* Correspondence: waritat@kwansei.ac.jp (T.W.); waritak@tottori-u.ac.jp (K.W.)
† These authors contributed equally to this work.

Abstract: Metastatic melanoma has a very poor prognosis. Statins, 3-hydroxy-3-methyl-glutaryl-coenzyme A reductase (HMGCR) inhibitors, are cholesterol-lowering agents with a potential for cancer treatment. The inhibition of HMGCR by statins, however, induces feedback, which paradoxically upregulates HMGCR expression via sterol regulatory element-binding protein-2 (SREBP2). Dipyridamole, an antiplatelet agent, is known to inhibit SREBP2 upregulation. We aimed to demonstrate the efficacy of statin–dipyridamole combination treatment in both human and spontaneously occurring canine melanoma cell lines. The half maximal inhibitory concentration (IC_{50}) of atorvastatin showed a 68–92% reduction when combined with dipyridamole, compared with that of atorvastatin alone. In some melanoma cell lines, cell proliferation was suppressed to almost zero by the combination treatment ($\geq$3 μM atorvastatin). Finally, the BRAF inhibitor, vemurafenib, further potentiated the effects of the combined statin–dipyridamole treatment in BRAF V600E mutation-bearing human melanoma cell lines. In conclusion, the inexpensive and frequently prescribed statin–dipyridamole combination therapy may lead to new developments in the treatment of melanoma and may potentiate the effects of vemurafenib for the targeted therapy of BRAF V600E-mutation bearing melanoma patients. The concordance between the data from canine and human melanoma cell lines reinforces this possibility.

Keywords: statin; drug repositioning; carcinostatic effect; mevalonate pathway; HMG-CoA reductase; dipyridamole; combination therapy; human melanoma; spontaneously occurring canine melanoma; comparative oncology

1. Introduction

Melanoma is an aggressive skin tumor responsible for most skin-cancer-related deaths globally [1]. There is a large interracial difference in the occurrence of melanoma, with the highest incidence in White populations (29.7 males and 19.1 females per 100,000), followed by Hispanics (4.4 males and 4.7 females per 100,000), Asians, and Black populations (1.1 males and 1.0 females per 100,000) [2]. In Japan, melanoma is a rare cancer usually diagnosed at a late stage compared to the time of diagnosis in Western countries [3]. Currently, the therapeutic options for melanoma include surgical resection, chemotherapy, radiotherapy, photodynamic therapy, immunotherapy, and targeted therapy [1]. Immune checkpoint inhibitor therapy targeting CTLA-4 or programmed cell death protein 1 (PD-1) and its ligand (PD-L1) and targeted therapy with kinase inhibitors (BRAF and mitogen-activated extracellular signal-regulated kinase (MEK) inhibitors) are the current standard treatments for melanoma [4]. However, there are two challenges: adverse events that can lead to skin and gastrointestinal toxicity, and reduced efficiency due to resistance to immune, chemo-, and targeted therapies [1]. This necessitates the search for additional therapy options.

Compactin (mevastatin), the first statin, was discovered by Dr. Akira Endo in Japan from the blue-green mold *Penicillium citrinum* Pen-51, isolated from a rice sample collected at a grain shop in Kyoto [5,6]. Thereafter, other statins (compactin analogs) were developed and are now used worldwide to treat hyperlipidemia. Statins function as 3-hydroxy-3-methyl-glutaryl-coenzyme A reductase (HMGCR) inhibitors and suppress cholesterol biosynthesis by specifically inhibiting HMGCR, the rate-limiting enzyme of the mevalonate pathway. This metabolic pathway is responsible for the synthesis of cholesterol and other important biomolecules, such as dolichols, which are crucial for glycosylation; ubiquinone, crucial for mitochondrial electron transport processes; and farnesyl pyrophosphate (FPP) and geranylgeranyl pyrophosphate (GGPP), which are essential for protein prenylation [7,8]. Therefore, the depletion of mevalonate pathway intermediates by statins interferes with the post-translational modification and activation of small guanosine triphosphatases (GTPases) (such as Ras, Rho, or Rac) and their downstream signaling, which affects cell proliferation and differentiation or leads to apoptosis [7]. Additionally, the mevalonate pathway supports tumorigenesis and is deregulated in human cancers [8]. Moreover, statins have been reported to have anticancer effects in different types of cancers, including lung, kidney, bladder, colon, breast, and prostate cancer [7,9–12]. Therefore, there is substantial interest in repurposing statins as therapeutic agents for cancer. Moreover, Jiang et al. suggested that because of their efficacy, statins may address the shortcomings of conventional cancer treatments and should be considered in the context of combined therapies for cancer [7].

However, the inhibition of HMGCR activity by statins paradoxically induces a feedback regulation in statin-treated cells, eventually resulting in the upregulation of HMGCR expression. The underlying mechanism involves the transcription of *HMGCR*, which is activated by sterol regulatory element binding protein-2 (SREBP2) [8]. As this homeostatic mechanism weakens the effectiveness of statins and creates the need to use higher doses for cancer inhibition, statins have yet to be successfully repurposed as cancer therapeutic drugs. Thus, for the successful use of statins in cancer therapy, the prevention of the homeostatic feedback loop that blunts statin efficacy may be required [13].

Our previous studies showed that atorvastatin is effective against all melanoma cells in both human [14] and spontaneously occurring canine melanoma cell lines [15,16]. Furthermore, plasma levels of atorvastatin, comparable to those used for the treatment of hypercholesterolemia, have been reported to inhibit the metastasis of human melanoma cells overexpressing RhoC in a xenograft model [17]. In addition, simvastatin and fluvastatin have been reported to inhibit tumor metastasis and growth by suppressing the Rho signaling pathway and to markedly improve the survival rate in a mouse melanoma model [18]. These findings highlight the need for further investigations of statins toward clinical applications in the treatment of metastatic melanoma.

In this study, we aimed to demonstrate that dipyridamole, an antiplatelet agent, potentiates the anticancer effects of statins against both human and spontaneously occurring canine melanoma by interfering with the statin-induced activation of SREBP2-driven HMGCR upregulation. Both statins and dipyridamole are currently approved drugs; therefore, our findings may contribute to the immediate advancement of their evaluation in clinical trials.

2. Materials and Methods

2.1. Cell Culture

Melanoma-derived SK-MEL-5 and MDA-MB-435 cells were obtained from the Division of Cancer Treatment and Diagnosis (DCTD) Tumor Repository (National Cancer Institute, Frederick, MD, USA). Three canine melanoma primary tumor cell lines, YCC, ITP, and HTR, established by Osaki et al. [19], were also used in this study. They tested negative for *Mycoplasma* using an e-Myco™ Mycoplasma PCR Detection Kit (iNtRON Biotechnology, Sungnam, Republic of Korea). The cell lines were cultured in RPMI 1640 medium (Thermo Fisher Scientific, Waltham, MA, USA) supplemented with 10% heat-inactivated fetal bovine serum (Biosera, Boussens, France) and penicillin/streptomycin (Fujifilm Wako Pure Chemical, Osaka, Japan; final concentration of 100 units/mL penicillin G and 100 µg/mL streptomycin) in a humidified incubator at 37 °C with 5% CO_2.

2.2. Reagents

Atorvastatin (Sigma-Aldrich, St. Louis, MO, USA) and dipyridamole (Sigma-Aldrich) were dissolved in dimethyl sulfoxide (DMSO; Fujifilm Wako Pure Chemical; final concentration of 0.1% in RPMI 1640 medium) at final concentrations of 0.3–30 µM and 1–100 µM, respectively. Vemurafenib, dissolved in 0.1% DMSO (Selleck Chemicals, Houston, TX, USA), was added to RPMI at final concentrations of 0.1–10 µM. DMSO was added to the control groups as the vehicle control at final concentrations of 0.2% and 0.3% in atorvastatin–dipyridamole combination treatment and atorvastatin–dipyridamole–vemurafenib combination treatments, respectively. Geranylgeranyl pyrophosphate ammonium salt solution (Sigma-Aldrich) was used at a final concentration of 20 µM with reference to the paper by Zhou et al. [20]. Methanol (final concentration, 1%; Fujifilm Wako Pure Chemical) was added to the control groups as the vehicle control; 0.3% DMSO and 1% methanol have no cytotoxic effects on human cancer cell lines [21]. All cell culture experiments were performed in triplicate.

2.3. Morphological Analysis by Optical and Fluorescence Microscopy

The cells were seeded in 6-well plates at a density of 1×10^5 cells/mL, incubated overnight prior to treatment with 3 µM dipyridamole, 10 µM atorvastatin, or their combination for 72 h, and then imaged using an Olympus IX71 microscope (Olympus, Tokyo, Japan).

Cultured cells were fixed with 2% paraformaldehyde (Nacalai Tesque, Kyoto, Japan) for 30 min and washed with phosphate-buffered saline (PBS). They were then permeabilized with 0.1% Triton-X-100 (Nacalai Tesque) for 15 min. After washing with PBS, the cells were treated with 2% bovine serum albumin for 15 min to block any non-specific proteins. Subsequently, 100 nM Acti-stain™ 488 phalloidin (PHDG1; Cytoskeleton, Denver, CO, USA) was used for F-actin staining. Following a PBS wash, the cells were subjected to nuclear staining using 5 µg/mL Hoechst 33342 (Dojindo, Kumamoto, Japan) for 15 min and mounted using Fluoromount/Plus™ (Diagnostic BioSystems, Pleasanton, CA, USA). Images were captured using a digital fluorescence microscope (BZ-X810; Keyence, Osaka, Japan).

2.4. Cell Proliferation Assay

The cells were seeded in 96-well plates at a density of 2.5×10^4 cells/mL and incubated overnight, prior to treatment with each reagent, for 72 h. Five different assays were performed: (1) single treatment with each concentration of dipyridamole, (2) treatment with each concentration of atorvastatin with (or without) 3 µM dipyridamole, (3) rescue experiment by GGPP against 10 µM atorvastatin and 3 µM dipyridamole combination treatment, (4) single treatment with each concentration of vemurafenib, and (5) combined treatment with 3 µM atorvastatin, 3 µM dipyridamole, and 0.1 or 0.3 µM vemurafenib. Absorbance was measured at 450 nm using an 800 TS microplate reader (BioTek, Winooski, VT, USA) and a Cell Counting Kit-8 (CCK-8, Dojindo). The IC_{50} values were calculated by constructing sigmoid curves based on cell viability using ImageJ software version 1.52a (National Institutes of Health, Bethesda, MD, USA).

2.5. RNA Extraction and Quantitative Real-Time Polymerase Chain Reaction (qRT-PCR)

Cells were seeded in 6-well plates and cultured until subconfluence. An ISOSPIN Cell and Tissue RNA kit (Nippon Gene, Tokyo, Japan) was used to extract total RNA for qRT-PCR from the cells 24 h after the addition of 1 μM and 10 μM atorvastatin and/or 3 μM dipyridamole in accordance with the manufacturer's instructions.

The RNA samples were treated with RNase-free DNase to eliminate genomic DNA contamination. cDNA was synthesized from 1 μg of RNA using the ReverTra Ace® qPCR RT Master Mix kit (Toyobo, Osaka, Japan). Expression levels of *HMGCR* were examined. The canine primer sets used for gene expression analysis were as follows: *HMGCR* forward 5′-GGAGAGCCTCTGAGTGGTTG-3′ and reverse 5′-TGTTCACTGCCACTTCCGTG-3′; *GAPDH* (internal reference) forward 5′-GGTAGTGAAGCAGGCATCGG-3′ and reverse 5′- TTACTCCTTGGAGGCCATGTG-3′. PCR was conducted using Applied Biosystems PowerUp SYBR Green Master Mix and a QuantStudio® 3 Real-Time PCR System (Thermo Fisher Scientific). The primer sets for humans and the PCR conditions have been described previously [20].

2.6. Western Blotting

The cells were seeded in 6-well plates and cultured until reaching subconfluence. Protein was extracted after 24 h of the addition of 10 μM atorvastatin, 3 μM dipyridamole, the drug combination, or 0.2% DMSO.

Western blotting was performed as described previously [20]. HMGCR protein levels were determined using an anti-HMGCR mouse monoclonal antibody (1:1000 dilution; AMAb90618; Atlas, Cambridge, UK). Anti-glyceraldehyde-3-phosphate dehydrogenase (GAPDH; 14C10) rabbit monoclonal antibody (1:1000 dilution, #2118; Cell Signaling Technology, Beverly, MA, USA) was used to detect GAPDH as an internal standard.

2.7. SEM Sample Preparation and Imaging

Cells treated with 5 μM atorvastatin alone or 3 μM dipyridamole in combination were imaged using SEM, as described below. Cells were cultured on plastic disks (Cell Disk LF1, Sumitomo Bakelite, Tokyo, Japan) and washed once with warm PBS. After aspirating the wash solution, cells were fixed with 2.5% glutaraldehyde diluted in PHEM buffer (pH 7.4; 60 mM PIPES, 25 mM HEPES, 10 mM EGTA, and 2 mM $MgCl_2$ in H_2O) at 25 °C for 30 min. Then, cells were washed with warm PHEM buffer for 5 min thrice, followed by post-fixation with 1% osmium solution dissolved in PHEM buffer for 30 min at 25 °C. After washing thrice with warm PHEM buffer for 5 min, the samples were dehydrated in an ascending ethanol series. Then, ethanol was replaced with 100% t-butyl alcohol, and the cell disks immersed in t-butyl alcohol were kept in the refrigerator (4 °C). Subsequently, the cells on the cell disks were lyophilized using a VFD-21 t-butanol freeze dryer (Vacuum Device, Ibaragi, Japan) and then coated with platinum/palladium (Pt/Pd) using a HITACHI E-1045 ion sputter coater (Hitachi High-Technologies, Tokyo, Japan). The cell surfaces were observed using a HITACHI SEM SU-8020 (Hitachi High-Technologies) at an accelerating voltage of 5 kV.

2.8. Statistical Analysis

Statistical analyses were performed using the Microsoft Excel add-in software (Bell Curve for Excel, version 4.02; Social Survey Research Information, Tokyo, Japan). Dunnett's test or a Tukey–Kramer post hoc test were used to compare cell viability and *HMGCR* mRNA expression levels in each atorvastatin-treated or combination atorvastatin- and dipyridamole-treated group with those of the controls. Statistical significance was set at p value < 0.05. All the experiments were repeated at least three times, independently.

3. Results

3.1. Dipyridamole Co-Treatment Augments the Cytostatic Effect of Atorvastatin in Both Human and Canine Melanoma Cell Lines

Regarding cell morphology after drug treatments, atorvastatin treatment alone induced cellular shrinkage and apoptosis-like morphological changes both in human and canine melanoma cell lines compared with those in sham-treated cells (Figure S1A,C). However, we observed no effect on cell morphology when cells were treated with dipyridamole alone (Figure S1B). A combined treatment with atorvastatin and dipyridamole induced more pronounced morphological changes than atorvastatin treatment alone (Figure S1C,D).

3.2. Half-Maximal Inhibitory Concentration (IC_{50}) Value of Dipyridamole Exceeds 16.85 µM

In the human melanoma cell lines MDA-MB-435 and SK-MEL-5, and canine melanoma cell line ITP, more than 10 µM dipyridamole had an inhibitory effect on cell proliferation (Figure S2A,B,D). In the canine melanoma cell lines HTR and YCC, dipyridamole treatment increased cell proliferation at lower concentrations; however, at higher concentrations, cell proliferation was inhibited (Figure S2C,E). IC_{50} values of dipyridamole for MDA-MD-435, SK-MEL-5, HTR, ITP, and YCC were 40.31, 29.77, 19.75, 16.85, and 29.81 µM, respectively (Figure S3).

3.3. Combined Atorvastatin and Dipyridamole Treatment Enhances the Cytostatic Effect in Both Human and Canine Melanoma Cell Lines Compared with Atorvastatin Treatment Alone

A significant decrease in cell proliferation was observed in the combination treatment group at lower concentrations of atorvastatin compared with that in the atorvastatin monotherapy group (Figure 1).

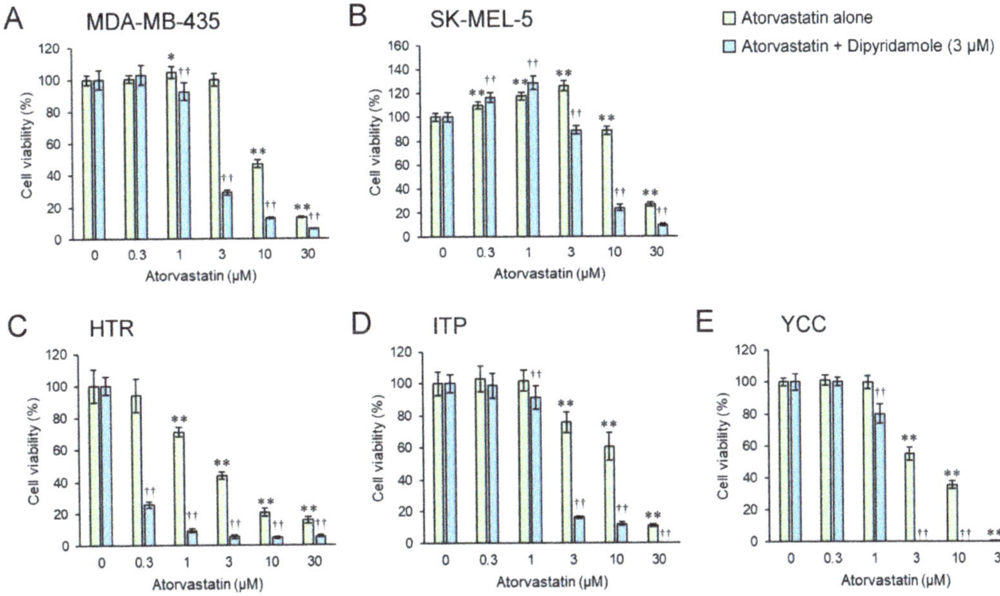

Figure 1. Enhancement of the growth inhibitory effect of atorvastatin on tumor cell lines by combination treatment with dipyridamole. Relative growth of human MDA-MB-435 (**A**) and SK-MEL-5 (**B**) and canine HTR (**C**), ITP (**D**), and YCC (**E**) melanoma cell lines is shown. Green and blue bars represent atorvastatin single treatment group and atorvastatin–dipyridamole combination treatment group, respectively. Values in DMSO control were set at 100%. Each value represents the mean ± SD (n = 3). Data were analyzed using a one-way analysis of variance (ANOVA) with Dunnett's test for multiple group comparisons. * $p < 0.05$, ** $p < 0.01$, †† $p < 0.01$ with respect to each control group.

The addition of dipyridamole reduced the concentration of atorvastatin required to significantly inhibit the cell proliferation of MDA-MB-435 cells, from 10 μM to 1 μM (1/10-fold), and of SK-MEL-5 cells from 10 μM to 3 μM (about 1/3-fold). In HTR cells, atorvastatin concentration reduced from 1 μM to 0.3 μM (about 1/3-fold), and in ITP and YCC cells from 3 μM to 1 μM (1/3-fold). The effects of atorvastatin alone or a combination of atorvastatin and dipyridamole depended on the cancer cell type. Notably, the addition of low concentrations of the drug increased the proliferation of some cells. In canine YCC cells, the combination of 3–30 μM atorvastatin and dipyridamole reduced cell proliferation to 0, while 30 μM atorvastatin alone reduced cell proliferation to 0. In ITP cells, the combination of 30 μM atorvastatin and dipyridamole reduced cell proliferation to zero. The IC_{50} values are shown in Table 1 and Figure S4.

Table 1. IC_{50} of atorvastatin.

Melanoma	IC_{50} Atorvastatin (μM)	IC_{50} Combination ¶ (μM)	Reduction (%)
MDA-MB-435	9.583	2.180	77
SK-MEL-5	21.769	5.618	74
HTR	2.286	0.184	92
ITP	14.466	1.715	88
YCC	3.507	1.117	68

¶: IC_{50} of atorvastatin in the combination.

3.4. Statin and/or Dipyridamole Affect Filopodia and Lamellipodia Formation

F-actin stress fibers are major contractile structures that are prominent in fibroblasts, smooth muscle cells, endothelial cells, and some cancer cell lines [22]. In many cancer cells with increased motility, F-actin stress fibers that form longitudinally across the cell body are often observed. At the periphery of the cell membrane, plasma membrane structures called filopodia and lamellipodia are formed, and cell migration occurs via protrusion at the front, mediated by these structures [23,24]. When F-actin was stained with phalloidin in MDA-MB-435 and SK-MEL-5 cells, more stress fibers were observed in MDA-MB-435 cells than in SK-MEL-5 cells (Figure S5A). The effects of statins and/or dipyridamole on the formation of filopodia and lamellipodia were found using a scanning electron microscope (SEM), especially in MDA-MB-435 cells (Figure S5B).

3.5. Atorvastatin Upregulates HMGCR mRNA Expression in a Dose-Dependent Manner While Dipyridamole Tends to Downregulate It

HMGCR expression increased upon statin treatment in a dose-dependent manner. However, the level of upregulation depended on the cancer cell type. Moreover, dipyridamole tended to downregulate *HMGCR* expression (Figure S6).

3.6. Dipyridamole Augments Atorvastatin's Anticancer Effect, Which Correlates with Its Attenuation of Statin-Induced Increase in HMGCR Expression

In all five human and canine melanoma cell lines, HMGCR protein expression at the steady state was not detected (extremely low level). The addition of atorvastatin alone drastically increased HMGCR protein expression, whereas the addition of dipyridamole alone did not increase its expression. However, dipyridamole significantly attenuated the statin-induced increase in HMGCR protein levels in all five atorvastatin co-treated cell lines (Figure 2).

3.7. Geranylgeranyl Pyrophosphate (GGPP) Rescues Cell Proliferation Inhibited by Dipyridamole Combination with Atorvastatin

The addition of GGPP attenuated the inhibitory effect of atorvastatin–dipyridamole co-treatment and significantly rescued ($p < 0.01$) cell proliferation in all cell lines examined: SK-MEL-5 and MDA-MB-435 (human melanoma), and YCC, ITP, and HTR (canine melanoma) (Figure 3). This also demonstrates that the decrease in the melanoma cell line viability by the statin–dipyridamole co-treatment is an on-target (i.e., HMGCR) effect on the mevalonate pathway.

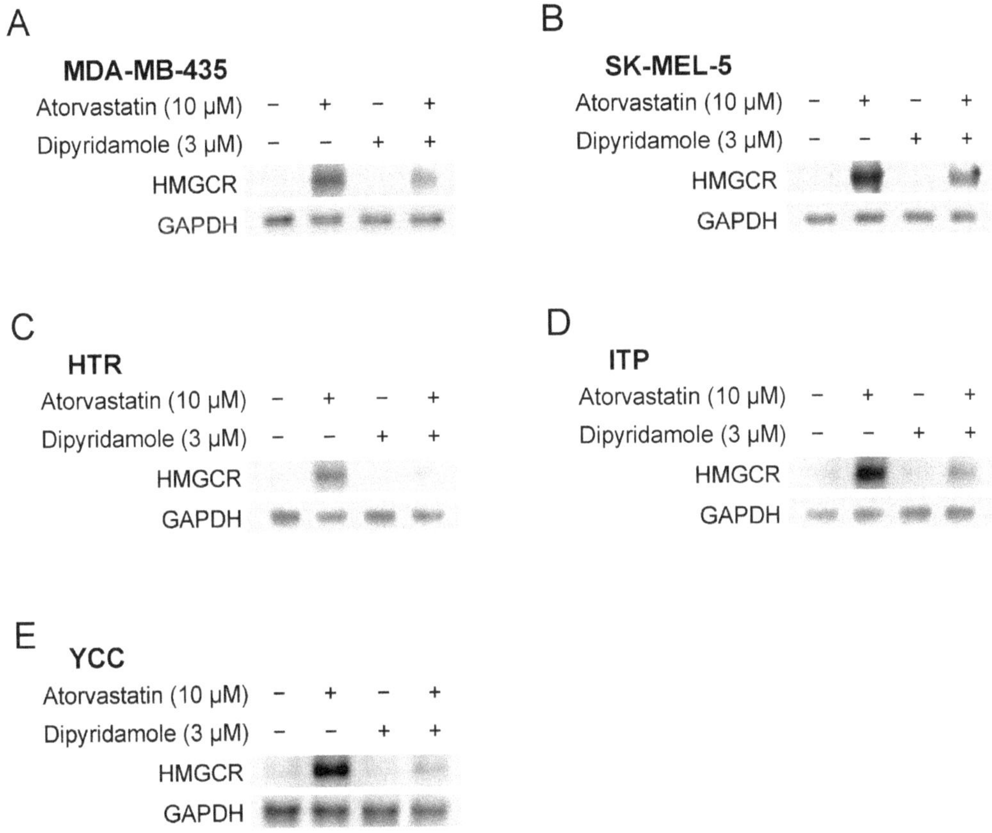

Figure 2. HMGCR expression after atorvastatin, dipyridamole, and their combination treatments. HMGCR protein expression in MDA-MB-435 (**A**), SK-MEL-5 (**B**), HTR (**C**), ITP (**D**), and YCC (**E**) cells was determined using Western blotting. From the left side: lane 1, vehicle control group; lane 2, 10 μM atorvastatin treatment group; lane 3, 3 μM dipyridamole treatment group; and lane 4, 10 μM atorvastatin plus 3 μM dipyridamole treatment group. The Western blot shown is representative of experiments performed in triplicate.

3.8. Vemurafenib Augments the Combined Inhibitory Effect of Statin and Dipyridamole

The MDA-MB-435 and SK-MEL-5 melanoma cells lines are known to harbor BRAF Val600Glu (V600E) mutations and to be sensitive to the BRAF inhibitor vemurafenib [25,26]. Indeed, vemurafenib treatment inhibited cell proliferation in a dose-dependent manner 72 h after the start of drug addition (Figure 4A,B). When used alone at a concentration that exhibited a 20–30% cytostatic effect on cell growth of the two human melanoma cell lines, vemurafenib did not augment the inhibitory effect on cell proliferation with atorvastatin alone, but it did so in the presence of atorvastatin and dipyridamole co-treatment (Figure 4C,D).

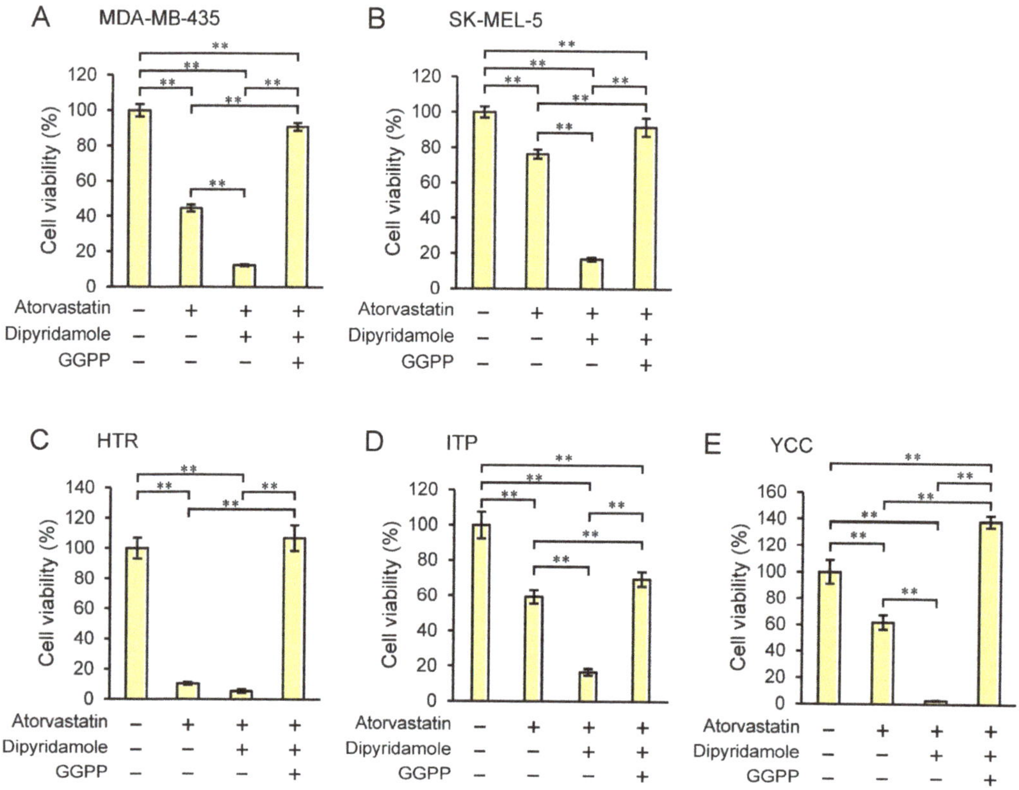

Figure 3. Rescue of atorvastatin- and/or dipyridamole-induced growth inhibition by GGPP. Relative growth of human (MDA-MB-435; (**A**) and SK-MEL-5; (**B**)) and canine (HTR; (**C**), ITP; (**D**), and YCC; (**E**)) melanoma cell lines in the presence or absence of exogenous geranylgeranyl pyrophosphate (GGPP). Values in vehicle control were set to 100%. Each value represents the mean ± SD (n = 3). Data were analyzed using one-way analysis of variance (ANOVA) with the Tukey–Kramer post hoc test for multiple group comparisons. ** $p < 0.01$.

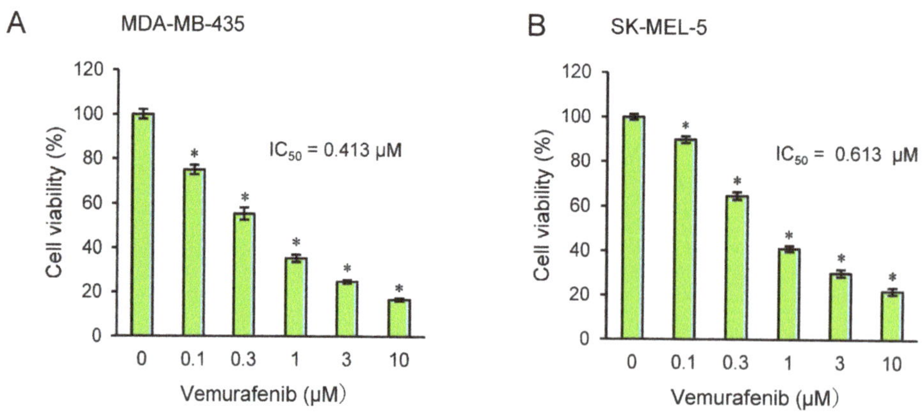

Figure 4. *Cont.*

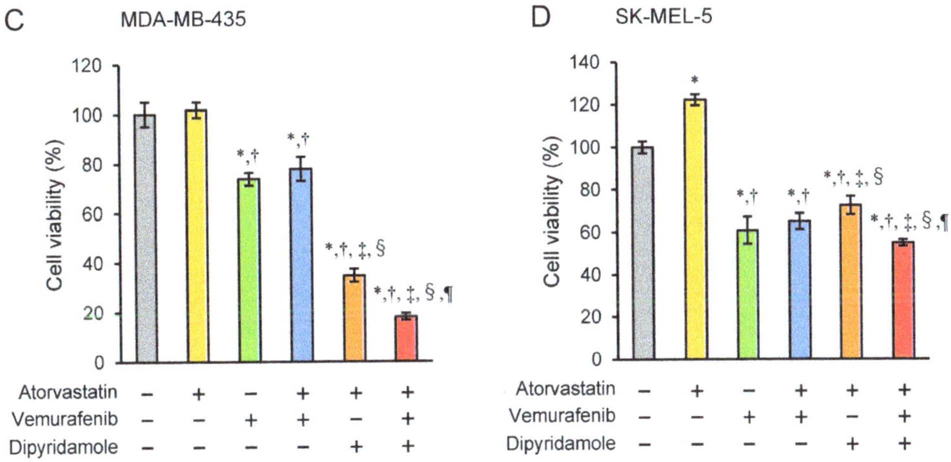

Figure 4. Enhancement of growth inhibitory effect of atorvastatin–dipyridamole combination on tumor cell lines by vemurafenib co-treatment. The relative growth of human melanoma cell lines 72 h after the start of drug treatment is shown for (**A**) vemurafenib single treatment of MDA-MB-435 cells and (**B**) vemurafenib single treatment of SK-MEL-5 cells, at the indicated drug concentrations. (**C**) Single or combined treatment with 0.1 μM vemurafenib, 3 μM atorvastatin, and 3 μM dipyridamole of MDA-MB-435 cells, and (**D**) single or combined treatment with 0.3 μM vemurafenib, 3 μM atorvastatin, and 3 μM dipyridamole of SK-MEL-5 cells at the 72 h time points are shown. Values in DMSO control were set at 100%. Each value represents the mean ± SD (n = 3). (**A**,**B**) Data were analyzed using one-way analysis of variance (ANOVA) with Dunnett's test for multiple group comparisons. * $p < 0.01$ with respect to each control group. (**C**,**D**) Control, atorvastatin, vemurafenib, atorvastatin+vemurafenib, atorvastatin+dipyridamole, and atorvastatin+vemurafenib+dipyridamole were indicated by grey, yellow, green, blue, orange, and red bars, respectively. Data were analyzed using one-way analysis of variance (ANOVA) with the Tukey–Kramer post hoc test for multiple group comparisons. * $p < 0.01$ (vs. control), † $p < 0.01$ (vs. atorvastatin), ‡ $p < 0.01$ (vs. vemurafenib), § $p < 0.01$ (vs. atorvastatin + vemurafenib), ¶ $p < 0.01$ (vs. atorvastatin + dipyridamole).

4. Discussion

Melanoma is curable when diagnosed early in its localized form. In contrast, metastatic melanoma has a very poor prognosis, and new strategies need to be explored by combining conventional chemo- and/or targeted therapies with new drugs to improve therapeutic outcomes [27]. However, Phase II and III clinical trials are expensive, and are a major hurdle to the development of new drugs. In contrast, the development of anticancer drugs through drug repositioning is much cheaper and may have a lower risk of failure [28]. Statins are such potential anticancer agents that target the mevalonate pathway [8].

To date, attempts have been made to augment the tumor-inhibitory effect of statins, which can be classified into three groups from the perspective of statin combination therapy. The first group of compounds includes those that exert their effects by interfering with the statin-induced activation of SREBP2-driven mevalonate pathway enzymes (including HMGCR). This group includes drugs that block the SREBP2-mediated feedback response by blocking SREBP2 processing (e.g., dipyridamole) [29,30] and HMGCR protein degraders (e.g., SR-12813) [20]. The second group includes drugs that likely exert their effects through alternative mechanism(s). Our own expression profile-based study identified BRAF inhibitors (e.g., dabrafenib), MEK inhibitors (e.g., selumetinib), Bcl-2/Bcl-x/Mcl-1 inhibitors (TW37), NF-κB inhibitors (piperlongumine), and HSP-90 inhibitors (elesclomol) as candidates for potentiating statins' inhibitory effects [31]. Other studies have shown additive or synergistic effects of combination therapy with statins, including with BRAF inhibitors [32,33], MEK inhibitors [34], and other inhibitors of the Ras-Raf-MEK-ERK pathway [35]. The third group includes those in which either group 1 and/or 2 may be relevant (e.g., nelfinavir, honokiol, and clotrimazole) [36]. Van Leeuwen et al. [36] expanded the number of agents similar to dipyridamole that augment the anticancer effect of fluvastatin, using computational pharmacogenomics, and suggested a strong need for further investigation of fluvastatin–nelfinavir, fluvastatin–honokiol, fluvastatin–clotrimazole, and fluvastatin–vemurafenib combinations.

In this study, we demonstrated the potential efficacy of the combination of atorvastatin and dipyridamole for the treatment of melanoma. The IC_{50} values of atorvastatin in both human and canine melanoma cell lines showed a 68–92% reduction when combined with dipyridamole compared with those of atorvastatin alone (Table 1 and Figure S4). Notably, in some melanoma cells, proliferation was suppressed to almost zero with the combination treatment (≥3 μM atorvastatin; Figure 1). The concentration of dipyridamole used in this study is close to the plasma levels in patients taking this drug [37,38]. By contrast, given that pharmacologically relevant concentrations of atorvastatin for treatment range from 0.1 to 0.3 μM [39], the 3-μM dose used herein is high; however, unlike in the treatment of dyslipidemia, it may be an acceptable concentration if it inhibits or kills cancer cells aggressively, in a single high dose, rather than being taken continuously. Collisson et al. [17] reported that in vitro, atorvastatin altered the morphology and Rho localization and attenuated RhoC signaling in human melanoma cells; however, in vivo, atorvastatin inhibited the invasion and metastasis of melanoma cells but did not affect their growth. As described above, they demonstrated that atorvastatin specifically inhibited metastasis in vivo rather than cell proliferation and stated that the potential clinical benefit of statin therapy did not correlate with the ability to kill cancer cells themselves. Collisson et al. [17] concluded that statins, at the levels routinely prescribed for hypercholesterolemia, may have specific antimetastatic effects. Based on their report and considering our results, at low concentrations of atorvastatin, which did not inhibit cell proliferation, it is possible that an anti-metastatic effect rather than an anti-cell death effect was in action. In fact, in MDA-MB-435, 5 μM atorvastatin single treatment barely inhibited cell proliferation (Figure S4); however, it affected the formation of filopodia and lamellipodia (Figure S5B, upper middle panel). In contrast, they were affected considerably by 5 μM atorvastatin and dipyridamole combination, inhibiting cell proliferation by approximately 80% (Figure S5B upper right panel). In SK-MEL-5, 5 μM atorvastatin single treatment slightly affected filopodia and lamellipodia formation (Figure S5B lower middle panel). As the atorvastatin concentration of 5 μM was almost the same as the IC_{50} of the combination treatment, cytoplasmic atrophy was evident and almost no filopodia or lamellipodia were observed (Figure S5B lower right panel). These results are not unexpected considering that the depletion of FPP and GGPP, the mevalonate pathway intermediates, by statins leads to interference with the post-translational modification and activation of Ras, Rho, or Rac [7,8]. Rho, Cdc42, and Rac regulate stress fibers, filopodia, and lamellipodia, respectively [40]. In our recent study, in which the inhibitory effects of various statins (atorvastatin, pitavastatin, fluvastatin, simvastatin, and rosuvastatin) on the cell proliferation of canine melanoma were investigated, we found that pitavastatin had the strongest inhibitory effect on cell proliferation [15]. If pitavastatin is combined with dipyridamole, lower statin concentrations may inhibit cancer cell proliferation. Additionally, the inhibition of cell proliferation by the combination of dipyridamole and atorvastatin was rescued by supplementation with GGPP, a metabolic intermediate of the mevalonate pathway, which showed that dipyridamole had an on-target effect on the mevalonate pathway (Figure 3). Notably, both statins and dipyridamole target the mevalonate pathway. However, statins induce HMGCR upregulation, whereas dipyridamole augments the antitumor effects of statins without inducing HMGCR upregulation (Figure 2).

The BRAF inhibitor vemurafenib is the standard treatment for unresectable or metastatic melanomas harboring activating BRAF V600E mutations [1]. However, its long-term efficacy is often reduced due to the invariable development of resistance. For melanoma treatment with BRAF inhibitors, metabolic changes, such as increased dependency on lipogenesis, have been suggested as adaptive mechanisms [41]. In addition, it has been reported that statin treatment increases the vulnerability of PGC1α-suppressed BRAF-inhibitor resistant melanomas [42], and it may be effective against melanomas that gradually develop resistance to vemurafenib. Indeed, we have found that vemurafenib further potentiated the effect of the combined statin–dipyridamole treatment on human melanoma cell lines (Figure 4). Wang et al. [43] reported that HMGCR expression was higher in vemurafenib-resistant melanoma cells and that the HMGCR level correlated well with vemurafenib resistance. They demonstrated that combined treatment with vemurafenib and physapubenolide enhanced sensitivity to vemurafenib by decreasing HMGCR expression. Therefore, this result (Figure 4) is medically relevant, and targeting SREBP2-driven mevalonate pathway upregulation may offer a new avenue for treating melanomas resistant to vemurafenib or to potentiate the effect of vemurafenib.

Furthermore, concomitant treatment with FDA-approved dacarbazine and simvastatin or fluvastatin suppressed both tumor growth and metastasis in murine models by attenuating the RhoA/RhoC pathway [44]. In colon cancer cells, dipyridamole augmented the cytotoxicity of the MEK1/2 inhibitor, trametinib, and was used to treat unresectable or metastatic malignant melanomas with BRAF mutations [1] through the dual targeting of the HMGCS1 and MEK pathways [45]. Based on this evidence, statins and dipyridamole are likely to be compatible therapeutic agents for advanced melanoma treatment.

Melanomas occur not only in humans, but also in many animals, including dogs, cats, horses, and pigs; however, they are more common in dogs than in other species [46]. Domestic dogs (*Canis lupus familiaris*) spontaneously develop melanoma and are exposed to environmental factors similar to those experienced by humans; they have a physiology similar to that of humans, indicating that dogs are excellent animal models for the development of novel therapies for melanoma [47]. Thus, comparative oncology, which compares humans with companion animals living in similar or shared environments, can provide useful insights into developmental mechanisms and treatments of human melanoma. Several studies, including ours, have shown that statins exert anticancer effects on canine tumors [16,48–50]. Furthermore, atorvastatin is well tolerated and has no apparent adverse effects or biochemical abnormalities in either healthy dogs or dogs with congestive heart failure [51]. Therefore, statins are considered suitable for cancer treatment in dogs. In addition, dipyridamole is more cytotoxic toward cancer cells than normal cells [52]. Given the lack of effective therapies for melanoma in dogs [47], statin–dipyridamole combination therapy may be a good treatment option, and the outcome from therapy in canines can be used as a reference for human melanoma treatment (Figure 5).

One limitation of this study is that the cytotoxicity of atorvastatin on hepatocytes, cardiomyocytes, or skeletal muscle cells was not evaluated. To apply statin therapy in the clinical setting, cytotoxic evaluation in normal cells is essential. Lipophilic statins, such as atorvastatin, lovastatin, cerivastatin, fluvastatin, and atorvastatin, decreased cell viability at increasing concentrations in human cardiomyocytes, murine skeletal muscle cells, cultured human hepatocytes, and primary rat hepatocytes, while hydrophilic statins (rosuvastatin and pravastatin) did not affect the viability [53–55]. In a rat skeletal muscle cell line, 100 μM atorvastatin showed cytotoxicity, while pravastatin (up to 1 mM) did not [56]. According to these reports, the concentrations of atorvastatin used this study (3 or 10 μM) do not seem to affect normal cells; however, it may be necessary to examine the efficacy of less cytotoxic hydrophilic statin and dipyridamole combination treatments in cancer cells.

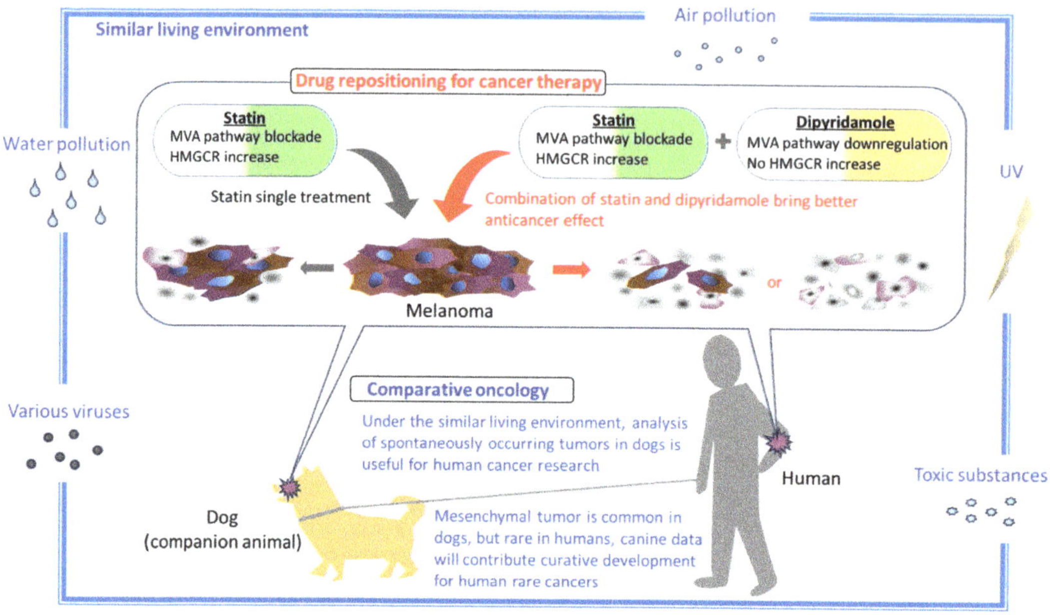

Figure 5. Comparative oncology: overview. The potential of the combination of statins and dipyridamole for cancer treatment through drug repositioning and the potential of comparative oncology in the analysis of spontaneously occurring cancers in domestic dogs that share the same living environment as humans are depicted. MVA pathway; mevalonate pathway.

5. Conclusions

Dipyridamole is a suitable potentiator of statins, and the following may be conceivable in statin–dipyridamole therapy for advanced melanoma: (1) the attenuation of metastasis formation with a well-tolerated statin-dipyridamole combination that can be safely administered on a long-term basis (with potential use as a postoperative adjuvant treatment), (2) the dual inhibition of distinct pathways compared to conventional therapeutic agents for melanoma, and (3) the use of statin–dipyridamole combination therapy in cases where conventional therapeutic agents cannot be applied.

Supplementary Materials: The following supporting information can be downloaded at: https://www.mdpi.com/article/10.3390/biomedicines12030698/s1, Figure S1: Changes in the morphology of dipyridamole-, atorvastatin-, and dipyridamole-and-atorvastatin-treated cells; Figure S2: Effect of dipyridamole treatment on growth of human and canine melanoma cells; Figure S3: Determination of half maximal inhibitory concentration (IC_{50}) value of dipyridamole on human and canine melanoma cells; Figure S4: Determination of IC_{50} value of atorvastatin in atorvastatin single treatment or combined treatment with dipyridamole in human and canine melanoma cells; Figure S5: Images of actin filaments, filopodia, and lamellipodia in human melanoma cells; Figure S6: Effect of atorvastatin and/or dipyridamole on *HMGCR* mRNA expression in human and canine melanoma cells.

Author Contributions: Conceptualization, T.W. and K.W.; Data curation, T.W., Z.N.O. and K.W.; Formal analysis, K.M., T.W. and K.W.; Funding acquisition, T.W. and K.W.; Investigation, N.I., T.W., M.N., K.S. and K.W.; Project administration, K.W.; Resources, T.W., T.O. and K.W.; Supervision, T.W., Z.N.O. and K.W.; Validation, N.I., K.M., T.W., J.T., T.I., Z.N.O. and K.W.; Visualization, N.I., K.M., T.W. and K.W.; Writing—original draft, N.I., K.M., T.W., Z.N.O. and K.W.; Writing—review and editing, N.I., K.M., T.W., J.T., T.O., T.I., Z.N.O. and K.W. All authors have read and agreed to the published version of the manuscript.

Funding: This research was supported by the Japan Society for the Promotion of Science KAKENHI (grant number JP20K07666) through a Grant-in-Aid for Scientific Research (C), and KAKENHI (grant number JP19H03514) through a Grant-in-Aid for Scientific Research (B).

Institutional Review Board Statement: Not applicable.

Informed Consent Statement: Not applicable.

Data Availability Statement: All relevant data supporting the key findings of this study are available within the article and its Supplementary Information files or from the corresponding author on reasonable request.

Acknowledgments: The authors thank Shiori Kamatani for her technical support.

Conflicts of Interest: The authors declare no potential competing interests.

References

1. Domingues, B.; Lopes, J.M.; Soares, P.; Populo, H. Melanoma treatment in review. *ImmunoTargets Ther.* **2018**, *7*, 35–49. [CrossRef]
2. Ward-Peterson, M.; Acuña, J.M.; Alkhalifah, M.K.; Nasiri, A.M.; Al-Akeel, E.S.; Alkhaldi, T.M.; Dawari, S.A.; Aldaham, S.A. Association between race/ethnicity and survival of melanoma patients in the united states over 3 decades: A secondary analysis of SEER data. *Medicine* **2016**, *95*, e3315. [CrossRef]
3. Yamazaki, N.; Kiyohara, Y.; Uhara, H.; Tsuchida, T.; Yoshida, A.; Yamada, T.; Komoto, A. Postmarketing surveillance of nivolumab plus ipilimumab combination therapy in Japanese patients with unresectable malignant melanoma. *J. Dermatol.* **2023**, *50*, 1108–1120. [CrossRef]
4. Dimitriou, F.; Frauchiger, A.L.; Urosevic-Maiwald, M.; Naegeli, M.C.; Goldinger, S.M.; Barysch, M.; Franzen, D.; Kamarachev, J.; Braun, R.; Dummer, R.; et al. Sarcoid-like reactions in patients receiving modern melanoma treatment. *Melanoma Res.* **2018**, *28*, 230–236. [CrossRef]
5. Endo, A. A historical perspective on the discovery of statins. *Proc. Jpn. Acad. Ser. B* **2010**, *86*, 484–493. [CrossRef]
6. Surma, S.; Mikhailidis, D.P.; Banach, M. Celebrating the 90th birthday of the scientist who discovered statins: Akira Endō. *Eur. Hear. J.* **2024**, *45*, 647–650. [CrossRef]
7. Jiang, W.; Hu, J.-W.; He, X.-R.; Jin, W.-L.; He, X.-Y. Statins: A repurposed drug to fight cancer. *J. Exp. Clin. Cancer Res.* **2021**, *40*, 241. [CrossRef]
8. Longo, J.; van Leeuwen, J.E.; Elbaz, M.; Branchard, E.; Penn, L.Z. Statins as anticancer agents in the era of precision medicine. *Clin. Cancer Res.* **2020**, *26*, 5791–5800. [CrossRef]
9. Amin, F.; Fathi, F.; Reiner, Ž.; Banach, M.; Sahebkar, A. The role of statins in lung cancer. *Arch. Med. Sci.* **2022**, *18*, 141–152. [CrossRef]
10. Lashgari, N.-A.; Roudsari, N.M.; Zadeh, S.S.T.; Momtaz, S.; Abbasifard, M.; Reiner, Ž.; Abdolghaffari, A.H.; Sahebkar, A. Statins block mammalian target of rapamycin pathway: A possible novel therapeutic strategy for inflammatory, malignant and neurodegenerative diseases. *Inflammopharmacology* **2023**, *31*, 57–75. [CrossRef]
11. Pun, N.T.; Jeong, C.-H. Statin as a potential chemotherapeutic agent: Current updates as a monotherapy, combination therapy, and treatment for anti-cancer drug resistance. *Pharmaceuticals* **2021**, *14*, 470. [CrossRef]
12. Zaky, M.Y.; Fan, C.; Zhang, H.; Sun, X.-F. Unraveling the anticancer potential of statins: Mechanisms and clinical significance. *Cancers* **2023**, *15*, 4787. [CrossRef]
13. Pandyra, A.; Penn, L.Z. Targeting tumor cell metabolism via the mevalonate pathway: Two hits are better than one. *Mol. Cell. Oncol.* **2014**, *1*, e969133. [CrossRef]
14. Warita, K.; Warita, T.; Beckwitt, C.H.; Schurdak, M.E.; Vazquez, A.; Wells, A.; Oltvai, Z.N. Statin-induced mevalonate pathway inhibition attenuates the growth of mesenchymal-like cancer cells that lack functional E-cadherin mediated cell cohesion. *Sci. Rep.* **2014**, *4*, 7593. [CrossRef]
15. Ishikawa, T.; Irie, N.; Tashiro, J.; Osaki, T.; Warita, T.; Warita, K.; Naito, M. Comparison of the anticancer effects of various statins on canine oral melanoma cells. *Veter-Comp. Oncol.* **2023**, *22*, 156–161. [CrossRef]
16. Ishikawa, T.; Osaki, T.; Sugiura, A.; Tashiro, J.; Warita, T.; Hosaka, Y.Z.; Warita, K. Atorvastatin preferentially inhibits the growth of high ZEB-expressing canine cancer cells. *Veter-Comp. Oncol.* **2022**, *20*, 313–323. [CrossRef]
17. Collisson, E.A.; Kleer, C.; Wu, M.; De, A.; Gambhir, S.S.; Merajver, S.D.; Kolodney, M.S. Atorvastatin prevents RhoC isoprenylation, invasion, and metastasis in human melanoma cells. *Mol. Cancer Ther.* **2003**, *2*, 941–948.
18. Tsubaki, M.; Takeda, T.; Kino, T.; Obata, N.; Itoh, T.; Imano, M.; Mashimo, K.; Fujiwara, D.; Sakaguchi, K.; Satou, T.; et al. Statins improve survival by inhibiting spontaneous metastasis and tumor growth in a mouse melanoma model. *Am. J. Cancer Res.* **2015**, *5*, 3186–3197. [PubMed]
19. Osaki, T.; Yokoe, I.; Sunden, Y.; Ota, U.; Ichikawa, T.; Imazato, H.; Ishii, T.; Takahashi, K.; Ishizuka, M.; Tanaka, T.; et al. Efficacy of 5-Aminolevulinic acid in photodynamic detection and photodynamic therapy in veterinary medicine. *Cancers* **2019**, *11*, 495. [CrossRef]

20. Zhou, Y.; Tashiro, J.; Kamatani, S.; Irie, N.; Suzuki, A.; Ishikawa, T.; Warita, K.; Oltvai, Z.N.; Warita, T. HMG-CoA reductase degrader, SR-12813, counteracts statin-induced upregulation of HMG-CoA reductase and augments the anticancer effect of atorvastatin. *Biochem. Biophys. Res. Commun.* **2023**, *677*, 13–19. [CrossRef]
21. Nguyen, S.T.; Nguyen, H.T.-L.; Truong, K.D. Comparative cytotoxic effects of methanol, ethanol and DMSO on human cancer cell lines. *Biomed. Res. Ther.* **2020**, *7*, 3855–3859. [CrossRef]
22. Tojkander, S.; Gateva, G.; Lappalainen, P. Actin stress fibers–assembly, dynamics and biological roles. *J. Cell Sci.* **2012**, *125*, 1855–1864. [CrossRef] [PubMed]
23. Rottner, K.; Stradal, T.E. Actin dynamics and turnover in cell motility. *Curr. Opin. Cell Biol.* **2011**, *23*, 569–578. [CrossRef]
24. Pandya, P.; Orgaz, J.L.; Sanz-Moreno, V. Modes of invasion during tumour dissemination. *Mol. Oncol.* **2017**, *11*, 5–27. [CrossRef] [PubMed]
25. Korch, C.; Hall, E.M.; Dirks, W.G.; Ewing, M.; Faries, M.; Varella-Garcia, M.; Robinson, S.; Storts, D.; Turner, J.A.; Wang, Y.; et al. Authentication of M14 melanoma cell line proves misidentification of MDA-MB-435 breast cancer cell line. *Int. J. Cancer* **2018**, *142*, 561–572. [CrossRef] [PubMed]
26. Yu, H.; Ma, M.; Yan, J.; Xu, L.; Yu, J.; Dai, J.; Xu, T.; Tang, H.; Wu, X.; Li, S.; et al. Identification of coexistence of BRAF V600E mutation and EZH2 gain specifically in melanoma as a promising target for combination therapy. *J. Transl. Med.* **2017**, *15*, 243. [CrossRef]
27. Mishra, H.; Mishra, P.K.; Ekielski, A.; Jaggi, M.; Iqbal, Z.; Talegaonkar, S. Melanoma treatment: From conventional to nanotechnology. *J. Cancer Res. Clin. Oncol.* **2018**, *144*, 2283–2302. [CrossRef] [PubMed]
28. Gupta, S.C.; Sung, B.; Prasad, S.; Webb, L.J.; Aggarwal, B.B. Cancer drug discovery by repurposing: Teaching new tricks to old dogs. *Trends Pharmacol. Sci.* **2013**, *34*, 508–517. [CrossRef]
29. Longo, J.; Mullen, P.J.; Yu, R.; van Leeuwen, J.E.; Masoomian, M.; Woon, D.T.; Wang, Y.; Chen, E.X.; Hamilton, R.J.; Sweet, J.M.; et al. An actionable sterol-regulated feedback loop modulates statin sensitivity in prostate cancer. *Mol. Metab.* **2019**, *25*, 119–130. [CrossRef]
30. Pandyra, A.; Mullen, P.J.; Kalkat, M.; Yu, R.; Pong, J.T.; Li, Z.; Trudel, S.; Lang, K.S.; Minden, M.D.; Schimmer, A.D.; et al. Immediate utility of two approved agents to target both the metabolic mevalonate pathway and its restorative feedback loop. *Cancer Res* **2014**, *74*, 4772–4782. [CrossRef]
31. Raghu, V.K.; Beckwitt, C.H.; Warita, K.; Wells, A.; Benos, P.V.; Oltvai, Z.N. Biomarker identification for statin sensitivity of cancer cell lines. *Biochem. Biophys. Res. Commun.* **2018**, *495*, 659–665. [CrossRef]
32. Baptista, D.; Ferreira, P.G.; Rocha, M. A systematic evaluation of deep learning methods for the prediction of drug synergy in cancer. *PLoS Comput. Biol.* **2023**, *19*, e1010200. [CrossRef]
33. Held, M.A.; Langdon, C.G.; Platt, J.T.; Graham-Steed, T.; Liu, Z.; Chakraborty, A.; Bacchiocchi, A.; Koo, A.; Haskins, J.W.; Bosenberg, M.W.; et al. Genotype-selective combination therapies for melanoma identified by high-throughput drug screening. *Cancer Discov.* **2013**, *3*, 52–67. [CrossRef]
34. Levine, B.D.; Cagan, R.L. Drosophila lung cancer models identify trametinib plus statin as candidate therapeutic. *Cell Rep.* **2016**, *14*, 1477–1487. [CrossRef]
35. Beckwitt, C.H.; Shiraha, K.; Wells, A. Lipophilic statins limit cancer cell growth and survival, via involvement of Akt signaling. *PLoS ONE* **2018**, *13*, e0197422. [CrossRef]
36. van Leeuwen, J.E.; Ba-Alawi, W.; Branchard, E.; Cruickshank, J.; Schormann, W.; Longo, J.; Silvester, J.; Gross, P.L.; Andrews, D.W.; Cescon, D.W.; et al. Computational pharmacogenomic screen identifies drugs that potentiate the anti-breast cancer activity of statins. *Nat. Commun.* **2022**, *13*, 6323. [CrossRef]
37. Guo, S.; Stins, M.; Ning, M.; Lo, E.H. Amelioration of inflammation and cytotoxicity by dipyridamole in brain endothelial cells. *Cerebrovasc. Dis.* **2010**, *30*, 290–296. [CrossRef]
38. Liu, Y.; Cone, J.; Le, S.N.; Fong, M.; Tao, L.; Shoaf, S.E.; Bricmont, P.; Czerwiec, F.S.; Kambayashi, J.; Yoshitake, M.; et al. Cilostazol and dipyridamole synergistically inhibit human platelet aggregation. *J. Cardiovasc. Pharmacol.* **2004**, *44*, 266–273. [CrossRef]
39. Bennaceur, K.; Atwill, M.; Al Zhrany, N.; Hoffmann, J.; Keavney, B.; Breault, D.; Richardson, G.; von Zglinicki, T.; Saretzki, G.; Spyridopoulos, I. Atorvastatin induces T cell proliferation by a telomerase reverse transcriptase (TERT) mediated mechanism. *Atherosclerosis* **2014**, *236*, 312–320. [CrossRef]
40. Nobes, C.D.; Hall, A. Rho, Rac, and Cdc42 GTPases regulate the assembly of multimolecular focal complexes associated with actin stress fibers, lamellipodia, and filopodia. *Cell* **1995**, *81*, 53–62. [CrossRef]
41. Talebi, A.; Dehairs, J.; Rambow, F.; Rogiers, A.; Nittner, D.; Derua, R.; Vanderhoydonc, F.; Duarte, J.A.G.; Bosisio, F.; Eynde, K.V.D.; et al. Sustained SREBP-1-dependent lipogenesis as a key mediator of resistance to BRAF-targeted therapy. *Nat. Commun.* **2018**, *9*, 2500. [CrossRef]
42. Liang, J.; Yu, D.; Luo, C.; Bennett, C.; Jedrychowski, M.; Gygi, S.P.; Widlund, H.R.; Puigserver, P. Epigenetic suppression of PGC1α (PPARGC1A) causes collateral sensitivity to HMGCR-inhibitors within BRAF-treatment resistant melanomas. *Nat. Commun.* **2023**, *14*, 3251. [CrossRef]
43. Wang, H.-Y.; Yu, P.; Chen, X.-S.; Wei, H.; Cao, S.-J.; Zhang, M.; Zhang, Y.; Tao, Y.-G.; Cao, D.-S.; Qiu, F.; et al. Identification of HMGCR as the anticancer target of physapubenolide against melanoma cells by in silico target prediction. *Acta Pharmacol. Sin.* **2022**, *43*, 1594–1604. [CrossRef]

44. Tsubaki, M.; Takeda, T.; Obata, N.; Kawashima, K.; Tabata, M.; Imano, M.; Satou, T.; Nishida, S. Combination therapy with dacarbazine and statins improved the survival rate in mice with metastatic melanoma. *J. Cell. Physiol.* **2019**, *234*, 17975–17989. [CrossRef] [PubMed]
45. Zhou, S.; Xu, H.; Tang, Q.; Xia, H.; Bi, F. Dipyridamole enhances the cytotoxicities of trametinib against colon cancer cells through combined targeting of HMGCS1 and MEK pathway. *Mol. Cancer Ther.* **2020**, *19*, 135–146. [CrossRef] [PubMed]
46. van der Weyden, L.; Patton, E.E.; A Wood, G.; Foote, A.K.; Brenn, T.; Arends, M.J.; Adams, D.J. Cross-species models of human melanoma. *J. Pathol.* **2016**, *238*, 152–165. [CrossRef]
47. Stevenson, V.B.; Klahn, S.; LeRoith, T.; Huckle, W.R. Canine melanoma: A review of diagnostics and comparative mechanisms of disease and immunotolerance in the era of the immunotherapies. *Front. Veter-Sci.* **2023**, *9*, 1046636. [CrossRef]
48. Torres, C.G.; Olivares, A.; Stoore, C. Simvastatin exhibits antiproliferative effects on spheres derived from canine mammary carcinoma cells. *Oncol. Rep.* **2015**, *33*, 2235–2244. [CrossRef] [PubMed]
49. Kobayashi, K.; Baba, K.; Kambayashi, S.; Okuda, M. Effect of simvastatin on cell proliferation and Ras activation in canine tumour cells. *Veter-Comp. Oncol.* **2021**, *19*, 99–108. [CrossRef] [PubMed]
50. Vigneau, A.; Rico, C.; Boerboom, D.; Paquet, M. Statins downregulateYAPandTAZand exert anti-cancer effects in canine mammary tumour cells. *Veter-Comp. Oncol.* **2022**, *20*, 437–448. [CrossRef] [PubMed]
51. Cunningham, S.; Rush, J.; Freeman, L. Short-term effects of atorvastatin in normal dogs and dogs with congestive heart failure due to myxomatous mitral valve disease. *J. Veter-Intern. Med.* **2013**, *27*, 985–989. [CrossRef]
52. Afrin, S.; Rahman, Y.; Sarwar, T.; Ansari, M.O.; Ahmed, S.; Alam Rizvi, M.; Shadab, G.H.A.; Tabish, M. Cytotoxic and genotoxic evaluation of dipyridamole and its alternative therapeutic potential in cancer therapy: An in vitro and in vivo approach. *J. Mol. Struct.* **2021**, *1249*, 131626. [CrossRef]
53. Kubota, T.; Fujisaki, K.; Itoh, Y.; Yano, T.; Sendo, T.; Oishi, R. Apoptotic injury in cultured human hepatocytes induced by HMG-CoA reductase inhibitors. *Biochem. Pharmacol.* **2004**, *67*, 2175–2186. [CrossRef]
54. Shu, N.; Hu, M.; Ling, Z.; Liu, P.; Wang, F.; Xu, P.; Zhong, Z.; Sun, B.; Zhang, M.; Li, F.; et al. The enhanced atorvastatin hepatotoxicity in diabetic rats was partly attributed to the upregulated hepatic Cyp3a and SLCO1B1. *Sci. Rep.* **2016**, *6*, 33072. [CrossRef]
55. Zhang, Q.; Qu, H.; Chen, Y.; Luo, X.; Chen, C.; Xiao, B.; Ding, X.; Zhao, P.; Lu, Y.; Chen, A.F.; et al. Atorvastatin induces mitochondria-dependent ferroptosis via the modulation of Nrf2-xCT/GPx4 axis. *Front. Cell Dev. Biol.* **2022**, *10*, 806081. [CrossRef]
56. Kaufmann, P.; Török, M.; Zahno, A.; Waldhauser, K.M.; Brecht, K.; Krähenbühl, S. Toxicity of statins on rat skeletal muscle mitochondria. *Cell. Mol. Life Sci.* **2006**, *63*, 2415–2425. [CrossRef] [PubMed]

biomedicines

Article

Cardioprotective Activity of Pharmacological Agents Affecting NO Production and Bioavailability in the Early Postnatal Period after Intrauterine Hypoxia in Rats

Olena Popazova [1,*], Igor Belenichev [2], Nina Bukhtiyarova [3], Victor Ryzhenko [4], Valentyn Oksenych [5,*] and Aleksandr Kamyshnyi [6]

1 Department of Histology, Cytology and Embryology, Zaporizhzhia State Medical and Pharmaceutical University, 69000 Zaporizhzhia, Ukraine
2 Department of Pharmacology and Medical Formulation with Course of Normal Physiology, Zaporizhzhia State Medical and Pharmaceutical University, 69000 Zaporizhzhia, Ukraine
3 Department of Clinical Laboratory Diagnostics, Zaporizhzhia State Medical and Pharmaceutical University, 69000 Zaporizhzhia, Ukraine
4 Department of Medical and Pharmaceutical Informatics and Advanced Technologies, Zaporizhzhia State Medical University, 69000 Zaporizhzhia, Ukraine
5 Broegelmann Research Laboratory, Department of Clinical Science, University of Bergen, 5020 Bergen, Norway
6 Department of Microbiology, Virology and Immunology, I. Horbachevsky Ternopil State Medical University, 46001 Ternopil, Ukraine
* Correspondence: popazova.ea@gmail.com (O.P.); valentyn.oksenych@uib.no (V.O.)

Abstract: Intrauterine hypoxia in newborns leads to a multifaceted array of alterations that exert a detrimental impact on the cardiovascular system. The aim of this research was to assess the cardioprotective effects of modulators of the nitric oxide (NO) system, including L-arginine, Thiotriazoline, Angiolin, and Mildronate, during the early postnatal period following intrauterine hypoxia. Methods: The study involved 50 female white rats. Pregnant female rats were given a daily intraperitoneal dose of 50 mg/kg of sodium nitrite starting on the 16th day of pregnancy. A control group of pregnant rats received saline instead. The resulting offspring were divided into the following groups: Group 1—intact rats; Group 2—rat pups subjected to prenatal hypoxia (PH) and daily treated with physiological saline; and Groups 3 to 6—rat pups exposed to prenatal hypoxia and treated daily from the 1st to the 30th day after birth. Nitrotyrosine levels, eNOS, iNOS, and NO metabolites were evaluated using ELISA; to measure the expression levels of iNOS mRNA and eNOS mRNA, a PCR test was utilized. Results: Angiolin enhances the expression of eNOS mRNA and boosts eNOS activity in the myocardium of rats with ischemic conditions. Arginine and particularly Thiotriazoline exhibited a consistent impact in restoring normal parameters of the cardiac nitroxidergic system following PH. Mildronate notably raised iNOS mRNA levels and notably reduced nitrotyrosine levels, providing further support for its antioxidative characteristics.

Keywords: prenatal hypoxia; cardioprotective; heat shock proteins; Angiolin; L-arginine; Thiotriazoline; Mildronate; eNOS; iNOS; nitrotyrosine

1. Introduction

Despite remarkable strides in both fundamental and clinical medicine, alongside advancements in the efficacy of perinatal care services, the prevalence of neonates who have encountered intrauterine hypoxia persists at unaltered rates. Moreover, in certain instances, there exists an alarming inclination towards its escalation. Intrauterine hypoxia experienced by newborns triggers a complex array of changes that exert an unfavorable impact on the central nervous system (CNS) and its regulatory influence on organs and systems, particularly the cardiovascular system [1]. At the core of cardiovascular disturbances following intrauterine hypoxia are disruptions in the mechanisms of neural and humoral regulation of heart and vascular function, as well as abnormalities in the conduction system (sinus tachy- and bradycardias, Hiss bundle branch blockade), transient neonatal pulmonary hypertension, prolonged persistence of fetal circulatory pathways, and impairment of cardiomyocyte metabolism [2]. Post-hypoxic cardiopathy serves as a risk factor for the development of cardiovascular pathologies (rhythm disorders, vascular dystonia, etc.) in subsequent age periods [3].

According to modern understanding, endothelial dysfunction and related disruptions in the NO system contribute to the development of numerous cardiovascular diseases. It is well-documented that fluctuations in NO levels in the body during pregnancy can result in classic symptoms of eclampsia, alterations in placental development, modifications in placental blood circulation, embryo- and fetopathies, intrauterine growth retardation, and fetal mortality [4]. NO may serve as a factor in both the pathogenesis and as a cyto- and organ-protective agent, particularly in terms of cardiovascular and endothelial protection [5,6]. Under prenatal hypoxic conditions, NO production increases, but concurrently, the synthesis of essential factors responsible for NO storage and transport decreases, resulting in NO deficiency in the heart and blood vessels. In prolonged prenatal hypoxia, reactive oxygen species (ROS) may impact the bioavailability of NO [7]. The increase in ROS during prenatal hypoxia and the disruption of the ROS/NO balance in the fetus result in heightened peripheral vasoconstriction, potentially leading to hypoxia in vital organs such as the heart and brain [8]. Prenatal hypoxia (PH) increases the expression of NADPH 1 homologue, which stimulates the production of superoxide. Superoxide can subsequently react with NO to form the stable peroxynitrite anion, thereby reducing the bioavailability of NO [9].

Hence, contemporary therapy for chronic fetoplacental insufficiency has incorporated L-arginine-based preparations (as a source for NO synthesis) and medications aimed at enhancing the bioavailability of NO [10,11]. Several studies have demonstrated the cardioprotective and endothelioprotective qualities of medications capable of enhancing both NO synthesis and its bioavailability. L-arginine, Thiotriazoline, Angiolin, and Mildronate are noteworthy in this context. L-arginine serves as a substrate for NO production in vascular endothelial cells, exhibiting antioxidant, cytoprotective, anti-hypoxic, and membrane-stabilizing attributes, and has been utilized in the management of gestosis and fetoplacental insufficiency [12].

Thiotriazoline (morpholinium 3-methyl-1,2,4-triazolyl-5-thioacetate) is a specific scavenger of NO and its cytotoxic forms. It increases NO bioavailability, protecting it from ROS. Thiotriazoline is also known for its anti-ischemic properties; it enhances the compensatory activation of the malate-aspartate shuttle mechanism, reduces the inhibition of oxidation processes in the Krebs cycle, and preserves intracellular ATP reserves. Thiotriazoline is employed in obstetric practice as part of a comprehensive approach in cases of threatened miscarriage [13].

Angiolin, also known as L-lysine 3-methyl-1,2,4-triazolyl-5-thioacetate, enhances the expression of VEGF and the density of proliferating endothelial cells within muscle-type vessels and microcirculatory channels. It boosts NO availability, elevates eNOS expression, and reduces the levels of peroxidation products during myocardial ischemia. Angiolin exhibits cardioprotective attributes in cases of myocardial ischemia, preserving mitochondrial ultrastructure and elevating ATP levels in the myocardium through the activation of the compensatory malate-aspartate shuttle mechanism [14].

Mildronate inhibits the conversion of gamma-butyrobetaine, a precursor of carnitine, which leads to the accumulation of gamma-butyrobetaine. This accumulation stimulates NO synthesis and has a positive impact on the endothelium of cardiac vessels [15]. Mildronate decreases the transport of long-chain fatty acids across mitochondrial membranes, which are mediated by carnitine, while it does not influence the metabolism of short-chain fatty acids. It also activates an alternative energy production system, involving glucose oxidation, and demonstrates anti-ischemic and cardioprotective characteristics [16].

Mildronate demonstrates anti-hypoxic properties in experimental cases of fetoplacental insufficiency [17].

Thus, the search for and development of approaches to pharmacotherapy targeting prenatal myocardial injury through modulation of the NO system is a pertinent task in contemporary pharmacology. The aforementioned rationale theoretically supports the potential of studying NO system modulators with diverse mechanisms of action—L-arginine, Thiotriazoline, Angiolin, and Mildronate as means of cardioprotection of posthypoxic cardiovascular system disorders in newborns.

The purpose of this study was to evaluate the cardioprotective activity of NO system modulators (L-arginine, Thiotriazoline, Angiolin, and Mildronate) in the early postnatal period after intrauterine hypoxia.

2. Materials and Methods

2.1. Description of Laboratory Animals and the PH Experimental Model

The research involved 50 female outbred white Wistar rats and 10 males, with weights ranging from 220 to 240 g and an age of approximately 4.5 months. These rats were procured from the vivarium of the Institute of Pharmacology and Toxicology at the National Medical Academy of Ukraine. They were housed in standard vivarium conditions, with temperatures maintained between 20 °C and 25 °C, humidity levels at 50–55%, and natural lighting; they were provided with a diet appropriate for this laboratory animal species and had access to water without restrictions. In this study, we utilized a model inducing chronic hematitic nitrite-induced prenatal hypoxia (PH) [14,18]. In order to establish a fixed pregnancy period, mature male rats were placed with virgin female rats with a ratio of 2 males per 4 females. The pregnancy timeline commenced upon the detection of spermatozoa in the vaginal smear (designated as day 1 of pregnancy). To induce hematitic hypoxia during the prenatal phase of development, pregnant female rats were subjected to daily intraperitoneal injections of sodium nitrite solution from day 16 to day 21 of pregnancy, at a dosage of 50 mg/kg, which induced a state of moderate hypoxia [18]. Pregnant rats in the control group were administered a physiological solution under the same conditions. The offspring was categorized into the following groups: group 1 consisted of intact, healthy rat pups born to females with physiologically normal pregnancies who were administered a physiological solution; group 2 encompassed pups from the control born after PH and daily administered a physiological solution; groups 3 to 6 consisted of pups after PH that received daily drugs treatments from postnatal day 1 to day 30. A portion of the rats was removed from the experiment on 30 days immediately after the end of administration of pharmacological agents, and a portion of the rats was removed 60 days after birth (30 days after administration of pharmacological agents)

The doses of L-arginine and Mildronate were taken from open literature sources. The doses of Thiotriazoline and Angiolin were calculated experimentally; these data are presented in the preclinical research report.

2.2. Justification for the Selected Drugs and Their Characteristics

We opted for medications with established experimental evidence demonstrating their capacity to regulate the nitric oxide (NO) system:

1. The intact group consisted of rats born from mothers with normal pregnancies, and they were administered a physiological solution.
2. The control group comprised rats born after experiencing intrauterine hypoxia, and they were given a physiological solution.
3. Thiotriazoline (Morpholinium-3-methyl-1,2,4- triazolyl-5-thioacetic acid) (2.5% solution for injections, "Arterium", Kyiv, Ukraine), metabolitotropic cardioprotector and antioxidant, 50 mg/kg, i/p [19].
4. Angiolin ([S]-2,6-diaminohexane acid 3-methyl-1,2,4-triazolyl-5-thioacecate) (substance, research, and production association "Farmatron", Zaporizhzhia, Ukraine), anti-ischemic, endothelium protective drug, 50 mg/kg, i/p [20].

5. L-arginine (42% solution for injection in vial, Tivortin, Yuria-pharm, Cherkasy, Ukraine), an NO precursor; it mitigates disruptions in the nitroxidergic system in ischemia, 200 mg/kg, i/p [21].
6. Mildronate (2-(2-carboxyethyl)-1,1,1-trimethylhydrazinium) (10% injection solution in ampoules, Grindex (Riga, Latvia), metabolitotropic agent, 100 mg/kg, i/p [22].

2.3. Anaesthesia

Under the administration of thiopental anesthesia (40 mg/kg), rats from all experimental groups were taken out of the study. Following this, blood samples were obtained from the celiac artery for subsequent analysis.

2.4. Preparation of Biological Material

The heart was rinsed with chilled 0.15 M KCl (4 °C) in a 1:10 ratio. After removing excess fat, connective tissue, and cutting out blood vessels and clots from internal cavities, the heart was washed again with 0.15 M KCl (4 °C) in a 1:10 ratio. Subsequently, it was pulverized in liquid nitrogen to achieve a powdery consistency. On a WT500 torsion balance (manufactured in Moscow, Russia), 100 mg of heart tissue, previously ground into a fine powder using liquid nitrogen, was accurately weighed. The powdered tissue was then thoroughly mixed with 10.0 mL of a medium maintained at 2 °C. This medium contained the following components in millimoles per liter (mmol/L): sucrose (250 mmol/L), Tris-HCl buffer (20 mmol/L), and EDTA (1 mmol/L), adjusted to a pH of 7.4. The homogenate was subsequently subjected to a pre-centrifugation step using a Sigma 3-30k refrigerated centrifuge (Osterode am Harz, Germany) at (+4 °C) for 7 min at 1000× *g* to remove large cell fragments. The resulting supernatant was carefully collected and then subjected to a second centrifugation step at (+4 °C) for 20 min at 17,000× *g* using the same Sigma 3-30k refrigerated centrifuge (Germany). The supernatant obtained from this step was collected and stored at −80 °C. The dense mitochondrial precipitate obtained after resuspension was utilized for further investigations. The determination of nitrotyrosine, iNOS, eNOS, and the concentration of NO metabolites (NOx) was carried out on the resuspended fraction.

The apex of the heart was placed in Bouin's fixative for 24 h. Following the standard process of tissue dehydration, and chloroform and paraffin impregnation, the myocardium was embedded in paraplast (McCormick, Hunt Valley, MD, USA). Serial histological sections, 5 μm thick, were prepared on a Microm-325 rotary microtome (Microm Corp., Munich, Germany). Subsequent to treatment with 0-xylene and ethanol, these sections were used for real-time PCR analysis.

2.5. Enzyme-Linked Immunosorbent Assay (ELISA)

Nitrotyrosine was assessed in the cytosol homogenate of the heart using the solid-phase immunoassay sandwich method of ELISA. The ELISA Kit (Catalog No. HK 501-02) from Hycult Biotech, Uden, Netherlands was used according to the instructions.

The activity of endothelial nitric oxide synthase (eNOS) in the cytosol was determined through enzyme immunoassay using the Cloud-Clone Corporation kit (Katy, TX, USA, #PAA868Ra01), according to the instructions.

The activity of inducible nitric oxide synthase (iNOS) in the cytosol was assessed through enzyme immunoassay using the MyBioSource kit (San Diego, CA, USA, #MBS023874), according to the instructions. These analyses were conducted on a complete plate enzyme immunoassay analyzer (SIRIO-S, Seac, Italy).

2.6. Biochemical Methods

The levels of NO metabolites (NOx) in the hearts were assessed using the Griess method. The supernatant obtained as above (1.0 mL) was deproteinized by adding 100 μL of 0.092 M zinc sulfate and 100 μL of 1 M NaOH, stirred, and left for 30–40 min. Then, it was centrifuged at 4000× *g* for 10 min (at 5 °C) using an Eppendorf™ 5430 G centrifuge (Hamburg, Germany). Subsequently, 100 μL of the resulting supernatant was transferred

of 38.8% compared to intact values. Nitrotyrosine concentration in the heart of 2-month-old rats after PH remained high and exceeded the values of healthy 2-month-old rats by 3.4 times.

Table 3. Effect of treatment on nitroxidergic system parameters in the cytosolic fraction of 2-month-old rat homogenates after prenatal hypoxia and treatment.

Experimental Groups	eNOS, pg/mL	iNOS, pg/mL	Nitrotyrosine, pg/mL	NO Metabolites (NOx), μmol/L
Intact (Rats born from rats with normal pregnancies) (n = 10)	31.2 ± 2.65	16.1 ± 1.42	14.1 ± 1.31	7.2 ± 0.67
PH (Rats with prenatal hypoxia) (control) (n = 10)	14.1 ± 1.54 [1]	33.7 ± 3.74 [1]	48.3 ± 3.88 [1]	4.4 ± 0.35 [1]
PH +L-arginine (n = 10)	26.2 ± 2.22 [1,*]	29.1 ± 2.32 [1]	40.2 ± 2.67 [1,*]	5.8 ± 0.44 *
PH + Thiotriazoline (n = 10)	21.2 ± 1.8 [1,*]	19.7 ± 2.23 *	28.1 ± 1.44 [1,*]	6.5 ± 0.57 *
PH + Angiolin (n = 10)	40.2 ± 3.65 [1,*]	16.7 ± 1.47 *	18.0 ± 2.05 *	6.9 ± 0.72 *
PH + Meldonium (n = 10)	18.4 ± 2.22 [1]	27.8 ± 4.77 [1]	40.3 ± 3.32 [1,*]	4.8 ± 0.53

Notes: [1]—$p \leq 0.05$ in relation to the intact group of animals; *—$p \leq 0.05$ in relation to the control group of animals.

Table 4. Expression of eNOS mRNA and iNOS mRNA in myocardial tissues of 2-month-old rats after prenatal hypoxia and treatment.

Experimental Groups	mRNA eNOS. u.e.	mRNA iNOS. u.e.
Intact (Rats born from rats with normal pregnancies) (n = 10)	1.000 ± 0.0078	1.000 ± 0.0076
PH (Rats with prenatal hypoxia) (control) (n = 10)	0.23 ± 0.0002 [1]	6.89 ± 0.0093 [1]
PH +L-arginine (n = 10)	0.718 ± 0.0002 [1,*]	3.90 ± 0.0022 [1,*]
PH + Thiotriazoline (n = 10)	2.770 ± 0.0113 [1,*]	3.011 ± 0.0021[1,*]
PH + Angiolin (n = 10)	5.410 ± 0.037 [1,*]	1.272 ± 0.0081[1,*]
PH + Meldonium (n = 10)	0.27 ± 0.0082 [1]	6.7103 ± 0.009 [1]

Notes: [1]—$p \leq 0.05$ in relation to the intact group of animals; *—$p \leq 0.05$ in relation to the control group of animals.

The course of administration of pharmacological preparations having properties of NO modulators during the 30-day period immediately after birth to post-PH rats influenced the indices of cardiac nitroxidergic system (Tables 1–4). Thus, immediately after discontinuation of the experimental therapy, the best indices were in the group receiving Angiolin. Angiolin administration leads to an increase in eNOS by 2.9 times and in eNOS mRNA by 32 times, and a decrease in iNOS by 50.4% and in iNOS mRNA by 3.8 times, in the heart of 1-month-old rats after PH compared to the group of 1-month-old rats after PH without treatment (control). The administration of Angiolin led to a notable 60% reduction in nitrotyrosine levels in the rat myocardium following prenatal hypoxia. Additionally, there was a substantial 81.2% increase in stable NO metabolites. This observation suggests that Angiolin effectively enhances both the production and bioavailability of NO. Administration of Thiotriazoline had a favorable effect on the state of the nitroxidergic system of the heart of 1-month-old PH rats. Thus, in this group immediately after the course administration of Thiotriazoline, there was an increase observed in eNOS by 50%, in eNOS mRNA by 15 times, and in stable metabolites of NO by 62.5%, and a decrease in iNOS by 22.5%, in iNOS mRNA by 73.8%, and in nitrotyrosine by 35%, in comparison with the control group. It can be concluded that Thiotriazoline, as well as its structural analog Angiolin, is able to increase NO production and its bioavailability. The effects of arginine on the indices of the nitroxidergic system of the heart of 1-month-old rats after PH were comparable to those of the group receiving Thiotriazoline. Immediately after course administration of meldonium to post-PH rats, no significant changes in nitrotyrosine concentration and eNOS mRNA expression were detected, and iNOS mRNA expression in the heart of this group was significantly higher than that in the control group.

The studies performed in the heart of 2-month-old animals after PH showed a persistent therapeutic effect after the use of NO modulators. Thus, as in the first observation. Angiolin application remained the most effective. In the heart of 2-month-old rats 1 month after 30-day Angiolin administration, eNOS increased by 2.85 times and eNOS mRNA by 23 times compared to control values, and iNOS decreased by 50% and iNOS mRNA by 81.5% compared to control values. Administration of Angiolin resulted in a 56.8% increase in stable NO metabolites.

The level of nitrotyrosine in the heart of this group did not differ significantly from that in the group of healthy 2-month-old rats. Arginine and, especially, Thiotriazoline also demonstrated a persistent effect on the normalization of the nitroxidergic system of the heart after PH. At 1 month after a course administration of Thiotriazoline, higher values compared with the control (eNOS by 50% and eNOS mRNA by 12 times) and lower values compared with the control (iNOS by 41.5% and iNOS mRNA by 56%) were observed. In this group, the concentration in the heart of stable NO metabolites was 47.7% higher, and the nitrotyrosine concentration in the heart was lower than that in the control group by 41.7%. One month after the course administration of meldonium, the indices of the nitroxidergic system did not differ from the control values. The only difference was a decrease in the level of nitrotyrosine in the heart of 2-month-old rats after PH.

Thus, we have established a positive effect of Angiolin, Thiotriazoline, and arginine on the indices of the nitroxidergic system of the heart of rats after PH, both at the end of the 30-day experimental treatment and one month after its cancellation (Figure 1).

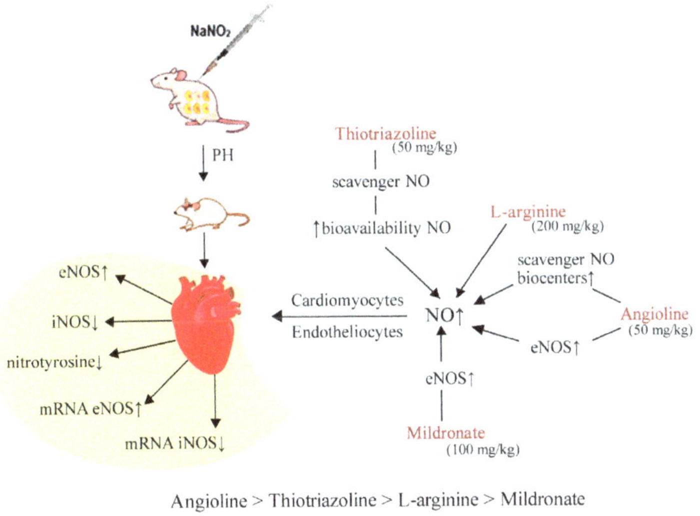

Figure 1. The cardiovascular system indicators in both the blood and heart of rats subjected to prenatal hypoxia and subsequent pharmacological modulation of the NO system.

4. Discussion

The revealed persistent disturbances of the nitroxidergic system of the heart after experimental PH consist of the suppression of eNOS expression by the increased expression of its inducible form, decreased NO bioavailability, and activation of nitrosative stress as evidenced by increased nitrotyrosine. (Figure 2). The disorders revealed by us are in line with modern views on the mechanisms of myocardial damage during ischemia and hypoxia, which have been established through experimental research and clinical observations [23,24]. PH is known to impair cardiac tolerance to ischemia/reperfusion, damage endothelium-dependent vasodilation/vasoconstriction mechanisms, and further contribute to cardiovascular pathologies such as hypertension, atherosclerotic vascular disease, and congestive heart failure [25]. There is evidence for decreased eNOS expression and activity in cadiomyocytes and endothelium and a risk of endothelial dysfunction after intrauterine hypoxia. Disruption of eNOS activity can be explained by altered interactions between eNOS and its regulatory partner proteins such as caveolin-1, calmodulin, and Hsp90. Alterations in phosphorylation and dephosphorylation of key serine and threonine residues in eNOS may also be involved in impaired eNOS activity [26,27]. Disturbances of endothelium-dependent vasodilation in coronary arteries of male and female offspring who underwent PH at the age of 4 and 9.5 months against the background of decreased eNOS and impaired function of SKCa and IKC channels were revealed [28]. Low eNOS values lead to impaired NO-dependent regulation of glutathione synthesis and reduced resistance to oxidative stress [29]. Decreased eNOS may be due to HIF-1a deficiency, as this factor activates eNOS expression by phosphorylation of a serine residue [30]. Increased iNOS expression was detected during the eNOS decrease after PH, which is aimed at compensating NO production [31]. High iNOS activity may be associated with cofactor deficiency and the release of superoxide and other reactive forms of NO [32].

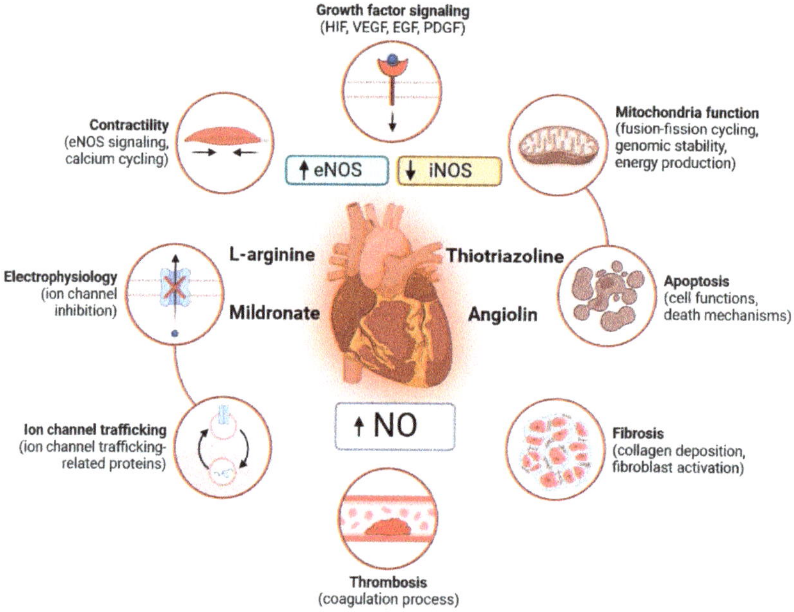

Figure 2. Indicators of the cardiovascular system in the blood and heart of rats subjected to prenatal hypoxia and subsequent pharmacological modulation.

However, under conditions of reduced thiol antioxidant deficiency, this leads to the formation of cytotoxic NO derivatives in "parasitic" reactions. Other researchers found that in preeclampsia, low activity of endothelial synthesis of NO and redox-dependent transformation of NO to peroxynitrite leads to a decrease in blood NO [5]. Such reactions can occur under conditions of L-arginine deficiency, antioxidant deficiency, mitochondrial dysfunction, and increased iNOS expression. Uncontrolled formation of cytotoxic derivatives of NO leads to nitrosylation of the most active parts of protein structures of ion channels, receptors, transmembrane pores, and signaling molecules, i.e., development of nitrosative stress.

A less important consequence of myocardial ischemia is the loss of such NO-mediated effects as suppression of cell proliferation and platelet aggregation, and, most importantly, inhibition of monocyte activation by the so-called adhesion molecules [33]. Nitrosative stress also leads to HSP70 deficiency in the cell, together with deprivation of the glutathione link of the thiol-disulfide system. Cytotoxic forms of NO lead not only to modification (reversible and irreversible) of macromolecules, including HSP70 itself, but also reduce the expression activity of genes encoding the synthesis of the latter [34,35]. The role of NO derivatives in suppressing gene activity and reducing the levels of various transcription factors has been demonstrated [36,37]. Apparently, excess forms of nitric oxide, such as peroxynitrite and nitrosonium ions, first nitrolyse the thiol–redox-dependent regions of these genes, then, at increasing concentrations, oxidize them [38,39]. All this justifies the use of pharmacological agents—modulators of the NO system—for myocardial protection after PH.

L-arginine is a common substrate for NO and polyamines (putrescine, spermine, and spermidine). NO and polyamines play an important role in reproduction, embryogenesis, reduction in neonatal mortality, and embryonic angiogenesis. NO regulates gene expression, protein synthesis, proliferation, growth, and differentiation of the fetus [40]. Therefore, the gaze of researchers and clinicians has been turned to the use of the NO substrate L-arginine to reduce the adverse effects of PH [12]. Our studies revealed a positive effect of arginine on NO system parameters in the heart of 1- and 2-month-old rats after PH.

However, the NO substrate was inferior to new molecules—Thiotriazoline and Angiolin. We speculate that in ischemia, NO formed from arginine under thiol antioxidant deficiency interacts with ROS and is converted to peroxynitrite [41]. In this regard, pharmacological agents combining the properties of positive modulators of NO and its transporters are promising.

Thiotriazoline is able to increase NO bioavailability in excess ROS. Thiotriazoline is an antioxidant and ROS scavenger, and NO increases the activity of glutathione-dependent enzymes and the level of reduced glutathione during myocardial ischemia. Thiotriazoline (10-5–10-7 M) in vitro reduced the levels of superoxide radicals and peroxynitrite due to the presence of a thiol group in its structure. Thiotriazoline prevents irreversible inactivation of the transcription factor NF-kB, protecting sensitive cysteine residues—Cys 252, Cys 154, and Cys 61 in its DNA-binding domains—from excess ROS. Thiotriazoline can participate in the restoration of these groups in the case of reversible inactivation, taking on the role of Redox Faktor-1. Thiotriazoline enhances the activation of expression of redox-sensitive genes that are essential for cellular defense against oxidative stress. Thiotriazoline reduces the intensity of nitrosative stress and increases eNOS activity [42,43].

Thiotriazoline increases the efficacy of arginine when co-administered. The pharmacological effect of the combination is due to a positive effect on the synthesis, transport, and bioavailability of NO and physiological functions of this molecular messenger [44]. In rats in which isadrin-pituitrin myocardial infarction was modeled, Thiotriazoline stimulated LDH in the direction of the formation of pyruvate from lactate, which eliminated lactic acidosis and normalized intracellular pH, and stimulated the Krebs cycle by increasing pyruvate [45]. In the same experimental mode, Thiotriazoline activated the malate-aspartate shunt in the myocardium in the acute period of myocardial infarction. Thiotriazoline administration (600 mg/day) to 8298 patients with II–III class stable angina pectoris reduced the number of weekly angina attacks by 46.32%, and in the control group by 33.24% (p = 0.028), respectively (p = 0.031), and increased exercise tolerance [46].

Experimental studies have established that Angiolin increases eNOS mRNA expression and eNOS activity in ischemic rat myocardium. Angiolin increases VEGF expression and the VEGF binding coefficient with vascular endothelium, as well as the density of endotheliocytes and proliferating endotheliocytes of the capillary network and vascular wall, and increases RNA concentration in endotheliocytes during hypoxia and circulatory ischemia [14]. Angiolin has a protective effect on NO and also increases its bioavailability; NO is an unstable, short-lived radical, and to prolong its "life", the formation of more stable S-nitrosol complexes with low molecular weight compounds (glutathione, cysteine) is envisaged, and with a deficiency of these compounds, NO bioavailability sharply decreases. With a deficiency of low-molecular thiols, NO under the action of ROS is transformed into peroxynitrite and can be the cause of initiation of nitrosative stress. Due to its chemical structure, Angiolin plays the role of a spin trap and can form a complex with NO [47]. Angiolin positively affects the state of myocardial nitroxidergic system in experimental ischemia—it increases NO synthesis by increasing eNOS expression, increases NO bioavailability, and reduces parasitic reactions by decreasing iNOS hyperactivity. The mechanism of the effect on eNOS expression can be explained in terms of Angiolin's effect on HSP70 and HIF-1a. Angiolin prolongs the "life time" of HIF-1a through HSP70-mechanisms. Angiolin also has a positive effect on the glutathione link thiol-disulfide system, which is conjugated with the NO system. It was revealed that in experimental myocardial ischemia, Angiolin increases the activity of glutathioreductase and glutathione peroxidase, and increases the concentration of reduced glutathione in the cytosol of rat myocardium [35]. HIF-1a is also known to increase eNOS and VEGF expression during hypoxia and ischemia [48]. Angiolin, due to its positive effect on the NO system, positively influenced cardio- and hemodynamics in experimental myocardial ischemia. Angiolin administration to rabbits with occlusion of the descending coronary artery led to restoration of left ventricular dysfunction, which was expressed in the increase in the left ventricular working index and left ventricular working stroke index, the increase in pressure in the left ventricle, and the decrease in total peripheral vascular resistance [14].

Mildronate (3-(2.2.2.2-trimethylhydrazine) propionate) reversibly blocks gamma-butyrobetaine hydroxylase, which catalyzes the conversion of gamma-butyrobetaine to carnitine, and thereby significantly inhibits the entry of carnitine, which provides transport of fatty acids across the membrane into muscle tissue cells. This effect of Mildronate is accompanied by a decrease in carnitine-dependent oxidation of free fatty acids (FFAs) and, consequently, leads to activation of glucose oxidation, which is more economical in conditions of ischemia. An important feature of the action of Mildronate, which distinguishes it from other drugs affecting myocardial metabolism, is the absence of accumulation of under-oxidized fatty acids inside mitochondria and an increase in NO production. This is due to the fact that Mildronate inhibits the hydroxylation of GBB and increases the intracellular pool of γ-butyrobetaine, whose esterification exhibits cholinomimetic properties. γ-butyrobetaine esters via acetylcholine receptors on endothelial cells can activate NOS [41]. Mildronate improves exercise tolerance and quality of life of patients, and positively affects the functional parameters of the heart-ejection fraction and systolic volume in myocardial ischemia [15]. Our studies confirmed the anti-hypoxic activity of Mildronate in PH. However, in this study, we did not find a significant positive effect of Mildronate on NO system parameters in the myocardium of animals undergoing PH. It was found that Mildronate significantly increased iNOS mRNA expression and significantly decreased nitrotyrosine concentration, which is more evidence of its antioxidative properties [49].

5. Conclusions

We observed that intrauterine hypoxia suppressed eNOS mRNA expression and eNOS activity, while increasing iNOS mRNA expression and iNOS activity in the myocardium of offspring at 1 and 2 months of age. Furthermore, this hypoxic condition resulted in reduced NO bioavailability and the activation of nitrosative stress in the neonatal myocardium. The results of our experimental study underscore the essential need for pharmacological interventions to correct myocardial NO system disorders in newborns. This represents a critical component of early and necessary cardioprotective measures following intrauterine hypoxia. While examining agents with reported NO-modulating properties, we discovered that not all of them had a positive impact on the myocardial NO system in newborns following experimental prenatal hypoxia (PH). Our study revealed that Thiotriazoline and Angiolin exhibited significant benefits by enhancing NO synthesis, improving bioavailability, and reducing nitrosative stress in the newborns' myocardium after PH. Our studies support further preclinical investigation of Angiolin as a potential cardioprotective agent following experimental prenatal hypoxia (PH). Additionally, the results indicate the potential for further preclinical and clinical research on Thiotriazoline, an authorized drug, as a treatment for cardiovascular pathologies resulting from intrauterine hypoxia.

Author Contributions: Conceptualization, O.P., I.B. and N.B.; methodology, I.B. and A.K.; software, O.P., I.B. and A.K; validation, O.P. and I.B.; formal analysis, A.K. and V.R.; investigation, O.P. and I.B.; data curation, O.P., I.B. and V.R.; N.B.; writing—original draft preparation, O.P., I.B., A.K. and N.B.; writing—review and editing, I.B., A.K. and V.O.; visualization, O.P. and V.R.; supervision, I.B., V.O. and A.K. All authors have read and agreed to the published version of the manuscript.

Funding: This research received no external funding.

Institutional Review Board Statement: Zaporizhzhia State Medical University Commission on Bioethics approved the experimental study (protocol No. 33 of 26 June 2021).

Informed Consent Statement: Not applicable.

Data Availability Statement: All the data generated during this research are included in the manuscript.

Conflicts of Interest: The authors declare no conflict of interest.

References

1. Rosa-Mangeret, F.; Benski, A.C.; Golaz, A.; Zala, P.Z.; Kyokan, M.; Wagner, N.; Muhe, L.M.; Pfister, R.E. 2.5 Million Annual Deaths-Are Neonates in Low- and Middle-Income Countries Too Small to Be Seen? A Bottom-Up Overview on Neonatal Morbi-Mortality. *Trop. Med. Infect. Dis.* **2022**, *7*, 64. [CrossRef] [PubMed]
2. Hutter, D.; Kingdom, J.; Jaeggi, E. Causes and mechanisms of intrauterine hypoxia and its impact on the fetal cardiovascular system: A review. *Int. J. Pediatr.* **2010**, *2010*, 401323. [CrossRef] [PubMed]
3. Immediate and long-term effects of posthypoxic myocardial ischemia in newborns. *Georgian Med. News* **2014**, *234*, 100–105. (In Russian)
4. Acauan Filho, B.J.; Pinheiro da Costa, B.E.; Ogando, P.B.; Vieira, M.C.; Antonello, I.C.; Poli-de-Figueiredo, C.E. Serum nitrate and NOx levels in preeclampsia are higher than in normal pregnancy. *Hypertens. Pregnancy* **2016**, *2*, 226–233. [CrossRef] [PubMed]
5. Khetsuriani, T.; Chabashvili, N.; Sanikidze, T. Role of endothelin-1 and nitric oxide level in pathogenesis preeclampsia. *Georgian Med. News* **2006**, *141*, 17–21. (In Russian)
6. Vural, P. Nitric oxide/endothelin-1 in preeclampsia. *Clin. Chim. Acta* **2002**, *317*, 65–70. [CrossRef]
7. Rood, K.; Lopez, V.; La Frano, M.R.; Fiehn, O.; Zhang, L.; Blood, A.B.; Wilson, S.M. Gestational Hypoxia and Programing of Lung Metabolism. *Front. Physiol.* **2019**, *10*, 1453. [CrossRef]
8. Kane, A.D.; Kothmann, E.; Giussani, D.A. Detection and response to acute systemic hypoxia. *BJA Educ.* **2020**, *20*, 58–64. [CrossRef]
9. Dikalova, A.E.; Góngora, M.C.; Harrison, D.G.; Lambeth, J.D.; Dikalov, S.; Griendling, K.K. Upregulation of Nox1 in vascular smooth muscle leads to impaired endothelium-dependent relaxation via eNOS uncoupling. *Am. J. Physiol. Heart Circ. Physiol.* **2010**, *299*, H673–H679. [CrossRef]
10. Duckitt, K.; Thornton, S.; O'Donovan, O.P.; Dowswell, T. Nitric oxide donors for treating preterm labour. *Cochrane Database Syst. Rev.* **2014**, *2014*, CD002860. [CrossRef]
11. Nazarov, S.B.; Ivanova, A.S.; Novikov, A.A. Effect of nitric oxide on physical development and erythropoiesis in the offspring of rats with impaired uteroplacental circulation. *Bull. Exp. Biol. Med.* **2013**, *154*, 737–739. [CrossRef]
12. Bednov, A.; Espinoza, J.; Betancourt, A.; Vedernikov, Y.; Belfort, M.; Yallampalli, C. L-Arginine Prevents Hypoxia-Induced Vasoconstriction in Dual-Perfused Human Placental Cotyledons. *Placenta* **2015**, *36*, 1254–1259. [CrossRef] [PubMed]
13. Shevchenko, A.O. Changes in the content of progesterone, insulin and cortisol in treatment course of pregnant women with the threat of preterm labor in chronic stress conditions *Zaporozh. Med. J.* **2018**, *20*, 334–338. [CrossRef]
14. Belenichev, I.F.; Mazur, I.A.; Abramov, A.V.; Kucherenko, L.I.; Bukhtiyarova, N.V.; Egorov, A.A.; Polyakova, E.N. The Endothelium-Protective Effect of 3-Methyl-1.2.4-Triazolyl-5-Thioacetate (S)-2.6-Diaminohexanic Acid (Lysinium): Effects on the Expression of Vascular Endothelial Growth Factor (VEGF) and the Characteristics of the Endotheliocytes of the Cerebral Vessels of Animals with Cerebral Ischemia. *Neurochem. J.* **2013**, *7*, 296–302.
15. Vilskersts, R.; Kigitovica, D.; Korzh, S.; Videja, M.; Vilks, K.; Cirule, H.; Skride, A.; Makrecka-Kuka, M.; Liepinsh, E.; Dambrova, M. Protective Effects of Meldonium in Experimental Models of Cardiovascular Complications with a Potential Application in COVID-19. *Int. J. Mol. Sci.* **2021**, *23*, 45. [CrossRef] [PubMed]
16. Kuka, J.; Vilskersts, R.; Cirule, H.; Makrecka, M.; Pugovics, O.; Kalvinsh, I.; Dambrova, M.; Liepinsh, E. The cardioprotective effect of mildronate is diminished after co-treatment with L-carnitine. *J. Cardiovasc. Pharmacol. Ther.* **2012**, *17*, 215–222. [CrossRef]
17. Krivtsova, E.I.; Pavlova, N.G.; Ponomarenko, Y.R.; Burmistrov, S.O.; Oparina, T.I.; Prokopenko, V.M.; Arutyunyan, A.V.; Konstantinova, N.N. Mechanism of mildronate effect on rabbit fetuses developing under conditions of placental insufficiency. *Bull. Exp. Biol. Med.* **1998**, *126*, 803–806. [CrossRef]

18. Sutovska, H.; Babarikova, K.; Zeman, M.; Molcan, L. Prenatal Hypoxia Affects Foetal Cardiovascular Regulatory Mechanisms in a Sex- and Circadian-Dependent Manner: A Review. *Int. J. Mol. Sci.* **2022**, *23*, 2885. [CrossRef]
19. Mukhina, I.V.; (Nizhnij Novgorod, Russia). Report on the Independent Preclinical Evaluation of the Specific Activity of the Dosage Forms of Thiotriazoline (2.5% Injection and Tablets). Unpublished internal report. 2009; 112p. (In Russian)
20. Kolesnik, Y.M.; (Zaporozhye, Ukraine). Report on Preclinical Study of Specific Biological Activity (Anti-Ischemic, Endothelio Protective) of the Drug Lisinium (Angiolin) at Parenteral Administration. Unpublished internal report. 2018; 125p. (In Ukranian)
21. Ghotbeddin, Z.; Basir, Z.; Jamshidian, J.; Delfi, F. Modulation of behavioral responses and CA1 neuronal death by nitric oxide in the neonatal rat's hypoxia model. *Brain Behav.* **2020**, *10*, e01841. [CrossRef]
22. Berlato, D.G.; de Bairros, A.V. Meldonium: Pharmacological, toxicological, and analytical aspects. *Toxicol. Res. Appl.* **2020**, *4*. [CrossRef]
23. Ferreiro, C.R.; Chagas, A.C.; Carvalho, M.H.; Dantas, A.P.; Jatene, M.B.; Bento De Souza, L.C.; Lemos Da Luz, P. Influence of Hypoxia on Nitric Oxide Synthase Activity and Gene Expression in Children with Congenital Heart Disease: A Novel Pathophysiological Adaptive Mechanism. *Circulation* **2001**, *103*, 2272–2276. [CrossRef]
24. Liu, J.; Gao, Y.; Negash, S.; Longo, L.D.; Raj, J.U. Long-term effects of prenatal hypoxia on endothelium-dependent relaxation responses in pulmonary arteries of adult sheep. *Am. J. Physiol. Lung Cell Mol. Physiol.* **2009**, *296*, L547–L554. [CrossRef] [PubMed]
25. Niu, Y.; Kane, A.D.; Lusby, C.M.; Allison, B.J.; Chua, Y.Y.; Kaandorp, J.J.; Nevin-Dolan, R.; Ashmore, T.J.; Blackmore, H.L.; Derks, J.B.; et al. Maternal Allopurinol Prevents Cardiac Dysfunction in Adult Male Offspring Programmed by Chronic Hypoxia During Pregnancy. *Hypertension* **2018**, *72*, 971–978. [CrossRef] [PubMed]
26. Patterson, A.J.; Zhang, L. Hypoxia and Fetal Heart Development. *Curr. Mol. Med.* **2010**, *10*, 653–666. [CrossRef] [PubMed]
27. Hauton, D.; Ousley, V. Prenatal Hypoxia Induces Increased Cardiac Contractility on a Background of Decreased Capillary Density. *BMC Cardiovasc. Disord.* **2009**, *9*, 1. [CrossRef]
28. Hula, N.; Liu, R.; Spaans, F.; Pasha, M.; Quon, A.; Kirschenman, R.; Cooke, C.-L.M.; Davidge, S.T. The Long-Term Effects of Prenatal Hypoxia on Coronary Artery Function of the Male and Female Offspring. *Biomedicines* **2022**, *10*, 3019. [CrossRef] [PubMed]
29. De Pascali, F.; Hemann, C.; Samons, K.; Chen, C.A.; Zweier, J.L. Hypoxia and reoxygenation induce endothelial nitric oxide synthase uncoupling in endothelial cells through tetrahydrobiopterin depletion and S-glutathionylation. *Biochemistry* **2014**, *53*, 3679–3688. [CrossRef]
30. Zhang, Z.; Yao, L.; Yang, J.; Wang, Z.; Du, G. PI3K/Akt and HIF 1 Signaling Pathway in Hypoxia Ischemia (Review). *Mol. Med. Rep.* **2018**, *18*, 3547–3554. [CrossRef]
31. Jung, F.; Palmer, L.A.; Zhou, N.; Johns, R.A. Hypoxic Regulation of Inducible Nitric Oxide Synthase via Hypoxia Inducible Factor-1 in Cardiac Myocytes. *Circ. Res.* **2000**, *86*, 319–325. [CrossRef]
32. Stamler, J.S. Redox Signaling: Nitrosylation and Related Target Interactions of Nitric Oxide. *Cell* **1994**, *78*, 931–936. [CrossRef]
33. Pérez-Torres, I.; Manzano-Pech, L.; Rubio-Ruíz, M.E.; Soto, M.E.; Guarner-Lans, V. Nitrosative Stress and Its Association with Cardiometabolic Disorders. *Molecules* **2020**, *25*, 2555. [CrossRef] [PubMed]
34. Dattilo, S.; Mancuso, C.; Koverech, G.; Di Mauro, P.; Ontario, M.L.; Petralia, C.C.; Calabrese, V. Heat Shock Proteins and Hormesis in the Diagnosis and Treatment of Neurodegenerative Diseases. *Immun. Ageing* **2015**, *12*, 20. [CrossRef] [PubMed]
35. Belenichev, I.F.; Aliyeva, O.G.; Popazova, O.O.; Bukhtiyarova, N.V. Involvement of Heat Shock Proteins HSP70 in the Mechanisms of Endogenous Neuroprotection: The Prospect of Using HSP70 Modulators. *Front. Cell Neurosci.* **2023**, *17*, 1131683. [CrossRef] [PubMed]
36. Bilous, I.I.; Pavlovych, L.L.; Kamyshnyi, A.M. Primary hypothyroidism and autoimmune thyroiditis alter the transcriptional activity of genes regulating neurogenesis in the blood of patients. *Endocr Regul* **2021**, *55*, 5–15. [CrossRef] [PubMed]
37. Topol, I.; Kamyshny, A. Study of expression of TLR2, TLR4 and transckription factor NF-kB structures of galt of rats in the conditions of the chronic social stress and modulation of structure of intestinal microflora. *Georgian Med. News* **2013**, *225*, 115–122.
38. Bogdan, C. Nitric Oxide and the Regulation of Gene Expression. *Trends Cell Biol.* **2001**, *11*, 66–75. [CrossRef]
39. Kröncke, K.D. Nitrosative Stress and Transcription. *Biol. Chem.* **2003**, *384*, 1365–1377. [CrossRef]
40. Hsu, C.N.; Tain, Y.L. Impact of Arginine Nutrition and Metabolism during Pregnancy on Offspring Outcomes. *Nutrients* **2019**, *11*, 1452. [CrossRef]
41. Suvorava, T.; Nagy, N.; Pick, S.; Lieven, O.; Rüther, U.; Dao, V.T.; Fischer, J.W.; Weber, M.; Kojda, G. Impact of eNOS-Dependent Oxidative Stress on Endothelial Function and Neointima Formation. *Antioxid. Redox Signal.* **2015**, *23*, 711–723. [CrossRef]
42. Zvyagintseva, T.V.; Myronchenko, S.I.; Kytsyuk, N.I.; Naumova, O.V. The Impact of Antioxidant-Enriched Ointments on Skin Morphology in Guinea Pigs Subjected to Local Ultraviolet Radiation: A Study in the Precarpathian Bulletin of the Shevchenko Scientific Society. *Pulse* **2019**, *6*, 64–72. [CrossRef]
43. Manischenkova, Y.; Shkala, L.; Dudich, T.; Litvinova, M.; Ivanova, M. Oxidative Stress in Patients with Diabetes Mellitus Type 2 Associated with Exacerbation of Chronic Pyelonephritis. *Int. J. Endocrinol.* **2022**, 19–22. [CrossRef]
44. Kucherenko, L.I.; Hromyleva, O.V.; Mazur, I.A.; Shishkina, S.V. Theoretical study about L-arginine complexes formation with thiotriazolin. *Zaporozhye Med. J.* **2017**, *19*, 108–112. [CrossRef]
45. Kastanayan, A.A.; Kartashova, E.A.; Zheleznyak, E.I. The effect of thiotriazoline on energy production in conditions ofchronic myocardial ischemia. *South Rus. J. Ther. Pract.* **2020**, *1*, 84–90. [CrossRef]

46. Kadin, D.V.; Chumak, B.A.; Filippov, A.E.; Shustov, S.B. Thiotriazoline in the Treatment of Stable Angina II-III Functional Class. *Kardiologiia* **2015**, *55*, 26–29. (In Russian) [CrossRef] [PubMed]
47. Kurutas, E.B. Theimportance of antioxidants which play the role in cellular response against oxidative/nitrosative stress: Current state. *Nutr. J.* **2015**, *15*, 71. [CrossRef]
48. Rodriguez-Miguelez, P.; Lima-Cabello, E.; Martínez-Flórez, S.; Almar, M.; Cuevas, M.J.; González-Gallego, J. Hypoxia-inducible Factor-1 Modulates the Expression of Vascular Endothelial Growth Factor and Endothelial Nitric Oxide Synthase Induced by Eccentric Exercise. *J. Appl. Physiol.* **2015**, *118*, 1075–1083. [CrossRef] [PubMed]
49. Gureev, A.P.; Sadovnikova, I.S.; Shaforostova, E.A.; Starkov, A.A.; Popov, V.N. Mildronate Protects Heart mtDNA from Oxidative Stress Toxicity Induced by Exhaustive Physical Exercise. *Arch. Biochem. Biophys.* **2021**, *705*, 108892. [CrossRef] [PubMed]

biomedicines

MDPI

Review

Novel Therapeutics for Type 2 Diabetes Mellitus—A Look at the Past Decade and a Glimpse into the Future

Ying Jie Chee [1,*] and Rinkoo Dalan [1,2]

1 Department of Endocrinology, Tan Tock Seng Hospital, Singapore 308433, Singapore; rinkoo_dalan@ttsh.com.sg
2 Lee Kong Chian School of Medicine, Nanyang Technological University, Singapore 308232, Singapore
* Correspondence: cheeyingjie_chee@ttsh.com.sg

Abstract: Cardiovascular disease (CVD) and kidney disease are the main causes of morbidity and mortality in type 2 diabetes mellitus (T2DM). Globally, the incidence of T2DM continues to rise. A substantial increase in the burden of CVD and renal disease, alongside the socioeconomic implications, would be anticipated. Adopting a purely glucose-centric approach focusing only on glycemic targets is no longer adequate to mitigate the cardiovascular risks in T2DM. In the past decade, significant advancement has been achieved in expanding the pharmaceutical options for T2DM, with novel agents such as the sodium-glucose cotransporter type 2 (SGLT2) inhibitors and glucagon-like peptide receptor agonists (GLP-1 RAs) demonstrating robust evidence in cardiorenal protection. Combinatorial approaches comprising multiple pharmacotherapies combined in a single agent are an emerging and promising way to not only enhance patient adherence and improve glycemic control but also to achieve the potential synergistic effects for greater cardiorenal protection. In this review, we provide an update on the novel antidiabetic agents in the past decade, with an appraisal of the mechanisms contributing to cardiorenal protection. Additionally, we offer a glimpse into the landscape of T2DM management in the near future by providing a comprehensive summary of upcoming agents in early-phase trials.

Keywords: type 2 diabetes mellitus; cardiovascular; renal; sodium-glucose co-transporter-2 inhibitors; glucagon-like peptide-1 receptor agonists; novel agents

1. Introduction

Individuals with type 2 diabetes mellitus (T2DM) have at two- to four-fold [1] increased risk of cardiovascular disease (CVD). Globally, nearly one-third of people with T2DM are affected by CVD [2]. CVD accounts for approximately half of all mortalities globally [3], disproportionately affecting individuals with T2DM to a much greater extent than individuals without T2DM. According to the United Kingdom Prospective Diabetes (UKPDS) Study follow-up data, fatal CVD is 70 times more frequent than microvascular complications after nine years of follow-up for T2DM [4].

Good glycemic control remains one of the fundamental cornerstones in managing T2DM, alongside cardiovascular risk reduction. Although intensive glycemic control is known to reduce microvascular and cardiovascular complications in type 1 DM [1,5], achieving satisfactory glycemic control alone is inadequate in lowering the cardiovascular burden in T2DM. As such, the US Food and Drug Administration and European Medicines Agency mandate that all new antidiabetic drugs be rigorously evaluated for cardiovascular safety and benefits through cardiovascular outcome trials [6].

The past decade witnessed the completion of the landmark cardiovascular outcome for sodium-glucose co-transporter-2 (SGLT2) inhibitors and glucagon-like peptide-1 (GLP-1) receptor agonists (GLP-1 RA). The SGLT2 inhibitor empagliflozin and the GLP-1 RA liraglutide were evaluated in the EMPA-REG [6] and LEADER [7] cardiovascular outcome trials (CVOTs), respectively. The significant cardiovascular risk reduction observed in these landmark trials established a new paradigm in T2DM management, shifting the traditional glucose-centric approach to one that emphasizes cardiovascular risk reduction. Although designed as antidiabetic agents, the cardiovascular and renal benefits conferred by SGLT2 inhibitors and GLP-1 RAs extended the indications to individuals with heart failure and kidney disease without diabetes [8–10]. Nearly a decade has passed since the release of the landmark EMPA-REG trial. In the past decade, the global use of SGLT2 inhibitors and GLP-1 RAs has increased. The DISCOVER study, which assessed global trends in SGLT2 inhibitor and GLP-1 RA prescriptions in more than 14,000 patients with T2DM from 37 countries, reported an increase in SGLT2 inhibitor and GLP-1 RA use from 10.8% to 16.1% over 8 years [11]. With the emergence of more CVOT data, the usage of SGLT2 inhibitors and GLP-1 RAs is expected to increase.

In the next decade, breaking new frontiers in discovering novel pathways and pharmaceutical targets for glucose-lowering pathways will be an important focus in reducing the global burden of T2DM. Given the vascular-centric nature of T2DM, with the process of atherosclerotic damage starting even before the development of diabetes [12], it will be crucial to understand the impact of these medications on the early atherosclerotic processes and progression over time. Novel antidiabetic agents will need to be rigorously evaluated through CVOTs. We scope the literature to review the evidence by which these medications can reverse the process of vascular dysfunction, and subsequent cardiorenal outcomes. This review aims to provide a comprehensive discussion of the past, present and future of T2DM management. We focus on the evidence proving cardiovascular and renal protection is conferred by the newer antidiabetic agents. We appraise the current landscape of novel antidiabetic agents that are currently awaiting further evaluation through well-designed CVOTs and offer insights into pharmaceutical targets for T2DM that are in early-phase clinical trials.

2. Materials and Methods

Our first goal is to appraise the literature for human and animal model studies that evaluate the efficacy and provide mechanistic insights into the cardiovascular and renal benefits of the relatively novel classes of antidiabetic medications available in the past decade. Our second goal is to provide an updated appraisal of candidate agents in early-phase trials with potential cardiovascular benefits. We searched MEDLINE using the following search terms:

Search terms 1—to identify novel agents:

("diabetes mellitus, type 2"[MeSH Terms] OR type 2 diabetes[Text Word] OR "ïnsulin resistance") AND ("novel agent*" OR "emerging treatment*" OR "emerging therapy*" OR "new agent" OR "new treatment*" OR "new therap*") to screen for novel agents in type 2 DM.

Search terms 2—to identify relevant human and animal studies on SGLT2 inhibitors and GLP-1 RAs:

For SGLT2 inhibitor: ("SGLT2 inhibitor" OR empaglifozin OR dapagliflozin OR canagliflozin OR ertugliflozin OR ipragliflozin OR sotagliflozin OR tofogliflozin) AND ("endothelial function" OR "flow-mediated dilation" OR "arterial stiffness" OR "pulse wave velocity" OR "cardio-ankle vascular index" OR "CAVI" OR "CRP" or "hsCRP" OR "C-reactive protein" OR "endothelial adhesion molecule" OR "thrombosis marker*" OR "thrombotic marker*" OR biomarker* OR interleukin)

For GLP-1 RAs: ("glucagon like peptide-1 receptor agonist" OR liraglutide OR semaglutide OR dulaglutide OR albiglutide OR exenatide OR lixisenatide OR tirzepatide) AND ("endothelial function" OR "flow mediated dilation" OR "arterial stiffness" OR "pulse wave velocity" OR "cardio-ankle vascular index" OR "CAVI" OR "CRP" or "hsCRP" OR "C-reactive protein" OR "endothelial adhesion molecule" OR "thrombosis marker*" OR "thrombotic marker*" OR biomarker* OR interleukin OR nephropathy OR renal OR kidney).

The timeline for all searches is restricted to 10 years.

We also searched for early-phase trials on novel antidiabetic agents on ClinicalTrials.gov. We only use the search term type 2 diabetes mellitus and apply additional filters to identify studies whose status is planned but not yet recruiting, recruiting, enrolling by invitation, and active, or not recruiting. We limited the age group to adults 18 years and above.

Our searches yielded the following:

Search terms 1 yielded 1936 results.

Search terms 2 (SGLT2 inhibitors) yielded 2788 results.

Search terms 3 (GLP-1 Ras) yielded 1381 results.

ClinialTrials.gov yielded 414 trials.

As this narrative review aims to comprehensively search the literature for updates in novel pharmacological therapies in T2DM and identify candidate agents in early-phase trials, we did not set the inclusion and exclusion criteria to limit the search. We summarize existing literature to provide an updated overview of the landscape of novel pharmacological therapies in T2DM with cardiovascular and renal benefits. We also discuss the mechanisms and candidate agents in early-phase trials.

3. SGLT2 Inhibitors

In 2015, the release of the EMPA-REG outcome trial demonstrated for the first time that a glucose-lowering agent, empagliflozin, an SGLT2 inhibitor, reduced cardiovascular mortality and heart failure hospitalization when given on top of standard care to patients with T2DM with CVD [6]. Since then, other SGLT2 inhibitors emerged in the market, including canagliflozin [13] and dapagliflozin [14], demonstrating similar class effects in terms of cardioprotection. The cardiovascular event curves begin to separate approximately 3–6 months after initiation of an SGLT2 inhibitor. Given the rapidity of cardiovascular risk reduction, it is postulated that there are other mechanisms beyond and independent of improvement in glycemic control.

The main SGLT2 inhibitors evaluated in cardiovascular outcome trials include empagliflozin (EMPA-REG) [6], canagliflozin (CREDENCE) [13], dapagliflozin (DECLARE-TIMI 58) [14] and ertugliflozin (VERTIS-CV) [15]. The EMPA-REG trial, which recruited individuals with T2DM and established CVD, reported a 14% relative risk reduction (hazard ratio (HR), 0.86; 95% confidence interval (CI), 0.74–0.99) in three-point major adverse cardiovascular events (MACE) comprising of cardiovascular mortality, nonfatal myocardial infarction or nonfatal stroke [6]. The therapeutic benefit of SGLT2 inhibitors in heart failure was first signaled in the EMPA-REG trial, which reported a significant reduction in heart failure hospitalizations by 35% (HR 0.65; 95% CI, 0.5–0.85) in the empagliflozin arm as a secondary outcome [6]. The CREDENCE [13] and DECLARE-TIMI 58 [14] trials validated this observation. Dedicated outcome trials focusing on heart failure patients were conducted to establish the efficacy of SGLT2 inhibitors in managing heart failure. The DAPA-HF trial, which enrolled 4744 patients with stable heart failure with a reduced ejection fraction (HFrEF), reported a reduction in the primary composite outcome of cardiovascular mortality and heart failure hospitalizations by 26% (HR 0.74; 95% CI, 0.65–0.85) [16]. The EMPEROR REDUCED trial, which evaluated empagliflozin, showed a 25% risk reduction (HR 0.75; 95% CI, 0.65–0.86) in the primary composite outcome of cardiovascular mortality and heart failure hospitalizations compared to placebo in individuals with HFrEF [17]. In heart failure with a preserved ejection fraction (HFpEF), SGLT2 inhibitors have shown similar benefits. The EMPEROR-Preserved trial, which investigated the efficacy of empagliflozin in patients with HFpEF and mildly reduced EF irrespective of diabetes, showed a 21% relative risk reduction in the primary composite outcome of cardiovascular mortality and heart failure hospitalizations (HR 0.79; 95% CI, 0.69–0.90) [18]. A similar result was reported in the DELIVER trial, which evaluated dapagliflozin and observed an 18% reduction in the primary composite outcome or worsening heart failure or cardiovascular death (HR 0.82; 95% CI, 0.73–0.92) and heart failure hospitalizations (HR 0.79; 95% CI, 0.69–0.91) [19]. The VERTIS-CV trial, which recruited individuals with T2DM and established CVD, showed that ertugliflozin was non-inferior to placebo in reducing MACE [15]. Figure 1 summarizes key cardiovascular outcome trials (CVOTs) with SGLT2 inhibitors.

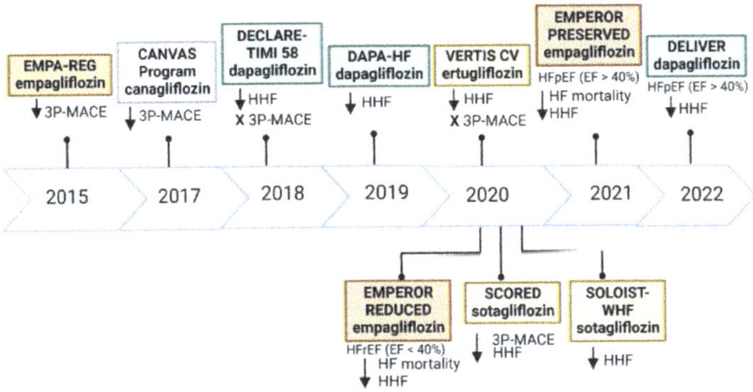

Figure 1. Key SGLT2 inhibitors cardiovascular outcome trials. Created with BioRender.com. 3P-MACE: 3-point major atherosclerotic cardiovascular events; HF: heart failure; HHF: hospitalization for heart failure; HFpEF: heart failure with preserved ejection fraction; HFrEF: heart failure with reduced ejection fraction.

Several mechanisms could explain the cardiovascular benefits of SGLT2 inhibitors. These include improvement in vascular dysfunction [20], inflammation [21], oxidative stress [22], and thrombosis [23]. In terms of cardiac markers, SGLT2 inhibitors reduce troponin I [24] and NT-proBNP [25,26]. The cardiovascular protection conferred by SGLT2 inhibitors is summarized in Figure 2 below.

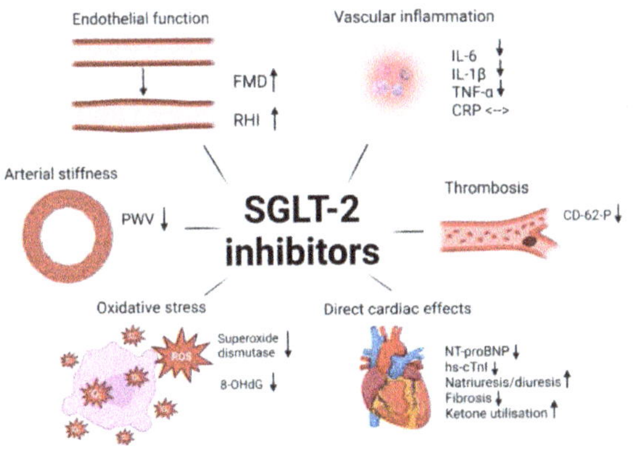

Figure 2. Summary of mechanisms of SGLT2 inhibitors in cardiovascular protection. Created with BioRender.com. FMD: flow-mediated dilation; RHI: reactive hyperaemia index; PWV: pulse wave velocity; IL: interleukin; TNR: tumor necrosis factor; 8-OHdG: 8-hydroxy-2′-deoxyguanosine; NT-proBNP: N-terminal pro b-type natriuretic peptide; hs-cTnI: high-sensitivity cardiac troponin T and I.

3.1. *Effects of SGLT2 Inhibitors on Vascular Function*

Subclinical vascular dysfunction, which includes endothelial dysfunction [27] and arterial stiffness [28], is an early process in atherosclerosis. The DEFENCE study, conducted in Japan, was one of the first to evaluate the effect of SGLT2 inhibitors on vascular function [29]. This randomized controlled trial (RCT) involved 80 patients with T2DM and found that dapagliflozin 5 mg daily for 16 weeks significantly improved flow-mediated dilation (FMD), a well-recognized marker of endothelial function [29], by 1.05% as compared to a 0.94% reduction in FMD in the metformin group ($p = 0.04$) for a subset of patients with baseline glycated haemoglobin (HbA1c) greater or equal to 7% [29]. The beneficial effect of SGLT2 inhibitors on FMD was summarized in a meta-analysis. Using dapagliflozin significantly increased FMD by 1.66% (95% CI, 0.56–2.76) [20]. The improvement in FMD was confirmed in another meta-analysis [30]. When compared to sulphonylureas, SGLT2 inhibition was associated with a higher FMD by a mean difference of 1.89% (95% CI, 0.1–3.75) [31]. Other SGLT2 inhibitors, including tofogiflozin and iprafliglozin, also improved FMD [32,33]. Additionally, the effect of SGLT2 inhibitors has been evaluated using the EndoPAT technology. SGLT2 inhibition increased the reactive hyperaemia index, which is a marker of peripheral microvascular function, from 0.45 to 0.66 ($p < 0.01$) only in the dapagliflozin group [34].

Apart from peripheral endothelial function, the coronary endothelial function is another key vascular bed that could impact cardiovascular outcomes, especially heart failure. Dysfunctional endothelium in the coronary microcirculation could impact cardiomyocyte health, and the resultant coronary microvascular dysfunction is a key determinant in HFpEF [35]. The improvement in coronary endothelial function by SGLT2 inhibitors was demonstrated in preclinical models. Empagliflozin and dapagliflozin improved cardiac microvascular endothelial cell function in mice exposed to ischaemic reperfusion injury, with a resultant increase in endothelium-dependent relaxation and reduction in reactive oxygen species and endothelial cell activation markers [36,37]. In addition, in mouse cardiomyocytes, SGLT2 inhibitors appear to demonstrate a class effect in which the Na^+/H^+ exchanger is inhibited, lowering Na flux into cardiomyocytes and promoting coronary vasodilation [38].

Endothelial dysfunction contributes to arterial stiffness, a pathophysiological process involving remodeling the elastic fibers in arteries and fibrosis of arterial walls [28]. Arterial stiffness can lead to atherosclerosis through increased shear stress, stimulating collagen deposition and extracellular matrix deposition in the arterial wall and accelerating the formation of atherosclerotic plaques [28]. Arterial stiffness can be measured using pulse wave velocity (PWV), which indicates the transit time of the arterial pressure waves in the large arteries, which increases in stiff arteries. Increased wall pressure could aggravate endothelial dysfunction, leading to a vicious cycle of endothelial dysfunction and arterial stiffening [28]. A 1 meter/second (m/s) increase in PWV increases the risk of cardiovascular events by 7% [39]. SGLT2 inhibition has been shown to improve arterial stiffness. A meta-analysis comparing the PWV between the SGLT2 inhibitors—dapagliflozin and empagliflozin—versus placebo found that SGLT2 inhibitors reduced PWV by 0.76 m/s [40], while an observational study with tofogliflozin showed a worsening of arterial stiffness in non-tofogliflozin but not in patients on tofogliflozin [41]. Further details of the impact of SGLT2 inhibitors on vascular function measurements are presented in Supplementary Table S1.

3.2. *Effects of SGLT2 Inhibitors on Mechanisms in Atherosclerosis*

1. SGLT2 inhibitors reduce vascular inflammation.

The amelioration of vascular inflammation by SGLT2 inhibitors has been demonstrated in animal studies. Dapagliflozin reduces inflammatory cytokines, including tumor necrosis factor-alpha (TNF-α), endothelial adhesion molecules and nuclear factor-kappa B (NF-kB) expression in mice [42]. Similar findings have also been observed in visceral adipose tissue of Zucker diabetic fatty rats, in which IL-1β, IL-6, TNF-a, and monocyte chemoattractant (MCP)-1 significantly reduced after 6 weeks of empagliflozin administration [43]. SGLT2 inhibition modulates NLRP3 inflammasome activity in humans, reducing IL-1β secretion [23,44–46]. Regarding the inflammatory cytokine, IL-6, a recent meta-analysis involving more than 5000 adult individuals with T2DM, the use of SGLT2 inhibitor reduced IL-6 by a mean of 1.04 and 1.3 compared to other antidiabetic medications [21]. Dapagliflozin use was also associated with a reduction in TNF-α [46]. However, the impact of SGLT2 inhibition on CRP is not clear. While Wang et al. found that CRP level was reduced by SGLT2 inhibitors [47], Buttice et al. did not find improvements in CRP or TNF-α in a meta-analysis comprising 38 RCTs investigating the effect of SGLT2 inhibition in inflammatory markers [48].

2. SGLT2 inhibitors attenuate oxidative stress and atherosclerosis

Oxidative stress plays a significant role in the atherosclerotic process and is closely associated with endothelial dysfunction. For instance, the endothelial adhesion molecule, vascular cell adhesion molecule 1 (VCAM-1), activates nicotinamide adenine dinucleotide phosphate (NADPH) oxidase 2, generating reactive oxygen species (ROS) [49] and rapidly induces matrix metalloproteinases (MMPs) [50]. The MMPs subsequently disrupt cell-to-cell adhesions and extracellular matrix [50], separating the intima from the blood vessel's medial lining, allowing smooth muscle cell migration and promoting atherosclerotic plaque formation [51]. Sustained exposure to excess ROS in the blood vessels, induced by mitochondria dysfunction, uncoupled nitric oxide synthase, myeloperoxidase, and NADPH oxidases [52], can induce endothelial dysfunction and drive inflammation further. SGLT2 inhibition has been shown to reduce leukocyte mitochondrial superoxide production [23,53], reduce NADPH and myeloperoxidase and increase the production of endogenous antioxidant glutathione [54]. The DEFENCE trial showed that 16 weeks of dapagliflozin reduced urine 8-hydroxy-2′-deoxyguanosine (8-OHdG), a marker of oxidative stress [29]. At the same time, studies on empagliflozin found increased mitochondrial superoxide dismutase activity, a key player in clearing ROS and reducing oxidative stress [23,53,55].

3. SGLT2 inhibitors reduce thrombosis

Platelet activation is a key process in promoting vascular inflammation through a sequential process involving rolling and firm adhesion of activated platelets to the endothelial surface [56–58]. These processes are mediated by specific receptors, such as P-selectin, and accelerate the recruitment of immune cells to the inflamed endothelium and subendothelial spaces to drive atherosclerosis [59]. Studies have shown that SGLT2 inhibitors reduce CD62-P antigen expression [23,60], a platelet activation marker stored in platelet granules that is rapidly mobilized to the cell surface upon activation [61]. This finding suggests a potential benefit of SGLT2 inhibitor in attenuating platelet activation, aggregation and atherothrombosis [62].

Supplementary Table S2 presents further information about selected studies evaluating the impact of SGLT2 inhibitors on specific biomarkers.

3.3. SGLT2 Inhibitors and Heart Failure

1. Clinical trials and cardiac markers

SGLT2 inhibitors have been consistently proven to reduce heart failure-related events. The hard clinical outcomes are supported by strong biochemical evidence demonstrating a significant reduction in N-terminal pro b-type natriuretic peptide (NT-proBNP), a marker of ventricular wall stress, cardiac remodelling and dysfunction [63]. SGLT2 inhibitors, dapagliflozin and canagliflozin, reduce NT-proBNP between 11 to 18.2% [24,25], with the reduction sustained for up to 6 years [64] (Supplementary Table S3). Postulated mechanisms of SGLT2 inhibitors include beneficial haemodynamic effects through diuresis and natriuresis, resulting in reduced cardiac preload, afterload [65] and reverse ventricular remodelling [66]. Furthermore, SGLT2 inhibitors may attenuate myocardial injury and subclinical cardiac damage [67], as evidenced by a significant reduction in high-sensitivity troponin I (hs-TnI) by empagliflozin [24] (Supplementary Table S3). Additionally, SGLT2 inhibition may provide direct cardioprotection through metabolic reprogramming, which shifts energy utilization from fatty acid and carbohydrates toward ketone body oxidation in myocardial cells, resulting in greater efficiency in generating energy in the myocardium [68]. Improvement in coronary microvascular endothelial function could also explain the beneficial effects of SGLT2 inhibition, specifically in HFpEF. In this first study comprising 16 patients, 4 weeks of dapagliflozin improved myocardial flow reserve, a marker of coronary microcirculation and vasodilation [69]. In other preclinical models, SGLT2 inhibitors reduced cardiac fibrosis by suppressing endothelial-to-mesenchymal transition by inhibiting TGF-beta/Smad signalling [70]. These processes, along with other mechanisms, such as reducing inflammation and oxidative stress, work synergistically to contribute to the beneficial effects of SGLT2 inhibition on the myocardium.

3.4. SGLT2 Inhibitors and the Kidneys

1. Clinical trials focusing on renal outcomes

The EMPA-KIDNEY trial, which involved patients with diabetic kidney disease, glomerular disease and hypertensive or renovascular disease, found that empagliflozin reduced kidney disease progression by 29% (HR 0.71; 95% CI, 0.62–0.81), with a 50% reduction in the rate of eGFR decline [71]. The CREDENCE trial recruited individuals with T2DM with or without CVD, but all had chronic kidney disease on stable maximally tolerated doses of an angiotensin-converting enzyme inhibitor or angiotensin receptor blocker. MACE was reduced by 32% (HR 0.68; 95% CI, 0.49–0.94) and 15% (HR 0.85; 95% CI, 0.69–1.06) in the primary and secondary prevention groups, respectively [13]. Canagliflozin was also associated with a relative risk reduction of 40% in doubling serum creatinine and a 32% reduction in reaching end-stage kidney disease [13]. The DECLARE-TIMI trial assigned patients with T2DM with or without CVD to dapagliflozin. Although dapagliflozin did not significantly lower MACE, there was a 17% reduction (HR 0.83; 95% CI, 0.73–0.95) in heart failure events [14]. On the other hand, the DAPA-CKD trial was terminated early due to efficacy. Dapagliflozin reduced the relative risk of sustained decline in renal function, end-stage kidney disease, or renal-related mortality by 39% (HR 0.61; 95% CI, 0.51–0.72) [72]. Figure 3 below summarizes the key renal outcome trials with SGLT2 inhibitors.

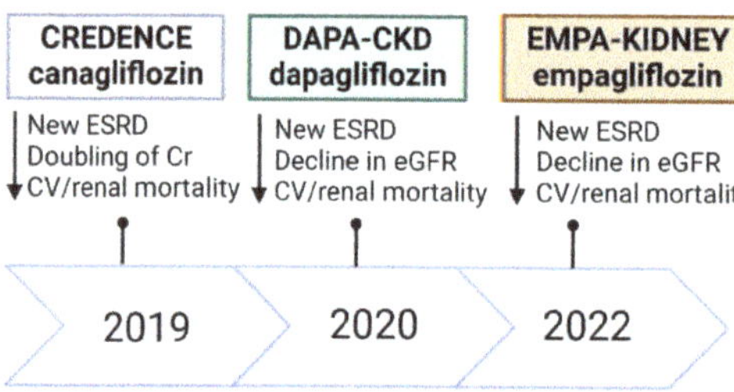

Figure 3. Key SGLT2 inhibitors renal outcome trials. Created with BioRender.com. ESRD: end stage renal disease; Cr: creatinine; CV: cardiovascular; eGFR: estimated glomerular filtration rate.

2. Mechanisms of SGLT2 inhibitors in renal protection.

Multiple pathophysiological processes contribute to the development of diabetic kidney disease (Figure 4). Oxidative stress, inflammation, and the increased release of growth-forming factors lead to podocyte damage, tubulointerstitial fibrosis and glomerulosclerosis [73]. These mechanisms, together with reduced sodium delivery to the glomerulus and altered tubuloglomerular feedback, induce glomerular efferent arteriolar vasoconstriction, increase intraglomerular pressure, and promote glomerulosclerosis [73]. SGLT2 inhibition blocks the reabsorption of sodium and glucose in the proximal tubules, restores sodium delivery to the macula densa, reverses efferent arteriolar vasoconstriction and relieves intraglomerular hypertension [73]. The benefits of SGTL2 inhibition have been validated through animal models and human studies that specifically measured changes in the glomerular and renal tubular injury markers (Supplementary Table S4). For example, SGLT2 inhibition has been shown to reduce urinary nephrin, a protein expressed in podocytes and a sensitive marker of podocyte injury [74]. Evidence suggests that increased urinary nephrin can be detected before albuminuria and is correlated with the severity of glomerular injury [75]. In addition, SGLT2 inhibition significantly increases transforming growth factor beta-1 (TGF-β) excretion [74]. TGF-β plays a crucial role in inducing hypertrophic response and is a key marker of renal fibrosis [76]. Another marker of renal fibrosis, MMP-7, is reduced by SGLT2 inhibition over 2 years [77]. Other markers studied include neutrophil gelatinase-associated lipocalin (NGAL), which is produced by neutrophils and released by injured renal tubular cells [78]. NGAL is significantly reduced by tofogliflozin, an SGLT2 inhibitor developed in Japan [79]. Another plasma biomarker is the liver-type fatty acid binding protein (L-FABP), secreted by renal proximal tubular cells in response to tissue hypoxia [80]. Canagliflozin use for 52 weeks has been shown to reduce urinary L-FABP significantly in T2DM individuals compared to non-users [81]. In terms of inflammatory markers, a post hoc analysis of the CANVAS trial showed a significant reduction in TNF receptors 1 and 2 [82], while other RCTs showed a reduction in IL-6 [21] and a proximal tubular injury marker [83], kidney injury molecule 1 [84,85]

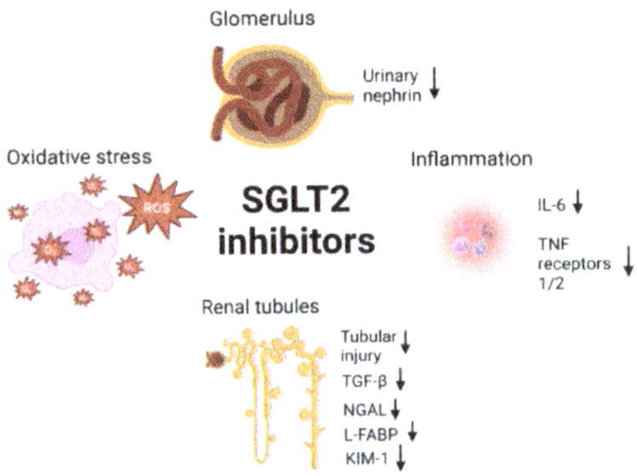

Figure 4. Mechanisms of renal protection by SGLT2 inhibitors. Created with BioRender.com. IL-6: interleukin-6; TNF: tumor necrosis factor: TGF-β: transforming growth factor β; NGAL: neutrophil gelatinase associated lipocalin; L-FABP: liver-type fatty acid binding protein; KIM-1: kidney injury molecule 1.

3.5. Adverse Effects Associated with SGLT2 Inhibitors

Particular caution needs to be taken when initiating SGLT2 inhibitors. Firstly, increased glucosuria predisposes to genitourinary infections. Meta-analyses reported a 2.9- to 3.3-fold increased risk for urogenital infections with SGLT2 inhibitors use in patients with T2DM [86]. Furthermore, the highest risk of genitourinary tract infections was reported to occur approximately in the first 28 days of initiation [87]. Fournier's gangrene, a rare but potentially fatal perineal soft tissue infection, was found to be associated with SGLT2 inhibitors [86]. Secondly, the risk of hypotension from volume depletion, especially with concomitant use of diuretics, needs to be monitored closely, especially in susceptible patients who have borderline low blood pressure at the time of initiation [88]. Thirdly, significant glucose-lowering with SGLT2 inhibitors reduces insulin and increases glucagon secretion. This altered insulin and glucagon balance promotes free fatty metabolism and ketone generation. The enhanced risk of euglycemic diabetic ketoacidosis (DKA) needs to be emphasized, especially during periods of acute illness, poor appetite or significant stress (e.g., undergoing invasive procedures), when it is prudent to withhold SGLT2 inhibitors temporarily [89].

3.6. Dual SGLT1 and SGLT2 Inhibitors

There is emerging interest in combining SGLT-1 and SGLT-2 inhibition for potential synergistic effects. Sotagliflozin is the first FDA-approved dual inhibitor of SGLT-1 and SGLT2. SGLT2 is expressed mainly in the early segments of the proximal tubule of the nephron and mediates the reabsorption of more than 90% of filtered glucose [90]. In contrast, SGLT1 is expressed predominantly in the epithelial cells of the brush border in the small intestine [90], mediating intestinal glucose reabsorption. SGLT1 is also located in the late proximal tubule in the nephron, where it reabsorbs 3% of filtered glucose in normoglycemic individuals [90]. However, in hyperglycemia, the amount of glucose reabsorbed by SGLT1 in the proximal tubule increases significantly, hence supporting the role of dual SGLT1 and SGLT2 inhibition (Figure 5) [91]. In the intestines, SGLT1 inhibition inhibits intestinal glucose absorption and increases glucose delivery to the distal gut, stimulating GLP-1 secretion and further reducing postprandial hyperglycemia [92].

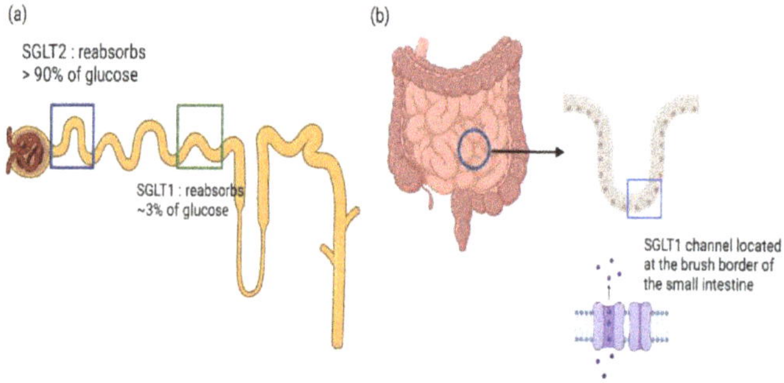

Figure 5. (**a**): Comparative differences in glucose reabsorption at proximal renal tubule between SGLT1 and SGLT2 receptors. (**b**): Main glucose reabsorption in the small intestine by SGLT1 receptors. Created with Biorender.com.

The main benefit of dual SGLT1 and SGLT2 inhibition is that it reduces heart failure events. The SCORED trial, which looked at the effects of sotagliflozin in more than 10,000 individuals with T2DM, chronic kidney disease and additional cardiovascular risk factors, demonstrated a reduction in the composite of cardiovascular mortality, heart failure hospitalizations and urgent visits by 26% (hazard ratio 0.74; 95% CI, 0.63–0.88) [93]. The SOLOIST-WHF trial, which recruited 1222 patients with T2DM who were recently hospitalized for decompensated heart failure, sotagliflozin users had reduced cardiovascular mortality and subsequent heart failure exacerbations by 33% (hazard ratio 0.67, 95% CI 0.52–0.85) [94] (Figure 1).

While SGLT2 inhibitors did not show a significant effect on stroke reduction, dual SGLT1 and SGLT2 inhibition was associated with a significant decrease in all-cause stroke by 34% (hazard ratio 0.66; 95% CI 0.48–0.91) and ischaemic stroke by 32% (hazard ratio 0.68; 95% CI 0.47 to 0.99) [95].

The incremental benefit of SGLT1 inhibition in neuroprotection could be attributable to a few postulated mechanisms. Firstly, SGLT1 is expressed in the brain and is increased in patients with T2DM. SGLT1 inhibition may reduce blood–brain barrier permeability and cerebral injury [96]. In the gut, SGLT1 inhibition increases glucose delivery to the distal intestine, alters the intestinal microbiome by increasing short-chain fatty acids and stimulating GLP-1 secretion, which has anti-atherogenic properties, reduces inflammation, thrombosis and oxidative stress, and stabilizes atherosclerotic plaques [97].

4. GLP-1 Receptor Agonist (GLP-1 RA)

The GLP-1 RA is another class of antidiabetic agent with cardiovascular and renal benefits. GLP-1 is an incretin hormone secreted from enteroendocrine L cells with pleiotropic effects on glucose regulation [98]. GLP-1 stimulates insulin secretion, inhibits glucagon release, promotes satiety and reduces gastric emptying [99]. In T2DM, the incretin effect is diminished but can be restored by GLP-1 infusion [100], making GLP-1 mimetics attractive agents to improve glycemic control. Moreover, GLP-1 affects systemic homeostasis by activating receptors in various organs, including the kidneys, heart, adipose tissue, liver and muscles [101]. GLP-1 receptors in the brain regulate food intake directly and indirectly through vagal afferents in the gut [102].

The first GLP-1 RA, exenatide, was approved for clinical use in 2004. Exenatide was derived from exendin, an endogenous GLP-1-like peptide secreted in the saliva of the lizard Heloderma suspectum (Gila monster) [103]. Endogenous GLP-1 has a short half-life of 2 min due to rapid degradation by DPP-4 [104]. With modifications to the amino acid structure, the half-life of exenatide is prolonged to 2.5 h [103]. Retaining more than 50% homology as endogenous GLP-1, exenatide enhances pancreatic beta-cell secretion and reduces postprandial hyperglycaemia [103]. Lixisenatide, another GLP-1 RA designed based on exendin-4, is modified at different amino acids, prolonging its half-life by up to 4 h [105]. Other GLP-1 RAs, specifically liraglutide and semaglutide, involved creating conjugates with long-chain fatty acid moieties to render the molecular size of the GLP-1 RAs too large to be filtered by the kidneys effectively, thereby reducing renal clearance and prolonging the half-life [106].

Currently, the most commonly used GLP 1 RAs for treating T2DM are liraglutide, semaglutide and dulaglutide. In addition to T2DM, liraglutide and semaglutide are also approved for treating obesity without T2DM. High-dose liraglutide (3 mg/day) was evaluated in the SCALE trial, a 56-week study involving more than 3700 patients with BMI ≥ 30 or ≥27 with at least one obesity-related complication, found a greater mean weight of 5.6 kg in the high dose liraglutide group compared to placebo [107]. The STEP trial, which evaluated the efficacy of semaglutide in weight loss, found a mean weight loss of nearly 15% at week 68 compared to 2.4% for placebo among individuals with obesity but without T2DM [108].

In terms of cardiovascular risk reduction, there appears to be a difference between the older formulations (exenatide, lisixenatide) and the newer generations (liraglutide, dulaglutide and semaglutide). Exenatide was not superior to placebo in reducing cardiovascular outcomes in patients with T2DM [109]. This was similar to lixisenatide, in which the rates of cardiovascular events were not significantly different from placebo among patients with T2DM and recent acute coronary syndrome [110]. However, liraglutide was the first GLP-1 RA to demonstrate positive cardiovascular benefits [7]. The LEADER trial, published in 2016, randomized more than 9300 patients with T2DM and high cardiovascular risk to liraglutide or placebo. Liraglutide was associated with a 13% relative risk reduction (HR 0.87; 95% CI, 0.78–0.97) in three-point MACE over 3.8 years of follow-up [7]. Following the LEADER trial, the SUSTAIN-6 trial [111], which assessed semaglutide, and the REWIND trial [112], which evaluated dulaglutide, both reported a significant reduction in major cardiovascular events in patients with type 2 DM at high cardiovascular risk. A meta-analysis of eight CVOTs reported a 14% reduction (HR 0.86; 95% CI, 0.80–0.93) in MACE, with separation of event curves approximately 12–18 months after initiation [113]. Figure 6 summarizes the key cardiovascular outcome trials for GLP-1 RAs.

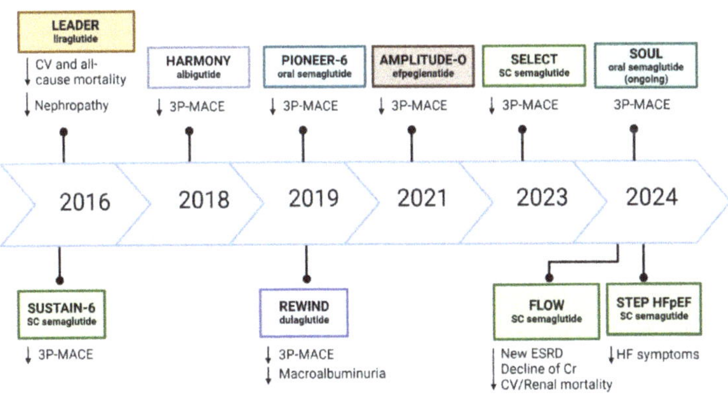

Figure 6. Key cardiovascular outcome trials for GLP-1 RAs. Created with BioRender.com. 3P-MACE: 3-point major atherosclerotic cardiovascular events; ESRD: end stage renal disease; CV: cardiovascular; HF: heart failure; HFpEF: heart failure with preserved ejection fraction.

GLP-1 RAs confer cardiovascular benefits through the following mechanisms: they improve vascular function [31,40], reduce inflammation [114,115], oxidative stress [11], thrombosis [115] and have direct effects on the heart. Figure 7 summarizes the cardiovascular benefits of GLP-1 RAs.

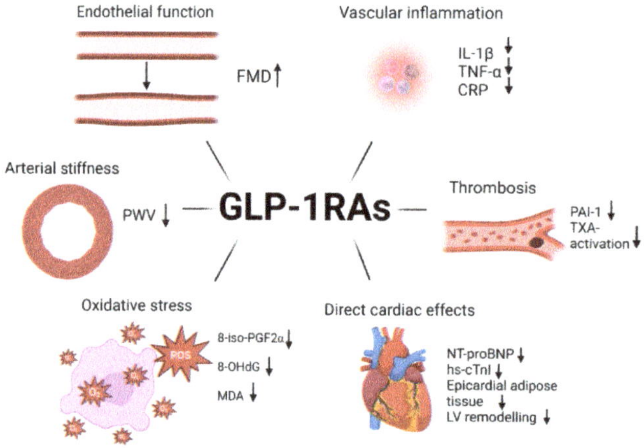

Figure 7. Mechanisms conferring cardiovascular protection by GLP-1 RAs. Created with BioRender.com. PWV: pulse wave velocity; PAI-1: plasminoagen activator inhibitor-1; TXA: thromboxane; TNF-α: tumor necrosis factor α; CRP: C-reactive protein; IL-1β: interleukin 1β; 8-iso-PGF2α: 8-iso-prostaglandin F2α; 8-OHdG: 8-hydroxy-2′-deoxyguanosine; MDA: malondialdehyde; hs-cTnI: high-sensitivity cardiac troponin I; NT-proBNP: N-terminal pro b-type natriuretic peptide; LV: left ventricle.

4.1. *Effects of GLP-1 RA on Endothelial Function and Arterial Stiffness*

A network meta-analysis comparing the efficacies of various antidiabetic agents found that GLP1-RAs increased FMD by a mean difference of 3.70 (95% CI 1.39–5.97) compared to lifestyle intervention [31]. In comparison with sulphonylureas and placebo, GLP-1 RAs also showed a significant improvement in FMD of 3.33 (95% CI 1.36–5.34) and 3.30 (95% CI 1.21–5.43), respectively [31]. The physiological improvement in FMD was supported by mechanistic insights revealing an improvement in endothelial function in human umbilical vein endothelial cells via the mTOR/Akt signaling pathway, promoting endothelial NOS activity and increasing NO production [116]. In addition, improvement in endothelial function could also be attributed to an increase in the regenerative capacity of the endothelium, as demonstrated by an increase in endothelial progenitor cells after 12 weeks of treatment with dulaglutide [117].

Regarding arterial stiffness, a network meta-analysis comparing different classes of antidiabetic agents revealed that only GLP-1 RAs improve arterial stiffness by reducing pulse wave velocity by a mean difference of 1.06 (95% CI −2.05 to −0.10) in individuals with abnormal glucose metabolism [40]. This improvement in arterial stiffness could be supported by positive changes in the extracellular matrix in the blood vessels, as demonstrated by an experimental study evaluating the effects of semaglutide on vascular structure in high-fat diet-induced obese mice, which revealed decreased levels of ECM proteins Coll5a1, Lama4 and Sparc [118].

The effects of GLP-1 RAs on endothelial function and arterial stiffness are summarized in Supplementary Table S5.

4.2. *Mechanisms of Cardiovascular Protection by GLP-1 RA*

1. Inflammation

Attenuating inflammation is a key protective mechanism of GLP-1 RAs. Contrary to SGLT2 inhibitors, GLP-1 RAs are associated with a stronger signal in reducing inflammation.

A meta-analysis showed significant reductions in CRP and TNF-alpha by GLP-1 RAs compared to standard antidiabetic agents or placebo, with a mean difference of −0.54 (95% CI, −0.75 to −0.34) and −0.39 (95% CI, −0.62 to −0.15) respectively [114]. Furthermore, a 180-day treatment with semaglutide or dulaglutide reduced IL-1β, suggesting possible beneficial effects on targeting the NLRP3 inflammasome pathway [119]. Liraglutide also reduces MCP-1 [115], which promotes the recruitment of monocytes and macrophages to the subendothelial layer [120]. VCAM-1, the endothelial cell surface adhesion that promotes migration across vessel walls [121], is significantly reduced by liraglutide [117,122]. Various evidence in preclinical models has also demonstrated the effects of GLP-1 RA in stabilizing atherosclerotic plaques through anti-inflammatory and anti-atherogenic mechanisms on endothelial cells, vascular smooth muscle cells, monocytes and macrophages [113].

2. Oxidative stress

Another cardioprotective mechanism of GLP1-RAs includes ameliorating oxidative stress, as demonstrated by a reduction in oxidative stress markers 8-OH-dG and 8-iso-PGF2a by liraglutide within 8 weeks [123]. Malondialdehyde (MDA), a compound derived from lipid peroxidation and a common biomarker to measure oxidative stress [104], was reduced by 0.84 (95% CI −1.61 to −0.06) compared to controls [124].

3. Thrombosis

GLP-1 RAs modulate thrombosis and fibrinolysis. In an RCT comparing liraglutide and sitagliptin (a DPP-4 inhibitor), plasminogen activator inhibitor 1 (PAI-1), an important player that inhibits fibrin clearance [115], was significantly reduced by liraglutide [115]. The reduction in PAI-I was observed as early as 2 weeks after initiating liraglutide and prior to weight loss [115]. In addition, it has been postulated that GLP-1 RAs may inhibit intra-arterial thrombus formation in mice by inhibiting platelet reactivity [125]. An RCT evaluating the antiplatelet effect of GLP-1 RAs found that liraglutide reduces thromboxane-dependent platelet activation, as reflected by the reduction in urinary excretion of U-11-dehydro-TXB_2, a metabolite of thromboxane A2 [126]. As GLP-1 receptors are widely distributed in the central nervous system and GLP-1 RAs can cross the blood–brain barrier, the aforementioned benefits of GLP-1 RAs could have significant neuroprotective effects [127] and could account for the 24% relative risk reduction in nonfatal stroke (HR 0.76; 95% CI, 0.61–0.95), a prespecified secondary outcome in the REWIND trial (dulaglutide) [128], and for the 39% (HR 0.61; 95% CI, 0.38–0.99) for nonfatal stroke in the SUSTAIN-6 trial (semaglutide) [111].

4.3. *Effects of GLP-1 RA on Heart Failure*

Emerging evidence supports the potential role of GLP-1 RA in heart failure (Figure 6). In a post hoc analysis of the REWIND trial, dulaglutide use was associated with a slower rise in NT-proBNP [128]. In the LIVE study, 241 individuals with HFrEF were randomized to liraglutide versus placebo for 24 weeks. In patients with T2DM, NT-proBNP decreased by 25% in the liraglutide group compared with placebo [129]. Liraglutide also reduced NT-proBNP significantly compared to metformin [130]. In the recent STEP-HFpEF trial looking at the effect of semaglutide in obese patients with HFpEF, semaglutide was associated with significant improvement in physical symptoms and exercise capacity, as well as a significant reduction in NT-proBNP by 25% [131]. The beneficial effects of GLP-1 RAs on HFpEF could be related to the alteration of epicardial adipose tissue (EAT) [132]. Evidence suggests that individuals with diastolic dysfunction have increased epicardial adipose tissue, which could lower peak oxygen consumption and worsen exercise tolerance [133]. Using liraglutide over 6 months, EAT thickness was significantly reduced from 9.6 to 6.26 mm versus no change in the metformin arm [134]. A reduction in EAT could attenuate left ventricular remodeling. Furthermore, reducing vascular inflammation, endothelial dysfunction, and oxidative stress could improve myocardial function [131]. Additionally, GLP-1 RAs inhibit the sodium-hydrogen exchanger 3 in proximal tubular cells to increase natriuresis and diuresis [135], contributing to favorable haemodynamic effects in heart failure. A summary of the impact of cardiovascular protection by GLP-1 RAs is presented in Supplementary Table S6.

4.4. Effects of GLP-1 RA on Renal Function

GLP-1 RAs reduced composite renal outcomes (development of macroalbuminuria, decline in renal function, renal replacement therapy or renal-related mortality) by 21% [136]. The mechanisms underpinning the benefits of GLP-1 RAs on renal outcomes could be attributed to the presence of GLP-1 receptors in the renal glomeruli and mesangial cells, attenuating the inflammatory response to advanced glycation end products and reducing the progression of diabetic kidney disease [137]. In addition, GLP-1 RAs reduce oxidative stress by upregulating cyclic adenosine monophosphate (cAMP) and increasing protein kinase A, reducing the apoptosis of kidney podocytes and slowing down renal glomerulosclerosis [138] (Figure 6). The activation of GLP-1 receptors in the kidneys leads to direct renal benefits. These include increased natriuresis, the reduction of vasoconstrictors such as angiotensin II and endothelin-1, and enhanced endothelium-dependent vasodilation [100]. The FLOW trial, a dedicated renal outcome trial that aimed to evaluate the efficacy of semaglutide in slowing the progression of renal impairment in individuals with T2DM and CKD, was prematurely terminated in October 2023 for efficacy [139]. The results were highly favorable. Among the 3533 participants with T2DM and CKD who were followed up for a median of 3.4 years, the risk of composite onset of end-stage renal disease—at least a 50% reduction in renal function or renal-related mortality—was reduced by 24% in the semaglutide group compared with placebo (HR 0.76; 95% CI 0.66–0.88) [140]. The SOUL trial is investigating the efficacy of oral semaglutide on combined cardiovascular and renal outcomes in 9650 individuals with T2DM [141]. The REMODEL trial, an ongoing mechanistic study investigating the effects of semaglutide on kidney oxygenation, inflammation and fibrosis, is planned to be completed by the end of 2024 (NCT04865770) (Figure 5) [142].

4.5. Adverse Effects Associated with GLP-1 RA

The most common adverse effect associated with GLP-1 RA is gastrointestinal intolerance, which tends to occur within one month of initiation [143]. More serious adverse effects include acute pancreatitis, which was reported to occur in approximately 3% of users [144]. The association between GLP-1 RA and thyroid cancer is unclear. While a nested case-control study reported a possible increased risk for all thyroid cancer by nearly 1.6 times and medullary thyroid cancer by 1.8 times [145], a recent cohort study did not show this association [146]. Regarding pancreatic cancer, GLP-1 RA is postulated to induce the proliferation of pancreatic islet cells and may stimulate pancreatic carcinogenesis in susceptible individuals [147]. However, there is a growing body of literature that suggests the lack of association between GLP-1 RA and pancreatic cancer [148]. With the increasing use of GLP-1 RA, long-term follow-up of data will provide more definitive evidence regarding cancer risks with GLP-1 RA.

4.6. Combination Agents with GLP-1

An emerging field in the pharmacological landscape for T2DM involves combining GLP-1 RAs with other agents. These include amylin analogue, GIP receptor agonist and glucagon receptor agonist.

1. GLP-1 + amylin analogue

One of these combinatory approaches involves a long-acting amylin analogue, cagrilintide, and semaglutide (CagriSema). This agent has recently shown more significant weight loss than the individual components. In a small exploratory trial involving 92 participants randomly assigned to CagriSema, semaglutide or cagrilintide, the mean change in HbA1c from baseline to week 32 was 2.2% for Cagrisema and weight loss of 15.6% for CagriSema versus 5.1% for semaglutide alone [149]. It has been postulated that amylin agonists could delay gastric emptying, reduce postprandial glucagon secretion, and improve insulin sensitivity synergistically when added to GLP1 receptor agonists [149].

2. GLP-1 + GIP receptor agonist (tirzepatide)

Unimolecular dual agonists have emerged as a promising strategy to enhance the metabolic effects of GLP-1 receptor agonists by combining them with other enteropancreatic hormones. An example of such a dual agonist agent is tirzepatide (LY3298176), which combines the agonist activities of GLP-1 and GIP receptors [150]. Tirzepatide has a greater affinity to GIP receptors and can be administered once weekly [150].

Tirzepatide has recently been extensively evaluated in phase 2 trials with either placebo (SURPASS-1) [151] or other active comparators, including semaglutide (SURPASS-2) [152], degludec (SURPASS-3) [153], glargine (SURPASS-4) [154] or add-on to basal insulin (SURPASS-5) [155]. At an incremental dose to a maximum of 15 mg per week, tirzepatide showed superiority in HbA1c and bodyweight reduction at 40 or 52 weeks. Ongoing studies are currently assessing the impact of switching GLP-1 RA to tirzepatide (SURPASS SWITCH: NCT05564039 and SURPASS SWITCH 2: NCT05706506). The use of tirzepatide in recently diagnosed T2DM is also being evaluated in the SURPASS-early trial (NCT05433584). Furthermore, the combination agent Cagrisema (cagrilintide and semaglutide) is compared against tirzepatide to determine the degree of HbA1c reduction (NCT062219690).

Apart from T2DM, tirzepatide is also extensively studied in patients with obesity without T2DM. In the SURMOUNT-1 trial, which recruited more than 2500 subjects with obesity but without T2DM to tirzepatide versus placebo, 91% (95% CI, 88–94) of participants were able to achieve at least 5% of weight loss versus 35% (95% CI, 30–39) with placebo [156]. More than 50% of participants who received the highest dose of tirzepatide could lose more than 20% of their weight, compared to just 3% in the placebo group [156]. The safety profile of tirzepatide was similar to GLP-1 receptor agonists, with mild to moderate gastrointestinal symptoms being the predominant adverse effects, which improved over time [156].

The cardiovascular benefits of GIP could be directly associated with the anti-atherogenic effects of GIP on human umbilical vein endothelial cells [157]. GIP reduces gene expression of advanced glycation end-product receptors and other pro-atherogenic molecules such as VCAM and PAI-I [158]. GIP also activates endothelial nitric oxide synthase, which synthesizes nitric oxide [157], a key vasodilator inhibiting vascular smooth muscle cell proliferation [159]. In addition, active GIP has also been shown to suppress inflammatory responses in macrophage foam cells, reduce expression of CD36, and promote anti-inflammatory and anti-oxidative stress effects by upregulating the cAMP pathway [160]. A post hoc analysis of the SURMOUNT-1 trial also showed a possible preferential reduction in triglyceride-rich lipoprotein [161]. All these actions contribute to atherosclerotic plaque stabilization in animal models [162].

Regarding the cardiovascular benefits of tirzepatide in humans, a meta-analysis comprising 4887 participants treated with tirzepatide reported a hazard ratio of 0.80 for four-component major adverse cardiovascular events and 0.80 for all-cause mortality (95% CI, 0.57–1.11) [163]. In a posthoc analysis of SURMOUNT-1, which recruited adults who were obese but without T2DM, tirzepatide use was associated with a significant reduction in predicted 10-year cardiometabolic risk score [164]. In terms of individual risk factors, tirzepatide leads to greater weight loss, improves glycemic control, and reduces blood pressure by up to 11.5 mmHg with the highest dose [165]. The ongoing SURPASS-CVOT trial will provide insights into the cardiovascular outcomes of tirzepatide against dulaglutide over 54 months of follow-up [166], while the SUMMIT trial will inform about the utility of tirzepatide in heart failure (NCT04847557).

In terms of renoprotection, tirzepatide was evaluated in the SURPASS-4 trial, in which subjects with CVD were recruited. The risk of a composite renal outcome, including progression to ESRD, new-onset macroalbuminuria and/or deterioration in renal function or renal-related mortality, was significantly reduced by 42% (hazard ratio 0.58; 95% CI 0.43–0.80) compared to glargine alone [167]. The molecular mechanisms in renoprotection have been primarily attributable to the direct effects of GLP1 receptor activation and the

The further evaluation of glimins in larger patient cohorts with longer follow-up is required to establish the additional cardiovascular and renal benefits beyond glucose-lowering.

2. Dual peroxisome proliferator-activated receptor (PPARα/γ) agonist

PPARs belong to the nuclear hormone receptor family essential to lipid and glucose metabolism [199]. Dual PPAR agonists combine the insulin-sensitizing effects of PPAR-alpha activation with the lipid-modifying properties of PPAR-gamma, making this agent potentially useful in treating diabetic dyslipidaemia. Aliglitazar, a dual PPAR agonist, had previously shown promising results in glucose-lowering. In a pooled analysis of data from 3 RCTs comprising 591 subjects, aliglitazar use was associated with a 1.08% reduction in HbA1c compared to 0.22% with placebo [200]. However, the development of aliglitazar was terminated after the AleCardio phase III trial showed a lack of efficacy and increased risk of heart failure, renal dysfunction and gastrointestinal haemorrhage [201]. On the other hand, saroglitazar, a newer dual PPAR agonist, has been approved for use in India since 2013 [202] and Mexico [203] following successful clinical trials. In the PRESS trials, saroglitzar was shown to reduce triglyceride by up to 45%, along with improvements in glycemic control [204,205]. Saroglitazar may address residual cardiovascular risks associated with high non-HDL cholesterol [206] and small, dense LDL cholesterol commonly observed in diabetic dyslipidaemia [207]. Given the potential role of saroglitazar in NAFLD, a phase 4 study that aims to recruit 1500 subjects with NAFLD with comorbidities such as T2DM, dyslipidaemia or metabolic syndrome was commenced in India in 2023 (NCT05872269) [208]. Although not reported to cause cardiovascular complications, it would be prudent to avoid or use dual PPAR agonists cautiously in patients with a history of congestive cardiac failure [209].

Apart from PPAR dual agonist, a pan-PPAR agonist targeting PPAR alpha/delta/gamma has been developed and recently approved for use in patients with T2DM and non-alcoholic steatohepatitis in China [210]. In a phase III trial, chiglitazar significantly improved insulin sensitivity and HOMA-IR compared to placebo or sitagliptin over 24 weeks of treatment [211]. Regarding lipid profiles, chiglitazar reduced triglycerides but increased LDL-cholesterol after 24 weeks of treatment [212]. A phase 3 trial is ongoing to assess the efficacy and safety of chglitazar as an add-on to metformin in China (NCT04807348) [213].

3. Glucokinase activator

Glucokinase is an enzyme that functions as a glucose sensor for stimulating insulin secretion and reducing fasting and postprandial glucose [214]. In T2DM, glucokinase expression is significantly reduced, resulting in an attenuated glucose sensitivity [215]. Therefore, glucokinase activators (GKAs) represent a novel class of antihyperglycemic agents that can potentially stimulate insulin secretion and promote hepatic glucose uptake in response to varying glycemic levels [216]. Partial, hepatoselective glucokinase activation reduces hypoglycemia risk [216].

Dorzagliatin, a mixed hepatopancreatic GKA, was shown to reduce HbA1c by 1.12% in the 75 mg twice-daily group compared to placebo [217]. There were no serious adverse events, and the incidence of adverse events or hypoglycemia was similar to that of the placebo [217]. Dorzaglipatin has progressed to a phase III trial, which showed that patients receiving dorzagliptin and metformin had a 1.07% decrease in HbA1c, compared to 0.5% for placebo [218]. However, dorzagliatin was associated with a significant elevation of triglycerides and body weight compared to placebo [219]. Further evaluation in longer clinical trials with active comparators is warranted to determine the long-term utility of GKAs.

PB-201 is a partial hepatopancreatic GKA that is investigated in clinical trials in China [220]. In a phase 1 trial, PB-201 100 mg twice daily reduced HbA1c by up to 1.9% [221]. In a phase 2 study, HbA1c levels reduction after 2 weeks of PB-201 was similar compared to sitagliptin [220]. PB-201 has progressed to phase 3, and an ongoing trial among 672 Chinese participants will aim to assess its safety and efficacy compared with vildagliptin and placebo over 24 weeks [220].

4. G-protein coupled receptor 40 (GPR40) agonist

The activation of GPR40 stimulates insulin secretion [222], making this a potential target for T2DM. Expressed in the pancreatic beta cells, the activation of GPR40 promotes glucose-dependent insulin secretion and ensures glucose concentration remains regulated in physiological concentrations while minimizing hypoglycemia [223]. Despite efficacy in postprandial glucose control comparable to glimepiride, earlier GPR 40 compounds such as fasiglifam (TAK-875) had been terminated due to idiosyncratic drug-induced liver injury [224]. It was postulated that fasiglifam inhibited biliary transporters, resulting in bile acid accumulation in the liver [225]. Furthermore, it was also postulated that mitochondrial dysfunction induced by the earlier GPR40 agents contributed to hepatic adverse effects [225].

CPL207280, the latest GPR40 agonist, was carefully designed to address potential safety concerns. In human hepatocyte cultures, CPL207280 had a negligible effect on hepatic mitochondria, and no deleterious hepatic effects were observed, suggesting the DILI observed with TAK-875 could be drug-specific and not a class-specific adverse effect [225]. In a phase 1 study, 14 days of CPL207280 administration was safe and well tolerated by healthy volunteers [226].

Figure 8 illustrates selected novel glucose-lowering agents. Supplementary Table S8 provides information on recently completed [220,226–232] and ongoing early-phase clinical trials involving novel glucose-lowering agents.

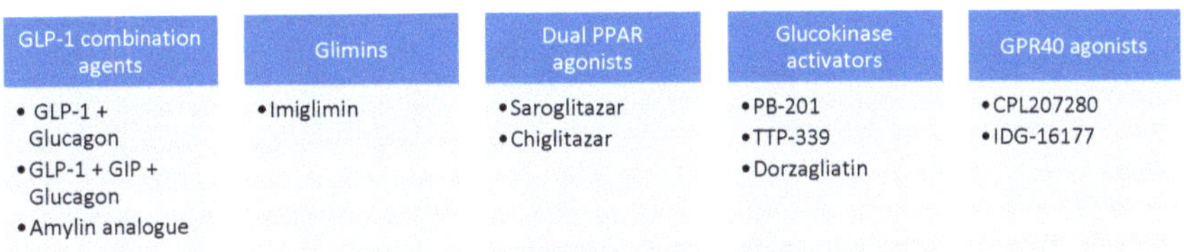

Figure 8. Novel glucose-lowering agents in early-phase clinical trials.

6. Future Directions and Conclusions

Looking back at the past decade, the release of the EMPA-REG trial results was a pivotal point that heralded a paradigm shift in the management of T2DM. The focus of T2DM management has shifted from a glucose-centric approach to one that comprehensively mitigates cardiovascular and renal risks. Over the past decade, there have been significant advances in the treatment of T2DM, with several new antidiabetic agents demonstrating robust cardiorenal benefits. The indications for these agents have since expanded to treat heart failure and kidney disease in patients without T2DM.

The management of T2DM is evolving rapidly, with more than 400 early-phase interventional studies registered on clinical trial platforms. In the coming decade, the focus will be on testing these novel agents via high-quality clinical trials with adequate participant retention and follow-up to assess their long-term efficacy. Trials that compare novel agents against placebo will be insufficient, and active comparators need to be carefully selected to meet the new standards of care in T2DM management. Intensive research into the synergistic effects of combination agents targeting different mechanisms in glycemic control and cardiorenal protection will yield further insight into the clinical efficacy and cost-effectiveness of such approaches.

Supplementary Materials: The following supporting information can be downloaded at: https://www.mdpi.com/article/10.3390/biomedicines12071386/s1, Table S1: Selected studies evaluating the effect of SGLT2 inhibitors on physiological vascular measurements; Table S2: Selected studies evaluating the effects of SGLT2 inhibitors on inflammatory, oxidative stress and thrombosis markers; Table S3: Selected studies evaluating the effect of SGLT2 inhibitors on cardiac biomarkers; Table S4: Selected studies of SGLT2 inhibitors and renal biomarkers; Table S5: Selected studies of GLP1-RAs and the effects on physiological vascular measurements; Table S6: Effects of GLP-1 RAs on vascular and cardiac biomarkers; Table S7: (a) Completed trials for tirzepatide in T2DM patients, (b) Tirzepatide trials for obesity, (c) Ongoing tirzepatide trials; Table S8: Selected ongoing early phase or recently completed trials involving novel antidiabetic agents. References [233–236] are cited in the supplementary materials.

Author Contributions: Conceptualization, Y.J.C. and R.D.; methodology, Y.J.C. and R.D.; data curation, Y.J.C.; writing—original draft preparation, Y.J.C.; writing—review and editing, Y.J.C. and R.D.; supervision, R.D. All authors have read and agreed to the published version of the manuscript.

Funding: This work is supported by the Transforming Vascular Health Program and the Personalized Cardiometabolic Risk Management Program funded by National Healthcare Group and Ng Teng Fong Foundation, respectively.

Institutional Review Board Statement: Not applicable.

Informed Consent Statement: Not applicable.

Data Availability Statement: No new data were created or analyzed in this study. Data sharing is not applicable to this article.

Conflicts of Interest: The authors declare no conflicts of interest.

References

1. Nathan, D.M.; Meigs, J.; Singer, D.E. The epidemiology of cardiovascular disease in type 2 diabetes mellitus: How sweet it is... or is it? *Lancet* **1997**, *350* (Suppl. 1), SI4–SI9. [CrossRef] [PubMed]
2. Lindstrom, M.; DeCleene, N.; Dorsey, H.; Fuster, V.; Johnson, C.O.; LeGrand, K.E.; Mensah, G.A.; Razo, C.; Stark, B.; Turco, J.V.; et al. Global Burden of Cardiovascular Diseases and Risks Collaboration, 1990–2021. *J. Am. Coll. Cardiol.* **2022**, *80*, 2372–2425. [CrossRef] [PubMed]
3. Einarson, T.R.; Acs, A.; Ludwig, C.; Panton, U.H. Prevalence of cardiovascular disease in type 2 diabetes: A systematic literature review of scientific evidence from across the world in 2007-2017. *Cardiovasc. Diabetol.* **2018**, *17*, 83. [CrossRef] [PubMed]
4. Turner, R.; Cull, C.; Holman, R. United Kingdom Prospective Diabetes Study 17: A 9-year update of a randomized, controlled trial on the effect of improved metabolic control on complications in non-insulin-dependent diabetes mellitus. *Ann. Intern. Med.* **1996**, *124 Pt 2*, 136–145. [CrossRef] [PubMed]
5. Diabetes Control and Complications Trial Research Group; Nathan, D.M.; Genuth, S.; Lachin, J.; Cleary, P.; Crofford, O.; Davis, M.; Rand, L.; Siebert, C. The effect of intensive treatment of diabetes on the development and progression of long-term complications in insulin-dependent diabetes mellitus. *N. Engl. J. Med.* **1993**, *329*, 977–986. [CrossRef] [PubMed]
6. Zinman, B.; Wanner, C.; Lachin, J.M.; Fitchett, D.; Bluhmki, E.; Hantel, S.; Mattheus, M.; Devins, T.; Johansen, O.E.; Woerle, H.J.; et al. Empagliflozin, Cardiovascular Outcomes, and Mortality in Type 2 Diabetes. *N. Engl. J. Med.* **2015**, *373*, 2117–2128. [CrossRef] [PubMed]
7. Marso, S.P.; Daniels, G.H.; Brown-Frandsen, K.; Kristensen, P.; Mann, J.F.E.; Nauck, M.A.; Nissen, S.E.; Pocock, S.; Poulter, N.R.; Ravn, L.S.; et al. Liraglutide and Cardiovascular Outcomes in Type 2 Diabetes. *N. Engl. J. Med.* **2016**, *375*, 311–322. [CrossRef] [PubMed]
8. Lo, C.W.H.; Fei, Y.; Cheung, B.M.Y. Cardiovascular Outcomes in Trials of New Antidiabetic Drug Classes. *Card. Fail. Rev.* **2021**, *7*, e04. [CrossRef] [PubMed]
9. Giaccari, A.; Pontremoli, R.; Filardi, P.P. SGLT-2 inhibitors for treatment of heart failure in patients with and without type 2 diabetes: A practical approach for routine clinical practice. *Int. J. Cardiol.* **2022**, *351*, 66–70. [CrossRef]
10. Roddick, A.J.; Wonnacott, A.; Webb, D.; Watt, A.; Watson, M.A.; Staplin, N.; Riding, A.; Lioudaki, E.; Kuverji, A.; El Kossi, M.; et al. UK Kidney Association Clinical Practice Guideline: Sodium-Glucose Co-transporter-2 (SGLT-2) Inhibition in Adults with Kidney Disease 2023 UPDATE. *BMC Nephrol* **2023**, *24*, 310. [CrossRef]
11. Arnold, S.V.; Tang, F.; Cooper, A.; Chen, H.; Gomes, M.B.; Rathmann, W.; Shimomura, I.; Vora, J.; Watada, H.; Khunti, K.; et al. Global use of SGLT2 inhibitors and GLP-1 receptor agonists in type 2 diabetes. Results from DISCOVER. *BMC Endocr. Disord.* **2022**, *22*, 111. [CrossRef] [PubMed]
12. Haffner, S.M.; Stern, M.P.; Hazuda, H.P.; Mitchell, B.D.; Patterson, J.K. Cardiovascular risk factors in confirmed prediabetic individuals. Does the clock for coronary heart disease start ticking before the onset of clinical diabetes? *JAMA* **1990**, *263*, 2893–2898. [CrossRef] [PubMed]
13. Mahaffey, K.W.; Jardine, M.J.; Bompoint, S.; Cannon, C.P.; Neal, B.; Heerspink, H.J.; Charytan, D.M.; Edwards, R.; Agarwal, R.; Bakris, G.; et al. Canagliflozin and Cardiovascular and Renal Outcomes in Type 2 Diabetes Mellitus and Chronic Kidney Disease in Primary and Secondary Cardiovascular Prevention Groups. *Circulation* **2019**, *140*, 739–750. [CrossRef] [PubMed]
14. Wiviott, S.D.; Raz, I.; Bonaca, M.P.; Mosenzon, O.; Kato, E.T.; Cahn, A.; Silverman, M.G.; Zelniker, T.A.; Kuder, J.F.; Murphy, S.A.; et al. Dapagliflozin and Cardiovascular Outcomes in Type 2 Diabetes. *N. Engl. J. Med.* **2019**, *380*, 347–357. [CrossRef] [PubMed]

15. Cannon, C.P.; Pratley, R.; Dagogo-Jack, S.; Mancuso, J.; Huyck, S.; Masiukiewicz, U.; Charbonnel, B.; Frederich, R.; Gallo, S.; Cosentino, F.; et al. Cardiovascular Outcomes with Ertugliflozin in Type 2 Diabetes. *N. Engl. J. Med.* **2020**, *383*, 1425–1435. [CrossRef] [PubMed]
16. McMurray, J.J.V.; Solomon, S.D.; Inzucchi, S.E.; Køber, L.; Kosiborod, M.N.; Martinez, F.A.; Ponikowski, P.; Sabatine, M.S.; Anand, I.S.; Bělohlávek, J.; et al. Dapagliflozin in Patients with Heart Failure and Reduced Ejection Fraction. *N. Engl. J. Med.* **2019**, *381*, 1995–2008. [CrossRef] [PubMed]
17. Packer, M.; Anker, S.D.; Butler, J.; Filippatos, G.; Pocock, S.J.; Carson, P.; Januzzi, J.; Verma, S.; Tsutsui, H.; Brueckmann, M.; et al. Cardiovascular and Renal Outcomes with Empagliflozin in Heart Failure. *N. Engl. J. Med.* **2020**, *383*, 1413–1424. [CrossRef]
18. Anker, S.D.; Butler, J.; Filippatos, G.; Ferreira, J.P.; Bocchi, E.; Böhm, M.; Brunner–La Rocca, H.-P.; Choi, D.-J.; Chopra, V.; Chuquiure-Valenzuela, E.; et al. Empagliflozin in Heart Failure with a Preserved Ejection Fraction. *N. Engl. J. Med.* **2021**, *385*, 1451–1461. [CrossRef] [PubMed]
19. Solomon, S.D.; McMurray, J.J.; Claggett, B.; de Boer, R.A.; DeMets, D.; Hernandez, A.F.; Inzucchi, S.E.; Kosiborod, M.N.; Lam, C.S.; Martinez, F.; et al. Dapagliflozin in Heart Failure with Mildly Reduced or Preserved Ejection Fraction. *N. Engl. J. Med.* **2022**, *387*, 1089–1098. [CrossRef]
20. Patoulias, D.; Papadopoulos, C.; Kassimis, G.; Vassilikos, V.; Karagiannis, A.; Doumas, M. Meta-Analysis Addressing the Effect of Sodium-Glucose Cotransporter 2 Inhibitors on Flow-Mediated Dilation in Patients With Type 2 Diabetes Mellitus. *Am. J. Cardiol.* **2022**, *165*, 133–135. [CrossRef]
21. Gohari, S.; Ismail-Beigi, F.; Mahjani, M.; Ghobadi, S.; Jafari, A.; Ahangar, H.; Gohari, S. The effect of sodium-glucose co-transporter-2 (SGLT2) inhibitors on blood interleukin-6 concentration: A systematic review and meta-analysis of randomized controlled trials. *BMC Endocr. Disord.* **2023**, *23*, 257. [CrossRef]
22. Schönberger, E.; Mihaljević, V.; Steiner, K.; Šarić, S.; Kurevija, T.; Majnarić, L.T.; Bilić Ćurčić, I.; Canecki-Varžić, S. Immunomodulatory Effects of SGLT2 Inhibitors-Targeting Inflammation and Oxidative Stress in Aging. *Int. J. Environ. Res. Public. Health* **2023**, *20*, 6671. [CrossRef]
23. Gohari, S.; Reshadmanesh, T.; Khodabandehloo, H.; Karbalaee-Hasani, A.; Ahangar, H.; Arsang-Jang, S.; Ismail-Beigi, F.; Dadashi, M.; Ghanbari, S.; Taheri, H.; et al. The effect of EMPAgliflozin on markers of inflammation in patients with concomitant type 2 diabetes mellitus and Coronary ARtery Disease: The EMPA-CARD randomized controlled trial. *Diabetol. Metab. Syndr.* **2022**, *14*, 170. [CrossRef]
24. Taheri, H.; Chiti, H.; Reshadmanesh, T.; Gohari, S.; Jalilvand, A.; Arsang-Jang, S.; Ismail-Beigi, F.; Ghanbari, S.; Dadashi, M.; Asgari, A.; et al. Empagliflozin improves high-sensitive cardiac troponin-I and high-density lipoprotein cholesterol in patients with type 2 diabetes mellitus and coronary artery disease: A post-hoc analysis of EMPA-CARD Trial. *J. Diabetes Metab. Disord.* **2023**, *22*, 1723–1730. [CrossRef] [PubMed]
25. Pascual-Figal, D.A.; Zamorano, J.L.; Domingo, M.; Morillas, H.; Nuñez, J.; Marcos, M.C.; Riquelme-Pérez, A.; Teis, A.; Santas, E.; Caro-Martinez, C.; et al. Impact of dapagliflozin on cardiac remodelling in patients with chronic heart failure: The DAPA-MODA study. *Eur. J. Heart Fail.* **2023**, *25*, 1352–1360. [CrossRef]
26. Januzzi, J.L., Jr.; Butler, J.; Jarolim, P.; Sattar, N.; Vijapurkar, U.; Desai, M.; Davies, M.J. Effects of Canagliflozin on Cardiovascular Biomarkers in Older Adults With Type 2 Diabetes. *J. Am. Coll. Cardiol.* **2017**, *70*, 704–712. [CrossRef]
27. Mudau, M.; Genis, A.; Lochner, A.; Strijdom, H. Endothelial dysfunction: The early predictor of atherosclerosis. *Cardiovasc. J. Afr.* **2012**, *23*, 222–231. [CrossRef] [PubMed]
28. Kim, H.L.; Kim, S.H. Pulse Wave Velocity in Atherosclerosis. *Front. Cardiovasc. Med.* **2019**, *6*, 41. [CrossRef]
29. Shigiyama, F.; Kumashiro, N.; Miyagi, M.; Ikehara, K.; Kanda, E.; Uchino, H.; Hirose, T. Effectiveness of dapagliflozin on vascular endothelial function and glycemic control in patients with early-stage type 2 diabetes mellitus: DEFENCE study. *Cardiovasc. Diabetol.* **2017**, *16*, 84. [CrossRef] [PubMed]
30. Wei, R.; Wang, W.; Pan, Q.; Guo, L. Effects of SGLT-2 Inhibitors on Vascular Endothelial Function and Arterial Stiffness in Subjects With Type 2 Diabetes: A Systematic Review and Meta-Analysis of Randomized Controlled Trials. *Front. Endocrinol.* **2022**, *13*, 826604. [CrossRef]
31. Wang, Y.; Yao, M.; Wang, J.; Liu, H.; Zhang, X.; Zhao, L.; Hu, X.; Guan, H.; Lyu, Z. Effects of Antidiabetic Drugs on Endothelial Function in Patients With Type 2 Diabetes Mellitus: A Bayesian Network Meta-Analysis. *Front. Endocrinol.* **2022**, *13*, 818537. [CrossRef]
32. Tochiya, M.; Makino, H.; Tamanaha, T.; Matsuo, M.; Hishida, A.; Koezuka, R.; Ohata, Y.; Tomita, T.; Son, C.; Miyamoto, Y.; et al. Effect of tofogliflozin on cardiac and vascular endothelial function in patients with type 2 diabetes and heart diseases: A pilot study. *J. Diabetes Investig.* **2020**, *11*, 400–404. [CrossRef] [PubMed]
33. Kang, S.M.; Yun, H.M.; Sohn, M.; Lim, S. Vascular and metabolic effects of ipragliflozin versus sitagliptin (IVS) in type 2 diabetes treated with sulphonylurea and metformin: IVS study. *Diabetes Obes. Metab.* **2023**, *25*, 1922–1931. [CrossRef]
34. Sugiyama, S.; Jinnouchi, H.; Kurinami, N.; Hieshima, K.; Yoshida, A.; Jinnouchi, K.; Nishimura, H.; Suzuki, T.; Miyamoto, F.; Kajiwara, K.; et al. The SGLT2 Inhibitor Dapagliflozin Significantly Improves the Peripheral Microvascular Endothelial Function in Patients with Uncontrolled Type 2 Diabetes Mellitus. *Intern. Med.* **2018**, *57*, 2147–2156. [CrossRef]
35. Salvatore, T.; Caturano, A.; Galiero, R.; Di Martino, A.; Albanese, G.; Vetrano, E.; Sardu, C.; Marfella, R.; Rinaldi, L.; Sasso, F.C. Cardiovascular Benefits from Gliflozins: Effects on Endothelial Function. *Biomedicines* **2021**, *9*, 1356. [CrossRef]

36. Cai, C.; Guo, Z.; Chang, X.; Li, Z.; Wu, F.; He, J.; Cao, T.; Wang, K.; Shi, N.; Zhou, H.; et al. Empagliflozin attenuates cardiac microvascular ischemia/reperfusion through activating the AMPKα1/ULK1/FUNDC1/mitophagy pathway. *Redox Biol.* **2022**, *52*, 102288. [CrossRef]
37. Ma, L.; Zou, R.; Shi, W.; Zhou, N.; Chen, S.; Zhou, H.; Chen, X.; Wu, Y. SGLT2 inhibitor dapagliflozin reduces endothelial dysfunction and microvascular damage during cardiac ischemia/reperfusion injury through normalizing the XO-SERCA2-CaMKII-coffilin pathways. *Theranostics* **2022**, *12*, 5034–5050. [CrossRef] [PubMed]
38. Uthman, L.; Baartscheer, A.; Bleijlevens, B.; Schumacher, C.A.; Fiolet, J.W.T.; Koeman, A.; Jancev, M.; Hollmann, M.W.; Weber, N.C.; Coronel, R.; et al. Class effects of SGLT2 inhibitors in mouse cardiomyocytes and hearts: Inhibition of Na^+/H^+ exchanger, lowering of cytosolic Na^+ and vasodilation. *Diabetologia* **2018**, *61*, 722–726. [CrossRef] [PubMed]
39. Ben-Shlomo, Y.; Spears, M.; Boustred, C.; May, M.; Anderson, S.; Benjamin, E.; Boutouyrie, P.; Cameron, J.; Chen, C.-H.; Cruickshank, J.K.; et al. Aortic pulse wave velocity improves cardiovascular event prediction: An individual participant meta-analysis of prospective observational data from 17,635 subjects. *J. Am. Coll. Cardiol.* **2014**, *63*, 636–646. [CrossRef]
40. Wang, J.; Wang, Y.; Wang, Y.; Li, Y.; Zhang, J.; Zhang, H.; Fu, X.; Guo, Z.; Yang, Y.; Kang, K.; et al. Effects of first-line antidiabetic drugs on the improvement of arterial stiffness: A Bayesian network meta-analysis. *J. Diabetes* **2023**, *15*, 685–698. [CrossRef]
41. Katakami, N.; Mita, T.; Yoshii, H.; Shiraiwa, T.; Yasuda, T.; Okada, Y.; Kurozumi, A.; Hatazaki, M.; Kaneto, H.; Osonoi, T.; et al. Tofogliflozin long-term effects on atherosclerosis progression and major clinical parameters in patients with type 2 diabetes mellitus lacking a history of cardiovascular disease: A 2-year extension study of the UTOPIA trial. *Cardiovasc. Diabetol.* **2023**, *22*, 143. [CrossRef] [PubMed]
42. Gaspari, T.; Spizzo, I.; Liu, H.; Hu, Y.; Simpson, R.W.; Widdop, R.E.; Dear, A.E. Dapagliflozin attenuates human vascular endothelial cell activation and induces vasorelaxation: A potential mechanism for inhibition of atherogenesis. *Diab Vasc. Dis. Res.* **2018**, *15*, 64–73. [CrossRef] [PubMed]
43. Aragón-Herrera, A.; Moraña-Fernández, S.; Otero-Santiago, M.; Anido-Varela, L.; Campos-Toimil, M.; García-Seara, J.; Román, A.; Seijas, J.; García-Caballero, L.; Rodríguez, J.; et al. The lipidomic and inflammatory profiles of visceral and subcutaneous adipose tissues are distinctly regulated by the SGLT2 inhibitor empagliflozin in Zucker diabetic fatty rats. *Biomed. Pharmacother.* **2023**, *161*, 114535. [CrossRef] [PubMed]
44. Yang, L.; Zhang, X.; Wang, Q. Effects and mechanisms of SGLT2 inhibitors on the NLRP3 inflammasome, with a focus on atherosclerosis. *Front. Endocrinol.* **2022**, *13*, 992937. [CrossRef] [PubMed]
45. Lee, S.-G.; Kim, S.H.; Kim, J.H.; Choi, E.; Cho, W.; Rim, J.H.; Hwang, I.; Lee, C.J.; Lee, M.; Oh, C.-M.; et al. SGLT2 inhibition modulates NLRP3 inflammasome activity via ketones and insulin in diabetes with cardiovascular disease. *Nat. Commun.* **2020**, *11*, 2127. [CrossRef]
46. Wang, C.; Qin, Y.; Zhang, X.; Yang, Y.; Wu, X.; Liu, J.; Qin, S.; Chen, K.; Xiao, W. Effect of Dapagliflozin on Indicators of Myocardial Fibrosis and Levels of Inflammatory Factors in Heart Failure Patients. *Dis. Markers* **2022**, *2022*, 5834218. [CrossRef] [PubMed]
47. Wang, D.; Liu, J.; Zhong, L.; Li, S.; Zhou, L.; Zhang, Q.; Li, M.; Xiao, X. The effect of sodium-glucose cotransporter 2 inhibitors on biomarkers of inflammation: A systematic review and meta-analysis of randomized controlled trials. *Front. Pharmacol.* **2022**, *13*, 1045235. [CrossRef] [PubMed]
48. Buttice, L.; Ghani, M.; Suthakar, J.; Gnanalingham, S.; Carande, E.; Kennedy, B.W.C.; Pitcher, A.; Gamble, J.H.P.; Ahmad, M.; Lewis, A.; et al. The effect of sodium-glucose cotransporter-2 inhibitors on inflammatory biomarkers: A meta-analysis of randomized controlled trials. *Diabetes Obes. Metab.* 2024; *ahead of print*. [CrossRef]
49. Cook-Mills, J.M.; Marchese, M.E.; Abdala-Valencia, H. Vascular cell adhesion molecule-1 expression and signaling during disease: Regulation by reactive oxygen species and antioxidants. *Antioxid. Redox Signal* **2011**, *15*, 1607–1638. [CrossRef] [PubMed]
50. Deem, T.L.; Cook-Mills, J.M. Vascular cell adhesion molecule 1 (VCAM-1) activation of endothelial cell matrix metalloproteinases: Role of reactive oxygen species. *Blood* **2004**, *104*, 2385–2393. [CrossRef]
51. Vacek, T.P.; Rehman, S.; Neamtu, D.; Yu, S.; Givimani, S.; Tyagi, S.C. Matrix metalloproteinases in atherosclerosis: Role of nitric oxide, hydrogen sulfide, homocysteine, and polymorphisms. *Vasc. Health Risk Manag.* **2015**, *11*, 173–183. [CrossRef]
52. Nowak, W.N.; Deng, J.; Ruan, X.Z.; Xu, Q. Reactive Oxygen Species Generation and Atherosclerosis. *Arter. Thromb. Vasc. Biol.* **2017**, *37*, e41–e52. [CrossRef] [PubMed]
53. Palma, F.R.; He, C.; Danes, J.M.; Paviani, V.; Coelho, D.R.; Gantner, B.N.; Bonini, M.G. Mitochondrial Superoxide Dismutase: What the Established, the Intriguing, and the Novel Reveal About a Key Cellular Redox Switch. *Antioxid. Redox Signal* **2020**, *32*, 701–714. [CrossRef] [PubMed]
54. Tsai, K.F.; Chen, Y.L.; Chiou, T.T.; Chu, T.H.; Li, L.C.; Ng, H.Y.; Lee, W.C.; Lee, C.T. Emergence of SGLT2 Inhibitors as Powerful Antioxidants in Human Diseases. *Antioxidants* **2021**, *10*, 1166. [CrossRef] [PubMed]
55. Iannantuoni, F.; de Marañon, A.M.; Diaz-Morales, N.; Falcon, R.; Bañuls, C.; Abad-Jimenez, Z.; Victor, V.M.; Hernandez-Mijares, A.; Rovira-Llopis, S. The SGLT2 Inhibitor Empagliflozin Ameliorates the Inflammatory Profile in Type 2 Diabetic Patients and Promotes an Antioxidant Response in Leukocytes. *J. Clin. Med.* **2019**, *8*, 1814. [CrossRef] [PubMed]
56. Gawaz, M.; Langer, H.; May, A.E. Platelets in inflammation and atherogenesis. *J. Clin. Investig.* **2005**, *115*, 3378–3384. [CrossRef] [PubMed]
57. Coenen, D.M.; Mastenbroek, T.G.; Cosemans, J.M.E.M. Platelet interaction with activated endothelium: Mechanistic insights from microfluidics. *Blood* **2017**, *130*, 2819–2828. [CrossRef]

58. Hamilos, M.; Petousis, S.; Parthenakis, F. Interaction between platelets and endothelium: From pathophysiology to new therapeutic options. *Cardiovasc. Diagn. Ther.* **2018**, *8*, 568–580. [CrossRef]
59. Nording, H.; Baron, L.; Langer, H.F. Platelets as therapeutic targets to prevent atherosclerosis. *Atherosclerosis* **2020**, *307*, 97–108. [CrossRef] [PubMed]
60. Kohlmorgen, C.; Gerfer, S.; Feldmann, K.; Twarock, S.; Hartwig, S.; Lehr, S.; Klier, M.; Krüger, I.; Helten, C.; Keul, P.; et al. Dapagliflozin reduces thrombin generation and platelet activation: Implications for cardiovascular risk reduction in type 2 diabetes mellitus. *Diabetologia* **2021**, *64*, 1834–1849. [CrossRef]
61. Hegazy, S.; Elsabaawy, M.; Eltabakh, M.; Hammad, R.; Bedair, H. CD62P (P-selectin) expression as a platelet activation marker in patients with liver cirrhosis with and without cholestasis. *Clin. Exp. Hepatol.* **2021**, *7*, 231–240. [CrossRef]
62. Wang, L.; Tang, C. Targeting Platelet in Atherosclerosis Plaque Formation: Current Knowledge and Future Perspectives. *Int. J. Mol. Sci.* **2020**, *21*, 9760. [CrossRef] [PubMed]
63. Weber, M.; Hamm, C. Role of B-type natriuretic peptide (BNP) and NT-proBNP in clinical routine. *Heart* **2006**, *92*, 843–849. [CrossRef] [PubMed]
64. Januzzi, J.L.; Xu, J.; Li, J.; Shaw, W.; Oh, R.; Pfeifer, M.; Butler, J.; Sattar, N.; Mahaffey, K.W.; Neal, B.; et al. Effects of Canagliflozin on Amino-Terminal Pro-B-Type Natriuretic Peptide: Implications for Cardiovascular Risk Reduction. *J. Am. Coll. Cardiol.* **2020**, *76*, 2076–2085. [CrossRef] [PubMed]
65. Joshi, S.S.; Singh, T.; Newby, D.E.; Singh, J. Sodium-glucose co-transporter 2 inhibitor therapy: Mechanisms of action in heart failure. *Heart* **2021**, *107*, 1032–1038. [CrossRef] [PubMed]
66. Gamaza-Chulián, S.; Díaz-Retamino, E.; González-Testón, F.; Gaitero, J.C.; Castillo, M.J.; Alfaro, R.; Rodríguez, E.; González-Caballero, E.; Martín-Santana, A. Effect of sodium-glucose cotransporter 2 (SGLT2) inhibitors on left ventricular remodelling and longitudinal strain: A prospective observational study. *BMC Cardiovasc. Disord.* **2021**, *21*, 456. [CrossRef] [PubMed]
67. Tang, O.; Matsushita, K.; Coresh, J.; Ndumele, C.; McEvoy, J.W.; Sharrett, A.R.; Hoogeveen, R.; Ballantyne, C.M.; Selvin, E. High-Sensitivity Cardiac Troponin I and T for Cardiovascular Risk Stratification in Adults With Diabetes. *Diabetes Care* **2020**, *43*, e144–e146. [CrossRef] [PubMed]
68. Maejima, Y. SGLT2 Inhibitors Play a Salutary Role in Heart Failure via Modulation of the Mitochondrial Function. *Front. Cardiovasc. Med.* **2020**, *6*, 186. [CrossRef] [PubMed]
69. Leccisotti, L.; Cinti, F.; Sorice, G.P.; D'amario, D.; Lorusso, M.; Guzzardi, M.A.; Mezza, T.; Gugliandolo, S.; Cocchi, C.; Capece, U.; et al. Dapagliflozin improves myocardial flow reserve in patients with type 2 diabetes: The DAPAHEART Trial: A preliminary report. *Cardiovasc. Diabetol.* **2022**, *21*, 173. [CrossRef] [PubMed]
70. Tian, J.; Zhang, M.; Suo, M.; Liu, D.; Wang, X.; Liu, M.; Pan, J.; Jin, T.; An, F. Dapagliflozin alleviates cardiac fibrosis through suppressing EndMT and fibroblast activation via AMPKα/TGF-β/Smad signalling in type 2 diabetic rats. *J. Cell Mol. Med.* **2021**, *25*, 7642–7659. [CrossRef]
71. EMPA-KIDNEY Collaborative Group. Impact of primary kidney disease on the effects of empagliflozin in patients with chronic kidney disease: Secondary analyses of the EMPA-KIDNEY trial. *Lancet Diabetes Endocrinol.* **2024**, *12*, 51–60. [CrossRef]
72. Heerspink, H.J.L.; Stefánsson, B.V.; Correa-Rotter, R.; Chertow, G.M.; Greene, T.; Hou, F.-F.; Mann, J.F.E.; McMurray, J.J.V.; Lindberg, M.; Rossing, P.; et al. Dapagliflozin in Patients with Chronic Kidney Disease. *N. Engl. J. Med.* **2020**, *383*, 1436–1446. [CrossRef]
73. Thomas, M.C.; Brownlee, M.; Susztak, K.; Sharma, K.; Jandeleit-Dahm, K.A.; Zoungas, S.; Rossing, P.; Groop, P.H.; Cooper, M.E. Diabetic kidney disease. *Nat. Rev. Dis. Primers* **2015**, *1*, 15018. [CrossRef] [PubMed]
74. Tian, Y.; Chen, X.M.; Liang, X.M.; Wu, X.B.; Yao, C.M. SGLT2 inhibitors attenuate nephrin loss and enhance TGF-β_1 secretion in type 2 diabetes patients with albuminuria: A randomized clinical trial. *Sci. Rep.* **2022**, *12*, 15695. [CrossRef] [PubMed]
75. Mesfine, B.B.; Vojisavljevic, D.; Kapoor, R.; Watson, D.; Kandasamy, Y.; Rudd, D. Urinary nephrin-a potential marker of early glomerular injury: A systematic review and meta-analysis. *J. Nephrol.* **2024**, *37*, 39–51. [CrossRef]
76. Sureshbabu, A.; Muhsin, S.A.; Choi, M.E. TGF-β signaling in the kidney: Profibrotic and protective effects. *Am. J. Physiol. Ren. Physiol.* **2016**, *310*, F596–F606. [CrossRef]
77. Heerspink, H.J.L.; Perco, P.; Mulder, S.; Leierer, J.; Hansen, M.K.; Heinzel, A.; Mayer, G. Canagliflozin reduces inflammation and fibrosis biomarkers: A potential mechanism of action for beneficial effects of SGLT2 inhibitors in diabetic kidney disease. *Diabetologia* **2019**, *62*, 1154–1166. [CrossRef] [PubMed]
78. Bolignano, D.; Donato, V.; Coppolino, G.; Campo, S.; Buemi, A.; Lacquaniti, A.; Buemi, M. Neutrophil gelatinase-associated lipocalin (NGAL) as a marker of kidney damage. *Am. J. Kidney Dis.* **2008**, *52*, 595–605. [CrossRef] [PubMed]
79. Ito, H.; Inoue, H.; Izutsu, T.; Matsumoto, S.; Antoku, S.; Yamasaki, T.; Mori, T.; Togane, M. Changes in the estimated glomerular filtration rate and predictors of the renal prognosis in Japanese patients with type 2 diabetes: A retrospective study during the 12 months after the initiation of tofogliflozin. *PLoS ONE* **2023**, *18*, e0292014. [CrossRef] [PubMed]
80. Noiri, E.; Doi, K.; Negishi, K.; Tanaka, T.; Hamasaki, Y.; Fujita, T.; Portilla, D.; Sugaya, T. Urinary fatty acid-binding protein 1: An early predictive biomarker of kidney injury. *Am. J. Physiol. Ren. Physiol.* **2009**, *296*, F669–F679. [CrossRef]
81. Takashima, H.; Yoshida, Y.; Nagura, C.; Furukawa, T.; Tei, R.; Maruyama, T.; Maruyama, N.; Abe, M. Renoprotective effects of canagliflozin, a sodium glucose cotransporter 2 inhibitor, in type 2 diabetes patients with chronic kidney disease: A randomized open-label prospective trial. *Diab Vasc. Dis. Res.* **2018**, *15*, 469–472. [CrossRef]

82. Sen, T.; Li, J.; Neuen, B.L.; Neal, B.; Arnott, C.; Parikh, C.R.; Coca, S.G.; Perkovic, V.; Mahaffey, K.W.; Yavin, Y.; et al. Effects of the SGLT2 inhibitor canagliflozin on plasma biomarkers TNFR-1, TNFR-2 and KIM-1 in the CANVAS trial. *Diabetologia* **2021**, *64*, 2147–2158. [CrossRef] [PubMed]
83. Song, J.; Yu, J.; Prayogo, G.W.; Cao, W.; Wu, Y.; Jia, Z.; Zhang, A. Understanding kidney injury molecule 1: A novel immune factor in kidney pathophysiology. *Am. J. Transl. Res.* **2019**, *11*, 1219–1229. [PubMed]
84. Liu, H.; Sridhar, V.S.; Lovblom, L.E.; Lytvyn, Y.; Burger, D.; Burns, K.; Brinc, D.; Lawler, P.R.; Cherney, D.Z.I. Markers of Kidney Injury, Inflammation, and Fibrosis Associated With Ertugliflozin in Patients With CKD and Diabetes. *Kidney Int. Rep.* **2021**, *6*, 2095–2104. [CrossRef] [PubMed]
85. Dekkers, C.C.J.; Petrykiv, S.; Laverman, G.D.; Cherney, D.Z.; Gansevoort, R.T.; Heerspink, H.J.L. Effects of the SGLT-2 inhibitor dapagliflozin on glomerular and tubular injury markers. *Diabetes Obes. Metab.* **2018**, *20*, 1988–1993. [CrossRef] [PubMed]
86. Nelinson, D.S.; Sosa, J.M.; Chilton, R.J. SGLT2 inhibitors: A narrative review of efficacy and safety. *J. Osteopath. Med.* **2021**, *121*, 229–239. [CrossRef] [PubMed]
87. Kang, M.; Heo, K.N.; Ah, Y.M.; Yang, B.R.; Lee, J.Y. Age- and sex-specific risk of urogenital infections in patients with type 2 diabetes treated with sodium-glucose co-transporter 2 inhibitors: A population-based self-controlled case-series study. *Maturitas* **2021**, *150*, 30–36. [CrossRef] [PubMed]
88. Toyama, T.; Neuen, B.L.; Jun, M.; Ohkuma, T.; Neal, B.; Jardine, M.J.; Heerspink, H.L.; Wong, M.G.; Ninomiya, T.; Wada, T.; et al. Effect of SGLT2 inhibitors on cardiovascular, renal and safety outcomes in patients with type 2 diabetes mellitus and chronic kidney disease: A systematic review and meta-analysis. *Diabetes Obes. Metab.* **2019**, *21*, 1237–1250. [CrossRef] [PubMed]
89. Donnan, J.R.; Grandy, C.A.; Chibrikov, E.; A Marra, C.; Aubrey-Bassler, K.; Johnston, K.; Swab, M.; Hache, J.; Curnew, D.; Nguyen, H.; et al. Comparative safety of the sodium glucose co-transporter 2 (SGLT2) inhibitors: A systematic review and meta-analysis. *BMJ Open* **2019**, *9*, e022577. [CrossRef] [PubMed]
90. Rieg, T.; Masuda, T.; Gerasimova, M.; Mayoux, E.; Platt, K.; Powell, D.R.; Thomson, S.C.; Koepsell, H.; Vallon, V. Increase in SGLT1-mediated transport explains renal glucose reabsorption during genetic and pharmacological SGLT2 inhibition in euglycemia. *Am. J. Physiol. Ren. Physiol.* **2014**, *306*, F188–F193. [CrossRef]
91. Rieg, T.; Vallon, V. Development of SGLT1 and SGLT2 inhibitors. *Diabetologia* **2018**, *61*, 2079–2086. [CrossRef]
92. Cefalo, C.M.A.; Cinti, F.; Moffa, S.; Impronta, F.; Sorice, G.P.; Mezza, T.; Pontecorvi, A.; Giaccari, A. Sotagliflozin, the first dual SGLT inhibitor: Current outlook and perspectives. *Cardiovasc. Diabetol.* **2019**, *18*, 20. [CrossRef] [PubMed]
93. Bhatt, D.L.; Szarek, M.; Pitt, B.; Cannon, C.P.; Leiter, L.A.; McGuire, D.K.; Lewis, J.B.; Riddle, M.C.; Inzucchi, S.E.; Kosiborod, M.N.; et al. Sotagliflozin in Patients with Diabetes and Chronic Kidney Disease. *N. Engl. J. Med.* **2021**, *384*, 129–139. [CrossRef] [PubMed]
94. Bhatt, D.L.; Szarek, M.; Steg, P.G.; Cannon, C.P.; Leiter, L.A.; McGuire, D.K.; Lewis, J.B.; Riddle, M.C.; Voors, A.A.; Metra, M.; et al. Sotagliflozin in Patients with Diabetes and Recent Worsening Heart Failure. *N. Engl. J. Med.* **2021**, *384*, 117–128. [CrossRef] [PubMed]
95. Aggarwal, R.; Bhatt, D.; Szarek, M.; Davies, M.; Banks, P.; Pitt, B.; Steg, P.G. Sotagliflozin Reduces Stroke Outcomes in Patients with Diabetes and Chronic Kidney Disease. *J. Am. Coll. Cardiol.* **2024**, *83* (Suppl. 13), 1733. [CrossRef]
96. Pitt, B.; Steg, G.; Leiter, L.A.; Bhatt, D.L. The Role of Combined SGLT1/SGLT2 Inhibition in Reducing the Incidence of Stroke and Myocardial Infarction in Patients with Type 2 Diabetes Mellitus. *Cardiovasc. Drugs Ther.* **2022**, *36*, 561–567. [CrossRef] [PubMed]
97. Pitt, B.; Bhatt, D.L.; Metra, M. Does SGLT1 inhibition add to the benefits of SGLT2 inhibition in the prevention and treatment of heart failure? *Eur. Heart J.* **2022**, *43*, 4754–4757. [CrossRef] [PubMed]
98. Müller, T.; Finan, B.; Bloom, S.; D'Alessio, D.; Drucker, D.; Flatt, P.; Fritsche, A.; Gribble, F.; Grill, H.; Habener, J.; et al. Glucagon-like peptide 1 (GLP-1). *Mol. Metab.* **2019**, *30*, 72–130. [CrossRef] [PubMed]
99. Mariam, Z.; Niazi, S.K. Glucagon-like peptide agonists: A prospective review. *Endocrinol. Diabetes Metab.* **2024**, *7*, e462. [CrossRef] [PubMed]
100. Bulum, T. Nephroprotective Properties of the Glucose-Dependent Insulinotropic Polypeptide (GIP) and Glucagon-like Peptide-1 (GLP-1) Receptor Agonists. *Biomedicines* **2022**, *10*, 2586. [CrossRef]
101. Andersen, A.; Lund, A.; Knop, F.K.; Vilsbøll, T. Glucagon-like peptide 1 in health and disease. *Nat. Rev. Endocrinol.* **2018**, *14*, 390–403. [CrossRef]
102. van Bloemendaal, L.; Kulve, J.S.T.; la Fleur, S.E.; Ijzerman, R.G.; Diamant, M. Effects of glucagon-like peptide 1 on appetite and body weight: Focus on the CNS. *J. Endocrinol.* **2014**, *221*, T1–T16. [CrossRef]
103. Bhavsar, S.; Mudaliar, S.; Cherrington, A. Evolution of exenatide as a diabetes therapeutic. *Curr. Diabetes Rev.* **2013**, *9*, 161–193. [CrossRef] [PubMed]
104. Kieffer, T.J.; McIntosh, C.H.; Pederson, R.A. Degradation of glucose-dependent insulinotropic polypeptide and truncated glucagon-like peptide 1 in vitro and in vivo by dipeptidyl peptidase IV. *Endocrinology* **1995**, *136*, 3585–3596. [CrossRef]
105. Barnett, A.H. Lixisenatide: Evidence for its potential use in the treatment of type 2 diabetes. *Core Evid.* **2011**, *6*, 67–79. [CrossRef]
106. Popoviciu, M.S.; Păduraru, L.; Yahya, G.; Metwally, K.; Cavalu, S. Emerging Role of GLP-1 Agonists in Obesity: A Comprehensive Review of Randomised Controlled Trials. *Int. J. Mol. Sci.* **2023**, *24*, 10449. [CrossRef]
107. Pi-Sunyer, X.; Astrup, A.; Fujioka, K.; Greenway, F.; Halpern, A.; Krempf, M.; Lau, D.C.; le Roux, C.W.; Violante Ortiz, R.; Jensen, C.B.; et al. A Randomized, Controlled Trial of 3.0 mg of Liraglutide in Weight Management. *N. Engl. J. Med.* **2015**, *373*, 11–22. [CrossRef] [PubMed]

108. Wilding, J.P.H.; Batterham, R.L.; Calanna, S.; Davies, M.; Van Gaal, L.F.; Lingvay, I.; McGowan, B.M.; Rosenstock, J.; Tran, M.T.D.; Wadden, T.A.; et al. Once-Weekly Semaglutide in Adults with Overweight or Obesity. *N. Engl. J. Med.* **2021**, *384*, 989–1002. [CrossRef]
109. Holman, R.R.; Bethel, M.A.; Mentz, R.J.; Thompson, V.P.; Lokhnygina, Y.; Buse, J.B.; Chan, J.C.; Choi, J.; Gustavson, S.M.; Iqbal, N.; et al. Effects of Once-Weekly Exenatide on Cardiovascular Outcomes in Type 2 Diabetes. *N. Engl. J. Med.* **2017**, *377*, 1228–1239. [CrossRef]
110. Pfeffer, M.A.; Claggett, B.; Diaz, R.; Dickstein, K.; Gerstein, H.C.; Køber, L.V.; Lawson, F.C.; Ping, L.; Wei, X.; Lewis, E.F.; et al. Lixisenatide in Patients with Type 2 Diabetes and Acute Coronary Syndrome. *N. Engl. J. Med.* **2015**, *373*, 2247–2257. [CrossRef] [PubMed]
111. Marso, S.P.; Bain, S.C.; Consoli, A.; Eliaschewitz, F.G.; Jódar, E.; Leiter, L.A.; Lingvay, I.; Rosenstock, J.; Seufert, J.; Warren, M.L.; et al. Semaglutide and Cardiovascular Outcomes in Patients with Type 2 Diabetes. *N. Engl. J. Med.* **2016**, *375*, 1834–1844. [CrossRef]
112. Gerstein, H.C.; Colhoun, H.M.; Dagenais, G.R.; Diaz, R.; Lakshmanan, M.; Pais, P.; Probstfield, J.; Riesmeyer, J.S.; Riddle, M.C.; Rydén, L.; et al. Dulaglutide and cardiovascular outcomes in type 2 diabetes (REWIND): A double-blind, randomised placebo-controlled trial. *Lancet* **2019**, *394*, 121–130. [CrossRef] [PubMed]
113. Marx, N.; Husain, M.; Lehrke, M.; Verma, S.; Sattar, N. GLP-1 Receptor Agonists for the Reduction of Atherosclerotic Cardiovascular Risk in Patients With Type 2 Diabetes. *Circulation* **2022**, *146*, 1882–1894. [CrossRef] [PubMed]
114. Bray, J.J.H.; Foster-Davies, H.; Salem, A.; Hoole, A.L.; Obaid, D.R.; Halcox, J.P.J.; Stephens, J.W. Glucagon-like peptide-1 receptor agonists improve biomarkers of inflammation and oxidative stress: A systematic review and meta-analysis of randomised controlled trials. *Diabetes Obes. Metab.* **2021**, *23*, 1806–1822. [CrossRef] [PubMed]
115. Mashayekhi, M.; Beckman, J.A.; Nian, H.; Garner, E.M.; Mayfield, D.; Devin, J.K.; Koethe, J.R.; Brown, J.D.; Cahill, K.N.; Yu, C.; et al. Comparative effects of weight loss and incretin-based therapies on vascular endothelial function, fibrinolysis and inflammation in individuals with obesity and prediabetes: A randomized controlled trial. *Diabetes Obes. Metab.* **2023**, *25*, 570–580. [CrossRef] [PubMed]
116. Wu, H.; Xiao, C.; Zhao, Y.; Yin, H.; Yu, M. Liraglutide Improves Endothelial Function via the mTOR Signaling Pathway. *J. Diabetes Res.* **2021**, *2021*, 2936667. [CrossRef] [PubMed]
117. Xie, D.; Li, Y.; Xu, M.; Zhao, X.; Chen, M. Effects of dulaglutide on endothelial progenitor cells and arterial elasticity in patients with type 2 diabetes mellitus. *Cardiovasc. Diabetol.* **2022**, *21*, 200. [CrossRef] [PubMed]
118. Yue, L.; Chen, S.; Ren, Q.; Niu, S.; Pan, X.; Chen, X.; Li, Z.; Chen, X. Effects of semaglutide on vascular structure and proteomics in high-fat diet-induced obese mice. *Front. Endocrinol.* **2022**, *13*, 995007. [CrossRef] [PubMed]
119. Hachuła, M.; Kosowski, M.; Ryl, S.; Basiak, M.; Okopień, B. Impact of Glucagon-Like Peptide 1 Receptor Agonists on Biochemical Markers of the Initiation of Atherosclerotic Process. *Int. J. Mol. Sci.* **2024**, *25*, 1854. [CrossRef] [PubMed]
120. Harrington, J.R. The role of MCP-1 in atherosclerosis. *Stem Cells* **2000**, *18*, 65–66. [CrossRef]
121. Pickett, J.R.; Wu, Y.; Zacchi, L.F.; Ta, H.T. Targeting endothelial vascular cell adhesion molecule-1 in atherosclerosis: Drug discovery and development of vascular cell adhesion molecule-1-directed novel therapeutics. *Cardiovasc. Res.* **2023**, *119*, 2278–2293. [CrossRef]
122. Chen, X.M.; Zhang, W.Q.; Tian, Y.; Wang, L.F.; Chen, C.C.; Qiu, C.M. Liraglutide suppresses non-esterified free fatty acids and soluble vascular cell adhesion molecule-1 compared with metformin in patients with recent-onset type 2 diabetes. *Cardiovasc. Diabetol.* **2018**, *17*, 53. [CrossRef] [PubMed]
123. Zhang, W.Q.; Tian, Y.; Chen, X.M.; Wang, L.F.; Chen, C.C.; Qiu, C.M. Liraglutide ameliorates beta-cell function, alleviates oxidative stress and inhibits low grade inflammation in young patients with new-onset type 2 diabetes. *Diabetol. Metab. Syndr.* **2018**, *10*, 91. [CrossRef] [PubMed]
124. Lankin, V.Z.; Tikhaze, A.K.; Melkumyants, A.M. Malondialdehyde as an Important Key Factor of Molecular Mechanisms of Vascular Wall Damage under Heart Diseases Development. *Int. J. Mol. Sci.* **2022**, *24*, 128. [CrossRef] [PubMed]
125. Thomas, M.C.; Coughlan, M.T.; Cooper, M.E. The postprandial actions of GLP-1 receptor agonists: The missing link for cardiovascular and kidney protection in type 2 diabetes. *Cell Metab.* **2023**, *35*, 253–273. [CrossRef] [PubMed]
126. Simeone, P.; Liani, R.; Tripaldi, R.; Di Castelnuovo, A.; Guagnano, M.T.; Tartaro, A.; Bonadonna, R.C.; Federico, V.; Cipollone, F.; Consoli, A.; et al. Thromboxane-Dependent Platelet Activation in Obese Subjects with Prediabetes or Early Type 2 Diabetes: Effects of Liraglutide- or Lifestyle Changes-Induced Weight Loss. *Nutrients* **2018**, *10*, 1872. [CrossRef] [PubMed]
127. Yang, X.; Qiang, Q.; Li, N.; Feng, P.; Wei, W.; Hölscher, C. Neuroprotective Mechanisms of Glucagon-Like Peptide-1-Based Therapies in Ischemic Stroke: An Update Based on Preclinical Research. *Front. Neurol.* **2022**, *13*, 844697. [CrossRef] [PubMed]
128. Gerstein, H.C.; Lee, S.F.; Paré, G.; Bethel, M.A.; Colhoun, H.M.; Hoover, A.; Lakshmanan, M.; Lin, Y.; Pirro, V.; Qian, H.R.; et al. Biomarker Changes Associated With Both Dulaglutide and Cardiovascular Events in the REWIND Randomized Controlled Trial: A Nested Case-Control Post Hoc Analysis. *Diabetes Care* **2023**, *46*, 1046–1051. [CrossRef]
129. Jorsal, A.; Kistorp, C.; Holmager, P.; Tougaard, R.S.; Nielsen, R.; Hänselmann, A.; Nilsson, B.; Møller, J.E.; Hjort, J.; Rasmussen, J.; et al. Effect of liraglutide, a glucagon-like peptide-1 analogue, on left ventricular function in stable chronic heart failure patients with and without diabetes (LIVE)-a multicentre, double-blind, randomised, placebo-controlled trial. *Eur. J. Heart Fail.* **2017**, *19*, 69–77. [CrossRef] [PubMed]
130. Lambadiari, V.; Pavlidis, G.; Kousathana, F.; Varoudi, M.; Vlastos, D.; Maratou, E.; Georgiou, D.; Andreadou, I.; Parissis, J.; Triantafyllidi, H.; et al. Effects of 6-month treatment with the glucagon like peptide-1 analogue liraglutide on arterial stiffness, left

ventricular myocardial deformation and oxidative stress in subjects with newly diagnosed type 2 diabetes. *Cardiovasc. Diabetol.* **2018**, *17*, 8. [CrossRef]
131. Butler, J.; Abildstrøm, S.Z.; Borlaug, B.A.; Davies, M.J.; Kitzman, D.W.; Petrie, M.C.; Shah, S.J.; Verma, S.; Abhayaratna, W.P.; Chopra, V.; et al. Semaglutide in Patients With Obesity and Heart Failure Across Mildly Reduced or Preserved Ejection Fraction. *J. Am. Coll. Cardiol.* **2023**, *82*, 2087–2096. [CrossRef]
132. Jalil, J.E.; Gabrielli, L.; Ocaranza, M.P.; MacNab, P.; Fernández, R.; Grassi, B.; Jofré, P.; Verdejo, H.; Acevedo, M.; Cordova, S.; et al. New Mechanisms to Prevent Heart Failure with Preserved Ejection Fraction Using Glucagon-like Peptide-1 Receptor Agonism (GLP-1 RA) in Metabolic Syndrome and in Type 2 Diabetes: A Review. *Int. J. Mol. Sci.* **2024**, *25*, 4407. [CrossRef] [PubMed]
133. Schulz, A.; Backhaus, S.J.; Lange, T.; Evertz, R.; Kutty, S.; Kowallick, J.T.; Hasenfuß, G.; Schuster, A. Impact of epicardial adipose tissue on cardiac function and morphology in patients with diastolic dysfunction. *ESC Heart Fail.* 2024; *ahead of print*. [CrossRef]
134. Iacobellis, G.; Mohseni, M.; Bianco, S.D.; Banga, P.K. Liraglutide causes large and rapid epicardial fat reduction. *Obes* **2017**, *25*, 311–316. [CrossRef] [PubMed]
135. Michos, E.D.; Bakris, G.L.; Rodbard, H.W.; Tuttle, K.R. Glucagon-like peptide-1 receptor agonists in diabetic kidney disease: A review of their kidney and heart protection. *Am. J. Prev. Cardiol.* **2023**, *14*, 100502. [CrossRef] [PubMed]
136. Sattar, N.; Lee, M.M.Y.; Kristensen, S.L.; Branch, K.R.H.; Del Prato, S.; Khurmi, N.S.; Lam, C.S.P.; Lopes, R.D.; McMurray, J.J.V.; Pratley, R.E.; et al. Cardiovascular, mortality, and kidney outcomes with GLP-1 receptor agonists in patients with type 2 diabetes: A systematic review and meta-analysis of randomised trials. *Lancet Diabetes Endocrinol.* **2021**, *9*, 653–662. [CrossRef] [PubMed]
137. Huang, L.; Ma, R.; Lin, T.; Chaudhari, S.; Shotorbani, P.Y.; Yang, L.; Wu, P. Glucagon-like peptide-1 receptor pathway inhibits extracellular matrix production by mesangial cells through store-operated Ca^{2+} channel. *Exp. Biol. Med.* **2019**, *244*, 1193–1201. [CrossRef] [PubMed]
138. Mima, A.; Nomura, A.; Fujii, T. Current findings on the efficacy of incretin-based drugs for diabetic kidney disease: A narrative review. *Biomed. Pharmacother.* **2023**, *165*, 115032. [CrossRef] [PubMed]
139. Gragnano, F.; De Sio, V.; Calabrò, P. FLOW trial stopped early due to evidence of renal protection with semaglutide. *Eur. Heart J. Cardiovasc. Pharmacother.* **2024**, *10*, 7–9. [CrossRef] [PubMed]
140. Perkovic, V.; Tuttle, K.R.; Rossing, P.; Mahaffey, K.W.; Mann, J.F.E.; Bakris, G.; Baeres, F.M.M.; Idorn, T.; Bosch-Traberg, H.; Lausvig, N.L.; et al. Effects of Semaglutide on Chronic Kidney Disease in Patients with Type 2 Diabetes. *N. Engl. J. Med.* 2024; *ahead of print*. [CrossRef]
141. McGuire, D.K.; Busui, R.P.; Deanfield, J.; Inzucchi, S.E.; Mann, J.F.E.; Marx, N.; Mulvagh, S.L.; Poulter, N.; Engelmann, M.D.M.; Hovingh, G.K.; et al. Effects of oral semaglutide on cardiovascular outcomes in individuals with type 2 diabetes and established atherosclerotic cardiovascular disease and/or chronic kidney disease: Design and baseline characteristics of SOUL, a randomized trial. *Diabetes Obes. Metab.* **2023**, *25*, 1932–1941. [CrossRef] [PubMed]
142. A Research Study to Find Out How Semaglutide Works in the Kidneys Compared to Placebo in People with Type 2 Diabetes Chronic Kidney Disease (the REMODELTrial) Identifier NCT04865770, U.S. National Library of Medicine. 2021. Available online: https://classic.clinicaltrials.gov/ct2/show/NCT04865770 (accessed on 3 April 2024).
143. Liu, L.; Chen, J.; Wang, L.; Chen, C.; Chen, L. Association between different GLP-1 receptor agonists and gastrointestinal adverse reactions: A real-world disproportionality study based on FDA adverse event reporting system database. *Front. Endocrinol.* **2022**, *13*, 1043789. [CrossRef]
144. Aldhaleei, W.A.; Abegaz, T.M.; Bhagavathula, A.S. Glucagon-like Peptide-1 Receptor Agonists Associated Gastrointestinal Adverse Events: A Cross-Sectional Analysis of the National Institutes of Health All of Us Cohort. *Pharmaceuticals* **2024**, *17*, 199. [CrossRef]
145. Bezin, J.; Gouverneur, A.; Pénichon, M.; Mathieu, C.; Garrel, R.; Hillaire-Buys, D.; Pariente, A.; Faillie, J.L. GLP-1 Receptor Agonists and the Risk of Thyroid Cancer. *Diabetes Care* **2023**, *46*, 384–390. [CrossRef] [PubMed]
146. Pasternak, B.; Wintzell, V.; Hviid, A.; Eliasson, B.; Gudbjörnsdottir, S.; Jonasson, C.; Hveem, K.; Svanström, H.; Melbye, M.; Ueda, P. Glucagon-like peptide 1 receptor agonist use and risk of thyroid cancer: Scandinavian cohort study. *BMJ* **2024**, *385*, e078225. [CrossRef] [PubMed]
147. Perfetti, R.; Zhou, J.; Doyle, M.E.; Egan, J.M. Glucagon-like peptide-1 induces cell proliferation and pancreatic-duodenum homeobox-1 expression and increases endocrine cell mass in the pancreas of old, glucose-intolerant rats. *Endocrinology* **2000**, *141*, 4600–4605. [CrossRef] [PubMed]
148. Dankner, R.; Murad, H.; Agay, N.; Olmer, L.; Freedman, L.S. Glucagon-Like Peptide-1 Receptor Agonists and Pancreatic Cancer Risk in Patients With Type 2 Diabetes. *JAMA Netw. Open* **2024**, *7*, e2350408. [CrossRef] [PubMed]
149. Frias, J.P.; Deenadayalan, S.; Erichsen, L.; Knop, F.K.; Lingvay, I.; Macura, S.; Mathieu, C.; Pedersen, S.D.; Davies, M. Efficacy and safety of co-administered once-weekly cagrilintide 2·4 mg with once-weekly semaglutide 2·4 mg in type 2 diabetes: A multicentre, randomised, double-blind, active-controlled, phase 2 trial. *Lancet* **2023**, *40*, 720–730. [CrossRef] [PubMed]
150. Kaneko, S. Tirzepatide: A Novel, Once-weekly Dual GIP and GLP-1 Receptor Agonist for the Treatment of Type 2 Diabetes. *Touchrev Endocrinol.* **2022**, *18*, 10–19. [CrossRef] [PubMed]
151. Rosenstock, J.; Wysham, C.; Frías, J.P.; Kaneko, S.; Lee, C.J.; Fernández Landó, L.; Mao, H.; Cui, X.; Karanikas, C.A.; Thieu, V.T. Efficacy and safety of a novel dual GIP and GLP-1 receptor agonist tirzepatide in patients with type 2 diabetes (SURPASS-1): A double-blind, randomised, phase 3 trial. *Lancet* **2021**, *398*, 143–155. [CrossRef] [PubMed]

152. Frías, J.P.; Davies, M.J.; Rosenstock, J.; Pérez Manghi, F.C.; Fernández Landó, L.; Bergman, B.K.; Liu, B.; Cui, X.; Brown, K.; SURPASS-2 Investigators. Tirzepatide versus Semaglutide Once Weekly in Patients with Type 2 Diabetes. *N. Engl. J. Med.* **2021**, *385*, 503–515. [CrossRef] [PubMed]
153. Ludvik, B.; Giorgino, F.; Jódar, E.; Frias, J.P.; Fernández Landó, L.; Brown, K.; Bray, R.; Rodríguez, Á. Once-weekly tirzepatide versus once-daily insulin degludec as add-on to metformin with or without SGLT2 inhibitors in patients with type 2 diabetes (SURPASS-3): A randomised, open-label, parallel-group, phase 3 trial. *Lancet* **2021**, *398*, 583–598. [CrossRef]
154. Del Prato, S.; Kahn, S.E.; Pavo, I.; Weerakkody, G.J.; Yang, Z.; Doupis, J.; Aizenberg, D.; Wynne, A.G.; Riesmeyer, J.S.; Heine, R.J.; et al. Tirzepatide versus insulin glargine in type 2 diabetes and increased cardiovascular risk (SURPASS-4): A randomised, open-label, parallel-group, multicentre, phase 3 trial. *Lancet* **2021**, *398*, 1811–1824. [CrossRef]
155. Dahl, D.; Onishi, Y.; Norwood, P.; Huh, R.; Bray, R.; Patel, H.; Rodríguez, Á. Effect of Subcutaneous Tirzepatide vs Placebo Added to Titrated Insulin Glargine on Glycemic Control in Patients With Type 2 Diabetes: The SURPASS-5 Randomized Clinical Trial. *JAMA* **2022**, *327*, 534–545. [CrossRef] [PubMed]
156. Jastreboff, A.M.; Aronne, L.J.; Ahmad, N.N.; Wharton, S.; Connery, L.; Alves, B.; Kiyosue, A.; Zhang, S.; Liu, B.; Bunck, M.C.; et al. Tirzepatide Once Weekly for the Treatment of Obesity. *N. Engl. J. Med.* **2022**, *387*, 205–216. [CrossRef] [PubMed]
157. Ding, L.; Zhang, J. Glucagon-like peptide-1 activates endothelial nitric oxide synthase in human umbilical vein endothelial cells. *Acta Pharmacol. Sin.* **2012**, *33*, 75–81. [CrossRef] [PubMed]
158. Ojima, A.; Matsui, T.; Maeda, S.; Takeuchi, M.; Yamagishi, S. Glucose-dependent insulinotropic polypeptide (GIP) inhibits signaling pathways of advanced glycation end products (AGEs) in endothelial cells via its antioxidative properties. *Horm. Metab. Res.* **2012**, *44*, 501–505. [CrossRef] [PubMed]
159. Tsihlis, N.D.; Oustwani, C.S.; Vavra, A.K.; Jiang, Q.; Keefer, L.K.; Kibbe, M.R. Nitric oxide inhibits vascular smooth muscle cell proliferation and neointimal hyperplasia by increasing the ubiquitination and degradation of UbcH10. *Cell Biochem. Biophys.* **2011**, *60*, 89–97. [CrossRef] [PubMed]
160. Mori, Y.; Matsui, T.; Hirano, T.; Yamagishi, S.I. GIP as a Potential Therapeutic Target for Atherosclerotic Cardiovascular Disease-A Systematic Review. *Int. J. Mol. Sci.* **2020**, *21*, 1509. [CrossRef] [PubMed]
161. Yu, D.; Shen, S.; Zhang, J.; Wang, Q. Effect of the Dual Glucose-Dependent Insulinotropic Peptide/Gulcagon-like Peptide 1 Receptor Agonist Tirzepatide on Lipid Profile and Waist Circumference: A Systematic Review and Meta-analysis. *Clin. Ther.* **2023**, *45*, 787–796. [CrossRef]
162. Nogi, Y.; Nagashima, M.; Terasaki, M.; Nohtomi, K.; Watanabe, T.; Hirano, T. Glucose-dependent insulinotropic polypeptide prevents the progression of macrophage-driven atherosclerosis in diabetic apolipoprotein E-null mice. *PLoS ONE* **2012**, *7*, e35683. [CrossRef] [PubMed]
163. Sattar, N.; McGuire, D.K.; Pavo, I.; Weerakkody, G.J.; Nishiyama, H.; Wiese, R.J.; Zoungas, S. Tirzepatide cardiovascular event risk assessment: A pre-specified meta-analysis. *Nat. Med.* **2022**, *28*, 591–598. [CrossRef]
164. Hankosky, E.R.; Wang, H.; Neff, L.M.; Kan, H.; Wang, F.; Ahmad, N.N.; Griffin, R.; Stefanski, A.; Garvey, W.T. Tirzepatide reduces the predicted risk of atherosclerotic cardiovascular disease and improves cardiometabolic risk factors in adults with obesity or overweight: SURMOUNT-1 post hoc analysis. *Diabetes Obes. Metab.* **2024**, *26*, 319–328. [CrossRef]
165. Lingvay, I.; Mosenzon, O.; Brown, K.; Cui, X.; O'Neill, C.; Fernández Landó, L.; Patel, H. Systolic blood pressure reduction with tirzepatide in patients with type 2 diabetes: Insights from SURPASS clinical program. *Cardiovasc. Diabetol.* **2023**, *22*, 66. [CrossRef] [PubMed]
166. Nicholls, S.J.; Bhatt, D.L.; Buse, J.B.; Prato, S.D.; Kahn, S.E.; Lincoff, A.M.; McGuire, D.K.; Nauck, M.A.; Nissen, S.E.; Sattar, N.; et al. Comparison of tirzepatide and dulaglutide on major adverse cardiovascular events in participants with type 2 diabetes and atherosclerotic cardiovascular disease: SURPASS-CVOT design and baseline characteristics. *Am. Heart J.* **2024**, *267*, 1–11. [CrossRef] [PubMed]
167. Heerspink, H.J.L.; Sattar, N.; Pavo, I.; Haupt, A.; Duffin, K.L.; Yang, Z.; Wiese, R.J.; Tuttle, K.R.; Cherney, D.Z.I. Effects of tirzepatide versus insulin glargine on kidney outcomes in type 2 diabetes in the SURPASS-4 trial: Post-hoc analysis of an open-label, randomised, phase 3 trial. *Lancet Diabetes Endocrinol.* **2022**, *10*, 774–785. [CrossRef] [PubMed]
168. Caruso, I.; Giorgino, F. Renal effects of GLP-1 receptor agonists and tirzepatide in individuals with type 2 diabetes: Seeds of a promising future. *Endocrine*, 2024; *ahead of print*. [CrossRef]
169. Rodriguez-Diaz, R.; Tamayo, A.; Hara, M.; Caicedo, A. The Local Paracrine Actions of the Pancreatic α-Cell. *Diabetes* **2020**, *69*, 550–558. [CrossRef] [PubMed]
170. Zeigerer, A.; Sekar, R.; Kleinert, M.; Nason, S.; Habegger, K.M.; Müller, T.D. Glucagon's Metabolic Action in Health and Disease. *Compr. Physiol.* **2021**, *11*, 1759–1783. [CrossRef] [PubMed]
171. Esler, W.P.; Bence, K.K. Metabolic Targets in Nonalcoholic Fatty Liver Disease. *Cell Mol. Gastroenterol. Hepatol.* **2019**, *8*, 247–267. [CrossRef] [PubMed]
172. Wewer Albrechtsen, N.J.; Holst, J.J.; Cherrington, A.D.; Finan, B.; Gluud, L.L.; Dean, E.D.; Campbell, J.E.; Bloom, S.R.; Tan, T.M.; Knop, F.K.; et al. 100 years of glucagon and 100 more. *Diabetologia* **2023**, *66*, 1378–1394. [CrossRef] [PubMed]
173. Hope, D.C.D.; Vincent, M.L.; Tan, T.M.M. Striking the Balance: GLP-1/Glucagon Co-Agonism as a Treatment Strategy for Obesity. *Front. Endocrinol.* **2021**, *12*, 735019. [CrossRef] [PubMed]

174. Parker, V.E.R.; Robertson, D.; Wang, T.; Hornigold, D.C.; Petrone, M.; Cooper, A.T.; Posch, M.G.; Heise, T.; Plum-Moerschel, L.; Schlichthaar, H.; et al. Efficacy, Safety, and Mechanistic Insights of Cotadutide, a Dual Receptor Glucagon-Like Peptide-1 and Glucagon Agonist. *J. Clin. Endocrinol. Metab.* **2020**, *105*, dgz047. [CrossRef]
175. Romero-Gómez, M.; Lawitz, E.; Shankar, R.R.; Chaudhri, E.; Liu, J.; Lam, R.L.H.; Kaufman, K.D.; Engel, S.S.; MK-6024 P001 Study Group. A phase IIa active-comparator-controlled study to evaluate the efficacy and safety of efinopegdutide in patients with non-alcoholic fatty liver disease. *J. Hepatol.* **2023**, *79*, 888–897. [CrossRef]
176. Alba, M.; Yee, J.; Frustaci, M.E.; Samtani, M.N.; Fleck, P. Efficacy and safety of glucagon-like peptide-1/glucagon receptor co-agonist JNJ-64565111 in individuals with obesity without type 2 diabetes mellitus: A randomized dose-ranging study. *Clin. Obes.* **2021**, *11*, e12432. [CrossRef] [PubMed]
177. le Roux, C.W.; Steen, O.; Lucas, K.J.; Startseva, E.; Unseld, A.; Hennige, A.M. Glucagon and GLP-1 receptor dual agonist survodutide for obesity: A randomised, double-blind, placebo-controlled, dose-finding phase 2 trial. *Lancet Diabetes Endocrinol.* **2024**, *12*, 162–173. [CrossRef] [PubMed]
178. Blüher, M.; Rosenstock, J.; Hoefler, J.; Manuel, R.; Hennige, A.M. Dose-response effects on HbA_{1c} and bodyweight reduction of survodutide, a dual glucagon/GLP-1 receptor agonist, compared with placebo and open-label semaglutide in people with type 2 diabetes: A randomised clinical trial. *Diabetologia* **2024**, *67*, 470–482. [CrossRef] [PubMed]
179. Sélley, E.; Kun, S.; Szijártó, I.A.; Kertész, M.; Wittmann, I.; Molnár, G.A. Vasodilator Effect of Glucagon: Receptorial Crosstalk Among Glucagon, GLP-1, and Receptor for Glucagon and GLP-1. *Horm. Metab. Res.* **2016**, *48*, 476–483. [CrossRef] [PubMed]
180. Petersen, K.M.; Bøgevig, S.; Holst, J.J.; Knop, F.K.; Christensen, M.B. Hemodynamic Effects of Glucagon: A Literature Review. *J. Clin. Endocrinol. Metab.* **2018**, *103*, 1804–1812. [CrossRef] [PubMed]
181. Carney, E.F. The renal glucagon receptor is essential to kidney metabolic and homeostatic functions. *Nat. Rev. Nephrol.* **2024**, *20*, 203. [CrossRef]
182. Parker, V.E.R.; Hoang, T.; Schlichthaar, H.; Gibb, F.W.; Wenzel, B.; Posch, M.G.; Rose, L.; Chang, Y.T.; Petrone, M.; Hansen, L.; et al. Efficacy and safety of cotadutide, a dual glucagon-like peptide-1 and glucagon receptor agonist, in a randomized phase 2a study of patients with type 2 diabetes and chronic kidney disease. *Diabetes Obes. Metab.* **2022**, *24*, 1360–1369. [CrossRef] [PubMed]
183. Coskun, T.; Urva, S.; Roell, W.C.; Qu, H.; Loghin, C.; Moyers, J.S.; O'Farrell, L.S.; Briere, D.A.; Sloop, K.W.; Thomas, M.K.; et al. LY3437943, a novel triple glucagon, GIP, and GLP-1 receptor agonist for glycemic control and weight loss: From discovery to clinical proof of concept. *Cell Metab.* **2022**, *34*, 1234–1247.e9. [CrossRef] [PubMed]
184. Rosenstock, J.; Frias, J.; Jastreboff, A.M.; Du, Y.; Lou, J.; Gurbuz, S.; Thomas, M.K.; Hartman, M.L.; Haupt, A.; Milicevic, Z.; et al. Retatrutide, a GIP, GLP-1 and glucagon receptor agonist, for people with type 2 diabetes: A randomised, double-blind, placebo and active-controlled, parallel-group, phase 2 trial conducted in the USA. *Lancet* **2023**, *402*, 529–544. [CrossRef]
185. Jastreboff, A.M.; Kaplan, L.M.; Frías, J.P.; Wu, Q.; Du, Y.; Gurbuz, S.; Coskun, T.; Haupt, A.; Milicevic, Z.; Hartman, M.L. Retatrutide Phase 2 Obesity Trial Investigators. Triple-Hormone-Receptor Agonist Retatrutide for Obesity—A Phase 2 Trial. *N. Engl. J. Med.* **2023**, *389*, 514–526. [CrossRef]
186. A Study of Retatrutide (LY3437943) in Participants with Obesity and Cardiovascular Disease (TRIUMPH-3). Identifier NCT05882045. U.S National Library of Medicine. 2023. Available online: https://classic.clinicaltrials.gov/ct2/show/NCT05882045 (accessed on 9 April 2024).
187. Pirags, V.; Lebovitz, H.; Fouqueray, P. Imeglimin, a novel glimin oral antidiabetic, exhibits a good efficacy and safety profile in type 2 diabetic patients. *Diabetes Obes. Metab.* **2012**, *14*, 852–858. [CrossRef] [PubMed]
188. Hozumi, K.; Sugawara, K.; Ishihara, T.; Ishihara, N.; Ogawa, W. Effects of imeglimin on mitochondrial function, AMPK activity, and gene expression in hepatocytes. *Sci. Rep.* **2023**, *13*, 746. [CrossRef] [PubMed]
189. Vial, G.; Chauvin, M.A.; Bendridi, N.; Durand, A.; Meugnier, E.; Madec, A.M.; Bernoud-Hubac, N.; Pais de Barros, J.P.; Fontaine, É.; Acquaviva, C.; et al. Imeglimin normalizes glucose tolerance and insulin sensitivity and improves mitochondrial function in liver of a high-fat, high-sucrose diet mice model. *Diabetes* **2015**, *64*, 2254–2264. [CrossRef]
190. Sanada, J.; Obata, A.; Fushimi, Y.; Kimura, T.; Shimoda, M.; Ikeda, T.; Nogami, Y.; Obata, Y.; Yamasaki, Y.; Nakanishi, S.; et al. Imeglimin exerts favorable effects on pancreatic β-cells by improving morphology in mitochondria and increasing the number of insulin granules. *Sci. Rep.* **2022**, *12*, 13220. [CrossRef]
191. Vinayagam, P.; Senathipathi, V.; Shivam, V.; Velraju, N. The role of Imeglimin in glycemic control, beta cell function and safety outcomes in patients with type 2 diabetes mellitus: A comprehensive meta-analysis. *Diabetes Epidemiol. Manag.* **2023**, *12*, 100164. [CrossRef]
192. Giruzzi, M. Imeglimin. *Clin. Diabetes* **2021**, *39*, 439–440. [CrossRef]
193. Singh, A.K.; Singh, A.; Singh, R.; Misra, A. Efficacy and safety of imeglimin in type 2 diabetes: A systematic review and meta-analysis of randomized placebo-controlled trials. *Diabetes Metab. Syndr.* **2023**, *17*, 102710. [CrossRef]
194. Konkwo, C.; Perry, R.J. Imeglimin: Current Development and Future Potential in Type 2 Diabetes. *Drugs* **2021**, *81*, 185–190. [CrossRef] [PubMed]
195. Detaille, D.; Vial, G.; Borel, A.L.; Cottet-Rouselle, C.; Hallakou-Bozec, S.; Bolze, S.; Fouqueray, P.; Fontaine, E. Imeglimin prevents human endothelial cell death by inhibiting mitochondrial permeability transition without inhibiting mitochondrial respiration. *Cell Death Discov.* **2016**, *2*, 15072. [CrossRef]

196. Uchida, T.; Ueno, H.; Konagata, A.; Taniguchi, N.; Kogo, F.; Nagatomo, Y.; Shimizu, K.; Yamaguchi, H.; Shimoda, K. Improving the Effects of Imeglimin on Endothelial Function: A Prospective, Single-Center, Observational Study. *Diabetes Ther.* **2023**, *14*, 569–579. [CrossRef]
197. Kitakata, H.; Endo, J.; Hashimoto, S.; Mizuno, E.; Moriyama, H.; Shirakawa, K.; Goto, S.; Katsumata, Y.; Fukuda, K.; Sano, M. Imeglimin prevents heart failure with preserved ejection fraction by recovering the impaired unfolded protein response in mice subjected to cardiometabolic stress. *Biochem. Biophys. Res. Commun.* **2021**, *572*, 185–190. [CrossRef] [PubMed]
198. Lachaux, M.; Soulié, M.; Hamzaoui, M.; Bailly, A.; Nicol, L.; Rémy-Jouet, I.; Renet, S.; Vendeville, C.; Gluais-Dagorn, P.; Hallakou-Bozec, S.; et al. Short-and long-term administration of imeglimin counters cardiorenal dysfunction in a rat model of metabolic syndrome. *Endocrinol. Diabetes Metab.* **2020**, *3*, e00128. [CrossRef] [PubMed]
199. Chigurupati, S.; Dhanaraj, S.A.; Balakumar, P. A step ahead of PPARγ full agonists to PPARγ partial agonists: Therapeutic perspectives in the management of diabetic insulin resistance. *Eur. J. Pharmacol.* **2015**, *755*, 50–57. [CrossRef] [PubMed]
200. Henry, R.R.; Buse, J.B.; Wu, H.; Durrwell, L.; Mingrino, R.; Jaekel, K.; El Azzouzi, B.; Andjelkovic, M.; Herz, M. Efficacy, safety and tolerability of aleglitazar in patients with type 2 diabetes: Pooled findings from three randomized phase III trials. *Diabetes Obes. Metab.* **2015**, *17*, 560–565. [CrossRef] [PubMed]
201. Lincoff, A.M.; Tardif, J.C.; Schwartz, G.G.; Nicholls, S.J.; Rydén, L.; Neal, B.; Malmberg, K.; Wedel, H.; Buse, J.B.; Henry, R.R.; et al. Effect of aleglitazar on cardiovascular outcomes after acute coronary syndrome in patients with type 2 diabetes mellitus: The AleCardio randomized clinical trial. *JAMA* **2014**, *311*, 1515–1525. [CrossRef] [PubMed]
202. Agrawal, R. The first approved agent in the Glitazar's Class: Saroglitazar. *Curr. Drug Targets* **2014**, *15*, 151–155. [CrossRef]
203. Bandyopadhyay, S.; Samajdar, S.S.; Das, S. Effects of saroglitazar in the treatment of non-alcoholic fatty liver disease or non-alcoholic steatohepatitis: A systematic review and meta-analysis. *Clin. Res. Hepatol. Gastroenterol.* **2023**, *47*, 102174. [CrossRef] [PubMed]
204. Pai, V.; Paneerselvam, A.; Mukhopadhyay, S.; Bhansali, A.; Kamath, D.; Shankar, V.; Gambhire, D.; Jani, R.H.; Joshi, S.; Patel, P. A Multicenter, Prospective, Randomized, Double-blind Study to Evaluate the Safety and Efficacy of Saroglitazar 2 and 4 mg Compared to Pioglitazone 45 mg in Diabetic Dyslipidemia (PRESS V). *J. Diabetes Sci. Technol.* **2014**, *8*, 132–141. [CrossRef] [PubMed]
205. Jani, R.H.; Pai, V.; Jha, P.; Jariwala, G.; Mukhopadhyay, S.; Bhansali, A.; Joshi, S. A multicenter, prospective, randomized, double-blind study to evaluate the safety and efficacy of Saroglitazar 2 and 4 mg compared with placebo in type 2 diabetes mellitus patients having hypertriglyceridemia not controlled with atorvastatin therapy (PRESS VI). *Diabetes Technol. Ther.* **2014**, *16*, 63–71. [CrossRef]
206. Shetty, S.R.; Kumar, S.; Mathur, R.P.; Sharma, K.H.; Jaiswal, A.D. Observational study to evaluate the safety and efficacy of saroglitazar in Indian diabetic dyslipidemia patients. *Indian. Heart J.* **2015**, *67*, 23–26. [CrossRef]
207. Siddiqui, M.S.; Parmar, D.; Sheikh, F.; Sarin, S.K.; Cisneros, L.; Gawrieh, S.; Momin, T.; Duseja, A.; Sanyal, A.J. Saroglitazar, a Dual PPAR α/γ Agonist, Improves Atherogenic Dyslipidemia in Patients With Non-Cirrhotic Nonalcoholic Fatty Liver Disease: A Pooled Analysis. *Clin. Gastroenterol. Hepatol.* **2023**, *21*, 2597–2605.e2. [CrossRef] [PubMed]
208. A Study to Evaluate the Safety Effectiveness of Saroglitazar 4mg in Patients with NAFLD with Comorbidities Identifier NCT05872269, U.S. National Library of Medicine. 2023. Available online: https://classic.clinicaltrials.gov/ct2/show/NCT05872269 (accessed on 10 April 2024).
209. Kalliora, C.; Drosatos, K. The Glitazars Paradox: Cardiotoxicity of the Metabolically Beneficial Dual PPARα and PPARγ Activation. *J. Cardiovasc. Pharmacol.* **2020**, *76*, 514–526. [CrossRef] [PubMed]
210. Wang, X.; Wang, Y.; Hou, J.; Liu, H.; Zeng, R.; Li, X.; Han, M.; Li, Q.; Ji, L.; Pan, D.; et al. Plasma proteome profiling reveals the therapeutic effects of the PPAR pan-agonist chiglitazar on insulin sensitivity, lipid metabolism, and inflammation in type 2 diabetes. *Sci. Rep.* **2024**, *14*, 638. [CrossRef] [PubMed]
211. Zhou, Y.; Wang, H.; Wang, Y.; Xu, X.; Li, F.; Zhou, J.; Shan, T.; Huang, R.; Cai, T.; Liu, X.; et al. Comparative Evaluation of Chiglitazar and Sitagliptin on the Levels of Retinol-Binding Protein 4 and Its Correlation With Insulin Resistance in Patients With Type 2 Diabetes. *Front. Endocrinol.* **2022**, *13*, 801271. [CrossRef] [PubMed]
212. Jia, W.; Ma, J.; Miao, H.; Wang, C.; Wang, X.; Li, Q.; Lu, W.; Yang, J.; Zhang, L.; Yang, J.; et al. Chiglitazar monotherapy with sitagliptin as an active comparator in patients with type 2 diabetes: A randomized, double-blind, phase 3 trial (CMAS). *Sci. Bull.* **2021**, *66*, 1581–1590. [CrossRef] [PubMed]
213. A Randomised Double-Blind Placebo Parallel Controlled Phase III Clinical Study to Evaluate the Efficacy and Safety of Chiglitazar Added to Metformin in Patients with Type 2 Diabetes Inadequately Controlled with Metformin Monotherapy (RECAM). Identifier NCT04807348. ICH Good Clinical Practice Network. 2021. Available online: https://ichgcp.net/clinical-trials-registry/NCT04807348 (accessed on 12 April 2024).
214. Matschinsky, F.M.; Wilson, D.F. The Central Role of Glucokinase in Glucose Homeostasis: A Perspective 50 Years After Demonstrating the Presence of the Enzyme in Islets of Langerhans. *Front. Physiol.* **2019**, *10*, 148. [CrossRef] [PubMed]
215. Haeusler, R.A.; Camastra, S.; Astiarraga, B.; Nannipieri, M.; Anselmino, M.; Ferrannini, E. Decreased expression of hepatic glucokinase in type 2 diabetes. *Mol. Metab.* **2014**, *4*, 222–226. [CrossRef] [PubMed]
216. Haddad, D.; Dsouza, V.S.; Al-Mulla, F.; Al Madhoun, A. New-Generation Glucokinase Activators: Potential Game-Changers in Type 2 Diabetes Treatment. *Int. J. Mol. Sci.* **2024**, *25*, 571. [CrossRef] [PubMed]
217. Zhu, D.; Gan, S.; Liu, Y.; Ma, J.; Dong, X.; Song, W.; Zeng, J.; Wang, G.; Zhao, W.; Zhang, Q.; et al. Dorzagliatin monotherapy in Chinese patients with type 2 diabetes: A dose-ranging, randomised, double-blind, placebo-controlled, phase 2 study. *Lancet Diabetes Endocrinol.* **2018**, *6*, 627–636. [CrossRef] [PubMed]

218. Zhu, D.; Zhang, Y.; Chen, L. 182-OR: A Novel Dual-Acting Glucokinase Activator (GKA) Dorzagliatin (HMS5552) Achieved Primary Efficacy Endpoint with Good Safety Profiles in T2DM Patients after 24 Weeks of Treatment in a Phase III Monotherapy Trial. *Diabetes* **2020**, *69* (Suppl. 1), 182-OR. [CrossRef]
219. Dutta, D.; Khandelwal, D.; Kumar, M.; Sharma, M. Efficacy and safety of novel dual glucokinase activator dorzagliatin in type-2 diabetes A meta-analysis. *Diabetes Metab. Syndr.* **2023**, *17*, 102695. [CrossRef] [PubMed]
220. Du, Y.; Gao, L.; Xiao, X.; Hou, X.; Ji, L. A multicentre, randomized, double-blind, parallel, active- and placebo-controlled Phase 3 clinical study of the glucokinase activator PB-201 in treatment-naive patients with type 2 diabetes mellitus: A study protocol. *Diabetes Obes. Metab.* **2023**, *25*, 649–655. [CrossRef] [PubMed]
221. Liu, D.; Du, Y.; Yao, X.; Wei, Y.; Zhu, J.; Cui, C.; Zhou, H.; Xu, M.; Li, H.; Ji, L. Safety, tolerability, pharmacokinetics, and pharmacodynamics of the glucokinase activator PB-201 and its effects on the glucose excursion profile in drug-naïve Chinese patients with type 2 diabetes: A randomised controlled, crossover, single-centre phase 1 trial. *EClinicalMedicine* **2021**, *42*, 101185. [CrossRef] [PubMed]
222. Usui, R.; Yabe, D.; Fauzi, M.; Goto, H.; Botagarova, A.; Tokumoto, S.; Tatsuoka, H.; Tahara, Y.; Kobayashi, S.; Manabe, T.; et al. GPR40 activation initiates store-operated Ca^{2+} entry and potentiates insulin secretion via the IP3R1/STIM1/Orai1 pathway in pancreatic β-cells. *Sci. Rep.* **2019**, *9*, 15562. [CrossRef] [PubMed]
223. Burant, C.F. Activation of GPR40 as a therapeutic target for the treatment of type 2 diabetes. *Diabetes Care* **2013**, *36* (Suppl. 2), S175–S179. [CrossRef] [PubMed]
224. Otieno, M.A.; Snoeys, J.; Lam, W.; Ghosh, A.; Player, M.R.; Pocai, A.; Salter, R.; Simic, D.; Skaggs, H.; Singh, B.; et al. Fasiglifam (TAK-875): Mechanistic Investigation and Retrospective Identification of Hazards for Drug Induced Liver Injury. *Toxicol. Sci.* **2018**, *163*, 374–384. [CrossRef] [PubMed]
225. Bazydlo-Guzenda, K.; Buda, P.; Mach, M.; Pieczykolan, J.; Kozlowska, I.; Janiszewski, M.; Drzazga, E.; Dominowski, J.; Ziolkowski, H.; Wieczorek, M.; et al. Evaluation of the hepatotoxicity of the novel GPR40 (FFAR1) agonist CPL207280 in the rat and monkey. *PLoS ONE* **2021**, *16*, e0257477. [CrossRef] [PubMed]
226. Bazydło-Guzenda, K.; Jarus-Dziedzic, K.; Gierczak-Pachulska, A.; Buda, P.; Rudzki, P.J.; Buś-Kwaśnik, K.; Juszczyk, E.; Tratkiewicz, E.; Rabczenko, D.; Segiet-Święcicka, A.; et al. First-in-human study of CPL207280, a novel G-protein-coupled receptor 40/free fatty acid receptor 1 agonist, in healthy volunteers after single and multiple administration. *Diabetes Obes. Metab.* **2024**, *26*, 1376–1385. [CrossRef]
227. Vella, A.; Freeman, J.L.R.; Dunn, I.; Keller, K.; Buse, J.B.; Valcarce, C. Targeting hepatic glucokinase to treat diabetes with TTP399, a hepatoselective glucokinase activator. *Sci. Transl. Med.* **2019**, *11*, eaau3441. [CrossRef]
228. Zhu, Z.; Li, Y.; Zheng, Q.; Adegbite, E.; Ross, S.; Telusca, L.; Jones, C.L.; Fenaux, M.; Xu, S.; Junaidi, M.K. An Open-Label, Active-Controlled Phase 2 Evaluation of Novel GLP-1 Analog Ecnoglutide in Adults with Obesity. *Diabetes* **2023**, *72* (Suppl. 1), 79-LB. [CrossRef]
229. Anwar, D.; Bao, Y.; Zhou, Y.; Chen, S.; Zhou, J.; Li, L.; Cheng, Z.; Dong, X.; Shi, X.; Su, X.; et al. Efficacy and Safety of Supaglutide as Add-on to Metformin in Patients with Type 2 Diabetes. *Diabetes* **2023**, *72* (Suppl. 1), 778-P. [CrossRef]
230. Chakravarthy, M.; Argüelles-Tello, F.A.; Sun, A.L.A.; Elliott, M.; Acosta, L.; Rankin, J.E.; Hansen, S.K. CT-388, A novel once-weekly dual GLP-1 and GIP receptor modulator, is safe, well-tolerated, and produces more than 8% weight loss in four weeks in overweight and obese adults. *Diabetes* **2023**, *72*, 75-LB. [CrossRef]
231. Ji, L.; Jiang, H.; An, P.; Deng, H.; Liu, M.; Li, L.; Feng, L.; Song, B.; Han-Zhang, H.; Ma, Q.; et al. IBI362 (LY3305677), a weekly-dose GLP-1 and glucagon receptor dual agonist, in Chinese adults with overweight or obesity: A randomised, placebo-controlled, multiple ascending dose phase 1b study. *EClinicalMedicine* **2021**, *39*, 101088. [CrossRef] [PubMed]
232. Ji, L.; Song, W.; Fang, H.; Li, W.; Geng, J.; Wang, Y.; Guo, L.; Cai, H.; Yang, T.; Li, H.; et al. Efficacy and safety of chiglitazar, a novel peroxisome proliferator-activated receptor pan-agonist, in patients with type 2 diabetes: A randomized, double-blind, placebo-controlled, phase 3 trial (CMAP). *Sci. Bull.* **2021**, *66*, 1571–1580. [CrossRef]
233. Rosenstock, J.; Frías, J.P.; Rodbard, H.W.; Tofé, S.; Sears, E.; Huh, R.; Fernández Landó, L.; Patel, H. Tirzepatide vs Insulin Lispro Added to Basal Insulin in Type 2 Diabetes: The SURPASS-6 Randomized Clinical Trial. *JAMA* **2023**, *330*, 1631–1640. [CrossRef]
234. Gao, L.; Lee, B.W.; Chawla, M.; Kim, J.; Huo, L.; Du, L.; Huang, Y.; Ji, L. Tirzepatide versus insulin glargine as second-line or third-line therapy in type 2 diabetes in the Asia-Pacific region: The SURPASS-AP-Combo trial. *Nat. Med.* **2023**, *29*, 1500–1510. [CrossRef]
235. Garvey, W.T.; Frias, J.P.; Jastreboff, A.M.; le Roux, C.W.; Sattar, N.; Aizenberg, D.; Mao, H.; Zhang, S.; Ahmad, N.N.; Bunck, M.C.; et al. Tirzepatide once weekly for the treatment of obesity in people with type 2 diabetes (SURMOUNT-2): A double-blind, randomised, multicentre, placebo-controlled, phase 3 trial. *Lancet* **2023**, *402*, 613–626. [CrossRef]
236. Aronne, L.J.; Sattar, N.; Horn, D.B.; Bays, H.E.; Wharton, S.; Lin, W.-Y.; Ahmad, N.N.; Zhang, S.; Liao, R.; Bunck, M.C.; et al. Continued Treatment With Tirzepatide for Maintenance of Weight Reduction in Adults With Obesity: The SURMOUNT-4 Randomized Clinical Trial. *JAMA* **2024**, *331*, 38–48. [CrossRef]

biomedicines

MDPI

Review

Diabetes and Stroke: Impact of Novel Therapies for the Treatment of Type 2 Diabetes Mellitus

Inês Henriques Vieira [1,*,†], Tânia Santos Carvalho [1,†], Joana Saraiva [1,2], Leonor Gomes [1,2] and Isabel Paiva [1]

1 Department of Endocrinology Diabetes and Metabolism, Hospitais da Universidade de Coimbra—ULS Coimbra, 3004-561 Coimbra, Portugal; 17690@ulscoimbra.min-saude.pt (T.S.C.)
2 Faculty of Medicine, Universidade de Coimbra, 3004-531 Coimbra, Portugal
* Correspondence: 11285@ulscoimbra.min-saude.pt
† These authors contributed equally to this work.

Abstract: Type 2 diabetes mellitus (T2DM) is a significant risk factor for stroke. Nevertheless, the evidence supporting stringent glycemic control to reduce macrovascular complications, particularly stroke, is not as clear as for microvascular complications. Presently, risk reduction strategies are based on controlling multiple risk factors, including hypertension, dyslipidemia, glycemia, smoking, and weight. Since 2008, new pharmacological therapies for treating T2DM have been required to undergo trials to ensure their cardiovascular safety. Remarkably, several novel therapies have exhibited protective effects against the combined endpoint of major cardiovascular events. Evidence from these trials, with stroke as a secondary endpoint, along with real-world data, suggests potential benefits in stroke prevention, particularly with glucagon-like peptide 1 receptor agonists. Conversely, the data on sodium–glucose cotransporter type 2 inhibitors remains more controversial. Dipeptidyl peptidase 4 inhibitors appear neutral in stroke prevention. More recent pharmacological therapies still lack significant data on this particular outcome. This article provides a comprehensive review of the evidence on the most recent T2DM therapies for stroke prevention and their impact on clinical practice.

Keywords: stroke; diabetes type 2; glucagon-like peptide 1 receptor agonists; sodium–glucose cotransporter type 2 inhibitors

1. Introduction

Stroke is the second most common cause of death and a leading cause of adult disability, affecting approximately 1.1 million inhabitants in the European Union every year [1].

In patients with diabetes mellitus (DM), the risk of stroke increases at least 1.5–3 times, with previous data reporting an increase of more than 4 times in men and 5 times in women. The risk of ischemic stroke escalates significantly with DM duration, with estimates indicating a 3% increased risk for each year of the disease, and a threefold higher risk among those with DM for over 10 years [2]. The prevalence of DM is more common in people with ischemic than hemorrhagic stroke—33 vs. 26%, respectively [3].

Most risk reduction strategies are based on controlling multiple risk factors, such as high blood pressure, dyslipidemia, glycemic control, smoking cessation, and weight loss. Currently, there are few therapies available that specifically target the risk of stroke [3].

In this narrative review, we sought to gather comprehensive data on the effect of the most recent non-insulin pharmacological therapies used in the treatment of diabetes on the risk of stroke and to translate it into recommendations for clinical practice. To this end, we performed a search on the PubMed database combining the medical subject heading (MESH) terms "Diabetes Mellitus, Type 2" and "Stroke". Articles with full text in English that provided information on the study question were selected based on their title and/or abstract. We prioritized articles published in the last 10 years; however, when particularly relevant or to provide context, older publications were also included. The bibliographies of the initially selected publications were also scanned, with the inclusion of other relevant texts. Additional research was conducted to provide context and to answer questions that emerged during the peer-review process.

2. Pathophysiology of Stroke in Diabetes Mellitus Patients

Due to its impact on atherosclerosis development, DM stands out as a major vascular risk factor. Nevertheless, unlike ischemic heart disease, where arteriosclerosis is key, stroke's pathogenic mechanisms are more complex. Only about 20–25% of all ischemic strokes are derived from atherosclerosis. Other significant mechanisms include cardioembolic origin (30%), small vessel disease (25%), and various rare causes, such as hypercoagulable states and inflammatory and noninflammatory vasculopathy. Furthermore, approximately 20% of strokes are hemorrhagic. DM heightens the risk of both ischemic and hemorrhagic strokes, underscoring the complexity of stroke prevention in this population [4].

In addition to its contribution to atherosclerosis, diabetes directly heightens the risk of cardioembolic events. It has been reported that, in atrial fibrillation (AF) patients, the presence of diabetes alone increases the risk of stroke by 4.0% a year [5].

The underlying pathophysiology of stroke and type 2 DM (T2DM) is also complicated by the association of other risk factors for stroke frequently seen in people with T2DM, such as hypertension and dyslipidemia [3].

At the microvascular level, four main mechanisms seem to predispose to stroke in patients with DM: acidosis, oxidative stress, inflammation, and changes in mitochondrial function. Theoretically, anaerobic conditions in areas of ischemia result in lactate accumulation, which can generate acidemia, which is exacerbated by hyperglycemia. However, it is still controversial whether it is acidemia per se or the combination of acidemia and hyperglycemia that causes harmful results [6].

Oxidative stress ensues when there is an imbalance between reactive oxygen species (ROS) production and the organism's antioxidant defenses, and is a major contributor to diabetes chronic complications. It may lead to cell death through several mechanisms, including protein denaturation, enzyme inactivation, and deoxyribonucleic acid and lipid damage by oxidation [7], contributing to vascular and endothelial damage [5]. In diabetes, several interplaying factors lead to an increase in oxidative stress, including the accumulation of glycolysis intermediates, generation of advanced glycation end products (AGEs), activation of protein kinase C (PKC), activation of the polyol and hexosamine pathways, and mitochondrial dysfunction [8,9].

AGEs, which can be generated when excess glucose interacts with the amino acid groups of plasma proteins, can also lead to structural and functional alterations in endothelial cells and blood vessels, and the activation of pro-inflammatory pathways [8]. Endothelial cells are particularly susceptible to hyperglycemia-induced damage. AGEs and excess ROS can also lead to a decrease in nitric oxide (NO) and a reduction in the activity of the endothelial NO synthase and consequent loss of the NO-dependent vasodilatory response, which is a hallmark of diabetic endothelial dysfunction [9].

Regarding inflammation, cytokines, such as tumor necrosis factor α (TNF-α) and interleukin 1β (IL-1β), lead to the expression of cell adhesion molecules on endothelial cells. This induces an increase in circulating polymorphonuclear leukocytes and the release of matrix metalloproteinases, which cause the disruption of the blood–brain barrier and edema [6].

A decrease in mitochondrial enzymatic activity decreases antioxidant defenses, thus increasing oxidative stress and potentiating the effect of ischemia [10].

3. Current Prevention Strategies

Current stroke prevention strategies in patients with T2DM are based on controlling each of the risk factors. Therefore, lifestyle measures are of primordial importance. Intensive blood pressure control has also been shown to reduce the risk of cerebrovascular damage in people with T2DM [11]. The presence of T2DM alone places patients in higher cardiovascular risk categories, leading to the recommendation for stricter control of the lipid profile [12,13].

Additionally, it is recommended to implement antithrombotic strategies when indicated or anticoagulation for those with a cardioembolic source [14,15]. For those with significant carotid stenosis, revascularization should be considered [16].

The hallmark study UK Prospective Diabetes Study (UKPDS) in patients with recent onset of T2DM demonstrated that improved glycemic control was associated with very early benefits in reducing microvascular complications. Conversely, no immediate effect on macrovascular complications was seen. In the 10-year analysis, benefits in reducing macrovascular complications started to emerge, but only in the metformin arm. Patients on insulin and sulphonylureas only had clear benefits at 20 years [17,18]. Trials such as Action to Control Cardiovascular Risk in Diabetes (ACCORD), Action in Diabetes and Vascular Disease: Preterax and Diamicron Modified Release Controlled Evaluation (ADVANCE), and Veterans Affairs Diabetes Trial (VADT) sought to analyze the impact of aggressive glycemic control on macrovascular events in people with several years of DM and established or high risk for cardiovascular disease (CVD). The results obtained did not favor the use of strict glycemic targets in this group of patients to optimize cardiovascular outcomes [19]. An important consideration is that the more intensive glycemic control in these studies was attained at the cost of a twofold increase in the risk of severe hypoglycemia, which is a potent marker of high absolute risk of cardiovascular events and mortality [20]. A metanalysis of individual participant data from these four studies demonstrated a significant reduction in myocardial infarctions and major CVD events as a whole, but no difference in stroke, heart failure, or mortality between intensive and less intensive glycemic control [21]. These landmark studies need to be considered with the important caveat that drugs such as sodium–glucose cotransporter type 2 inhibitors (SGLT2is) and glucagon-like peptide 1 receptor agonists (GLP1-Ra) were not in clinical use at the time.

One might pose the following question: could stroke prevention depend not only on the degree of glycemic control, but also on the choice of antihyperglycemic drugs? This issue will be explored in subsequent sections of this text.

4. New Antihyperglycemic Drugs and Influence on Stroke

The treatment algorithm recommended for T2DM has undergone important changes in recent years. Until 2017, the American Diabetes Association (ADA) recommended the use of metformin as the first-line and a selection of the following drugs based on factors such as effectiveness, cost, and adverse effects [22]. In 2018, the ADA and the European Association for the Study of Diabetes (EASD) published a consensus report in which it was recommended, after metformin, preference for SGLT2is and GLP1-Ra in patients with established cardiovascular disease or chronic kidney disease [23]. In recent years, data have emerged to support the benefit of these two groups of drugs, even in patients not treated with metformin [24]. In this context, in 2022, the ADA and the EASD published a new consensus in which they recommend that drugs such as SGLT2is and GLP1-Ra can be used as first-line therapies in patients with established or high risk for CVD, independently of the background use of metformin [25].

The changes observed in the diabetes treatment algorithm largely result from the various cardiovascular outcome trials that have been mandatory according to the Food and Drug Administration since 2008. The initial aim of these trials was to demonstrate the cardiovascular safety of drugs for the treatment of DM before their introduction to the market. However, data have emerged demonstrating the cardiovascular and renal benefits of drugs such as GLP1-Ra and SGLT2is, justifying their preference [26]. In these trials, the following are frequently assessed: the risk of the three-point composite outcome of major cardiovascular events (3P-MACE)—non-fatal myocardial infarction, non-fatal stroke, and cardiovascular death, the risk of hospitalization for heart failure (HF), and risk of adverse renal events. Therefore, stroke is evaluated as a primary outcome only in conjunction with other events, not allowing the benefits of this outcome to be so directly inferred [27].

4.1. Glucagon-like Peptide 1 Receptor Agonists (GLP1-Ra)

Glucagon-like peptide-1 (GLP-1) is a peptide predominantly produced in enteroendocrine L cells in the distal ileum and colon. Its plasma levels increase within minutes after food ingestion. The GLP-1 receptor (GLP1-R) is expressed in the α and β cells of pancreatic islets, in the central and peripheral nervous system, heart, kidney, lung, and gastrointestinal tract. The activation of this receptor increases insulin release in a glucose-dependent manner, promotes resistance to apoptosis, increases β-cell survival, inhibits glucagon secretion, delays gastric emptying, diminishes food intake, and promotes greater glucose elimination through neural mechanisms [28].

Most of these drugs have demonstrated cardiovascular benefits, and are currently recommended as one of the preferred groups in people with T2DM and established or high risk of CVD and/or chronic kidney disease (CKD) [25].

As previously mentioned, in cardiovascular outcome trials (CVOTs), the composite of major cardiovascular events (3P-MACE) is frequently used. Several clinical trials to date have demonstrated a protective effect of GLP1-Ra regarding major cardiovascular events, namely LEADER (Liraglutide Effect and Action in Diabetes: Evaluation of Cardiovascular Outcome Results), SUSTAIN-6 (Semaglutide Unabated Sustainability in Treatment of Type 2 Diabetes 6), Harmony Outcomes with Albiglutide, REWIND (Researching Cardiovascular Events With a Weekly Incretin in Diabetes) with dulaglutide, and the AMPLITUDE-O trial (Effect of Efpeglenatide on Cardiovascular Outcomes) [29–33]. CVOTs with Lixisenatide, Exenatide, and oral semaglutide have so far demonstrated non-inferiority [34–36]. In these trials, the effect on the risk of stroke was also specifically reported as a secondary outcome, with the SUSTAIN 6 and REWIND studies showing a statistically significant reduction in the risk of fatal and non-fatal stroke (hazard ratio 0.61, CI 0.38–0.99 and 0.76 CI 0.62–0.94, respectively) [30,32]. In most of the remaining trials, there was also a trend toward a reduction in the risk of stroke, although without reaching statistical significance [3].

Several metanalyses were performed that provided data on GLP1-Ra's influence on the risk of stroke. In a network metanalysis from 2019, GLP1-Ra (vs. placebo) was shown to significantly reduce non-fatal stroke (OR = 0.88, 95% CI (0.77, 0.99), $p = 0.002$) [37]. In 2020, Malhotra et al. found that GLP-1Ra could reduce nonfatal strokes (OR 0.84; 95% CI (0.76–0.94)) and all strokes (OR 0.84; 95% CI (0.75–0.93), $p = 0.001$) [38]. Subsequent metanalyses performed by Grewal et al. and Palmer et al. also corroborated a beneficial effect of GLP1-Ra on stroke prevention [39,40]. Wei et al. reported that a 17% reduction in the risk of stroke with GLP1-Ra (vs. placebo) (RR = 0.83, 95% CI (0.73, 0.95), $p = 0.005$) was at the cost of ischemic stroke (RR = 0.83, 95% CI (0.73, 0.95), $p = 0.008$) reduction, with no effect on hemorrhagic stroke (RR = 0.83, 95% CI (0.57, 1.20), $p = 0.31$) [41].

Most data suggest the prevention of recurrent stroke, but there are also data on primary prevention. A retrospective cohort study based on an insurance database in Thailand (1998 to 2018) sought to evaluate the effect of GLP1-Ra on the prevention of ischemic stroke in the Asian population with T2DM without established CVD. The authors conclude that prolonged use and higher doses of GLP-1-Ra were associated with a reduced risk of hospitalization for ischemic stroke among Asian patients with T2DM who did not have established atherosclerotic CVD [42].

A post hoc analysis of the SUSTAIN 6 and the PIONEER trials also supported semaglutide's ability to reduce the risk of first stroke. This effect was mainly attributed to the reduction in small vessel occlusion [43].

Several mechanisms have been proposed for the neuroprotection conferred by GLP1-Ra, namely a neuroprotective effect with increases in neurogenesis and angiogenesis and decreases in apoptosis, oxidative stress, neuroinflammation, excitotoxicity, and the area of infarction [44]. Beneficial effects on atherosclerotic plaque have been supported by several preclinical studies [45,46], as well as by data suggesting that liraglutide decreases the medial thickness of the carotid intimal layer [47]. There also seems to be a role in the reduction in reactive oxygen species production and oxidative stress [41]. Preclinical studies suggest that liraglutide decreases inflammation in endothelial cells through calcium and AMP-activated protein kinase mechanisms and increases the expression of antioxidant genes downstream of protein kinase A and cAMP response element-binding protein [41]. GLP1-Ra was also shown to lead to a decrease in the inflammatory macrophage activation molecule sCD163, a decrease in the levels of TNF-α and IL-6 (pro-inflammatory), and an increase in adiponectin (anti-inflammatory) [48]. There may be an additional contribution to increasing neuronal energy supply through the positive regulation of GLUT4 involved in the supply of metabolic energy to fire neurons [41]. Recent metanalysis showed that the overall reduction in cardiovascular events with GLP1-Ra seems to be mediated in part by decreases in hemoglobin A1C [49,50]. In addition to all these effects, there are indirect benefits through action on various cardiovascular risk parameters, namely the modest improvement in lipid profile and blood pressure and a significant effect on weight [3].

When considering the introduction of GLP1-Ra, it is essential to take into account potential side effects that may limit their use. The side effects of GLP1Ra encompass gastrointestinal disturbances, pancreatitis, gallbladder disease, increased heart rate, and potential increased risk of medullary thyroid cancer (only documented in rodents) [51,52]. Recently, some concerns have been raised regarding its use in patients with HF with reduced ejection fraction (HF-rEF), which may be related to its effect on heart rate [53].

4.2. Sodium–Glucose Cotransporter Type 2 Inhibitors (SGLT2is)

Glucose only begins to be excreted in the urine when a glycemia threshold of around 180 mg/dL is exceeded, with a linear increase in glycosuria beyond this concentration. This threshold for glycosuria increases in patients with T2DM. SGLTs are responsible for transporting glucose across epithelial cells by active transport. The SGLT2 isoform is mainly found in the proximal convoluted tubule, being responsible for the reabsorption of over 90% of filtered glucose. Additionally, it is also found in much lower concentrations in the brain, liver, thyroid, and skeletal muscle. The pharmacological blockade of these transporters leads to an increase in glycosuria, allowing the excretion of 50–60% of filtered glucose [54,55].

Studies on cardiovascular outcomes have demonstrated the effectiveness of SGLT2is in reducing the incidence of hospitalizations for HF and the 3P-MACE composite, and most evidence suggests that the benefit on 3P-MACE may be limited to people with established CVD [56]. In general, observational studies have demonstrated the benefit of SGLT2is in both the primary and secondary prevention of 3P-MACE events, whereas RCTs have not, which is likely attributed to the different conditions of these types of studies [57].

Several mechanisms have been proposed for the cardiorenal benefits of SGLT2is, namely decreased blood pressure; modest weight loss; improvement of cardiac energy metabolism; prevention of inflammation, ischemia–reperfusion injury, and adverse cardiac remodeling; and inhibition of the sympathetic nervous system [58]. The decrease in glucose and sodium reabsorption achieved by the inhibition of SGLT2 leads to a decrease in HbA1c and global glucotoxicity. There is also a local effect of reducing glucose overload in tubular cells, which enhances the production of erythropoietin with consequent better oxygenation. With the increase in sodium excretion, there is an improvement in the reduction of intra-glomerular pressure, a reduction in albuminuria, preservation of glomerular filtration rate, and a decrease in blood pressure. The increased excretion of glucose enhances the negative caloric balance that leads to weight loss and the excretion of uric acid [55].

In the main CVOTs with SGLT2i, the impact on stroke risk has been reported [59]. In early CVOTs, such as Empagliflozin Cardiovascular Outcome Event Trial in Type 2 Diabetes Mellitus Patients (EMPA-REG) [60], Canagliflozin Cardiovascular Assessment Study (CANVAS) [61], Dapagliflozin Effect on CardiovascuLAR Events (DECLARE-TIMI) [62], and Ertugliflozin Efficacy and Safety Cardiovascular Outcomes Trial (VERTIS CV) [63], there was a neutral effect on the risk of total stroke and no fatal stroke. In EMPA-REG, there was actually a tendency toward a higher risk of stroke without statistical significance (HR 1.18, CI 0.89–1.56). In this regard, it should be noted that, more recently, the observational cohort study in 11 countries, EMPagliflozin comparative effectiveness and Safety (EMPRISE), was published, which even suggests that empagliflozin may be associated with an 18% reduction in the risk of stroke compared with dipeptidyl peptidase 4 inhibitors (DPP4is) [64]. More recent data derived from the EMPRISE study have shown a similar risk of the composite outcome myocardial infarction or stroke when compared with GLP1-RA. The risk of stroke was evaluated as a secondary outcome and there was no statistically significant difference (HR 1.08, IC 0.95–1.22 for SGLT2i) [65]. Thus, although it has been proposed that there may be a contribution of the effect of hypotension and hemoconcentration justifying an increased risk of stroke with SGLT2i [59], it is more likely that it is an effect of chance.

Some authors argue that these CVOTs may have insufficient statistical power to test the effect of SGLT2i on reducing stroke risk, given that they mainly included patients with DM with established CVD other than stroke. Furthermore, nonfatal stroke is typically considered a component of the 3P-MACE composite outcome, rather than the primary outcome [59]. Other authors, however, suggest that SGLT2i reduces the 3P-MACE in a way unrelated to antiatherogenic effects, as there seem to be no discernible effects on MI or stroke incidence [66].

In a metanalysis published in April 2023, 36 clinical trials that reported on the effect of SGLT2is on the occurrence of stroke were taken into account, and no statistically significant difference was found between patients under SGLT2i vs. the control group, (RR: 0.97; 95% CI, 0.89–1.07, $p = 0.56$), even though SGLT2i use was associated with a statistically significant reduction in the risk of AF (RR: 0.87; 95% CI, 0.76–0.99, $p = 0.03$) [67]. A previous metanalysis also indicated neutrality of SGLT2i regarding stroke [37,40].

Lui et al. evaluated a population-based retrospective cohort of people with T2DM identified from Hong Kong electronic health records between 2008 and 2020. Patients who received SGLT2i or GLP-1RA were matched by propensity score matching. The authors did not find a significant difference between the SGLT2i and GLP1-Ra groups. They found, however, that patients with a history of stroke seemed to benefit more from the use of GLP1-Ra. There was a significantly higher risk of ischemic stroke among people on SGLT2is compared with GLP1-Ra users (HR 1.53, 95% CI 1.01–2.33, $p = 0.044$; IRR 1.52, 95% CI 1.02–2.27, $p = 0.041$). The risks of hemorrhagic stroke and cardioembolic stroke were similar for the groups treated with both pharmacological groups [68].

Regarding hemorrhagic stroke, there are data from two meta-analyses attributing a 50% reduction in the risk of hemorrhagic stroke to patients on SGLT2i vs. placebo [69,70]. There are several theoretical explanations for a possible benefit of SGLT2is on the risk of hemorrhagic stroke: a beneficial effect of blood pressure reduction, [68] increased low-density lipoprotein (LDL) cholesterol and triglycerides, reduced overload of small vessels and microhemorrhages, and "cerebrorenal" interaction [59]. A 4–10 mmHg reduction in systolic blood pressure has indeed been observed among both hypertensive and normotensive patients with T2DM using SGLT2is [71]. Some studies have suggested a relationship between a reduction in LDL and a higher risk of hemorrhagic stroke, but this is highly controversial and not supported by more recent analyses [72]. A beneficial effect of SGLT2is on kidney outcomes has been demonstrated consistently in several clinical trials and real-world studies [73]. There are several traditional risk factors shared between CKD and cerebrovascular disease. Uremia and changes in phosphocalcium metabolism can contribute to vascular medial calcification and endothelial damage, and CKD can precipitate certain stroke risk factors, such as AF [59].

A recent comprehensive metanalysis analyzed the differential effect of SGLT2is and GLP-1Ra on the risk of stroke. The authors report that, even though data from RCTs and CVOTs mostly favor GLP1-Ra, data from observational studies do not support a difference in the risk of stroke between the two pharmacological classes. Differences in study populations and lack of head-to-head comparisons in RCTs were suggested as potential explanatory factors. As such, the authors conclude that it is not linear whether, in the real-life setting, GLP-1Ra should be prioritized over SGLT2is for stroke prevention [74].

It is also worth considering that SGLT2is may be beneficial in stroke prevention in specific populations, such as those with HF with reduced ejection fraction (HF rEF), AF, and more severe CKD. Among patients with HF-rEF but not with preserved ejection fraction (HFpEF), the initiation of SGLT2i versus DPP4i was associated with a lower risk of myocardial infarction or stroke (HR: 0.86 [0.75. 0.99]). In comparison with GLP1-Ra, this superiority of SGLT2is was not demonstrated [56]. In a nationwide database from Taiwan, medication with SGLT2is in T2DM patients with AF and without previous cardiovascular events was associated with a lower incidence of stroke and dementia [75]. A recent metanalysis of 10 RCTs suggested that the effects of SGLT2is on stroke, HF, and cardiovascular death prevention was greater for patients with more severe CKD. Stroke risk reduction was only found in patients with a lower glomerular filtration rate (GFR), while in patients with a GFR >80 mL/min/1.73 m^2, a higher risk was found in patients under SGLT2i vs. placebo [76].

It is also important to mention a metanalysis by Sayour et al., which sought to evaluate whether there was an influence of SGLT2 receptor selectivity on cardiovascular outcomes. The authors concluded that, in high-CV-risk T2DM patients, dual SGLT2/1 inhibition reduced stroke risk, but had limited additional benefits [77].

To conclude this section, it is paramount to be aware of the potential disadvantages of this drug class when contemplating their introduction to patients with T2DM. Side effects of SGLT2i include elevated ketone body levels and euglycemic ketoacidosis (rare in T2DM), genital mycotic infections, volume depletion, acute kidney injury, and possibly, although controversial, Fournier gangrene. Canagliflozin may also increase the risk of lower-extremity amputation and bone fractures, although such effects have not been reported with other SGLT2is [52,78,79].

4.3. *Dipeptidyl Peptidase 4 Inhibitors (DPP4is)*

Dipeptidyl peptidase 4 is an enzyme that breaks down incretin hormones, such as GLP1 and glucose-dependent insulinotropic polypeptide (GIP). DPP4is work by blocking this enzyme, thus preventing the breakdown of incretin hormones. GLP1 is believed to be the major player in mediating the therapeutic effect of DPP4is [80].

These drugs have also been subjected to cardiovascular outcome trials, but generally demonstrating neutral results [81,82].

Regarding stroke specifically, the metanalyses carried out to date have, as expected, corroborated the neutrality of these drugs in the risk of stroke, highlighting the beneficial effect of GLP1-Ra [83,84]. Although DPP4is have a similar mechanism of effect to GLP1-Ra, these drugs do not cross the blood–brain barrier, do not induce an increase in plasma GLP1, and have a weak effect on reducing infarct volume [83].

4.3.1. Tirzepatide

Tirzepatide is a dual GLP-1 and GIP receptor agonist, approved by the Food and Drug Administration (FDA) and later by the European Medicines Agency (EMA) for T2DM [58,85].

The tirzepatide versus insulin glargine in type 2 diabetes and increased cardiovascular risk: a randomized, open-label, parallel-group, multicenter, phase 3 trial (SURPASS-4) has been completed, demonstrating a great reduction in HbA1c, less risk of hypoglycemia, and cardiovascular safety with tirzepatide vs. glargine [86]. SURPASS-CVOT is still ongoing and will be able to better clarify the advantages of this drug and its impact on CVD [87].

4.3.2. Finerenone

Finerenone is a non-steroidal mineralocorticoid receptor antagonist that has demonstrated cardiovascular benefit in patients with T2DM and risk of CVD. It is currently recommended by the ADA in people with CKD to reduce the risk of CVD and the progression of kidney disease in those with albuminuria [88].

Although the drug has effectively shown a benefit in the 3P-MACE composite outcome in the Finerenone in Chronic Kidney Disease and Type 2 Diabetes: Combined FIDELIO-DKD and FIGARO-DKD Trial Programme Analysis (FIDELITY) pooled analysis, it has not yet been shown to specifically prevent stroke [89,90].

Table 1 provides a summary of the evidence regarding the more recently introduced therapies, that underwent CVOTs, on 3P-MACE in general and on stroke in particular.

Table 1. Summary of data on the effect on major adverse cardiovascular events and stroke from novel therapies for the treatment of type 2 diabetes mellitus.

	Effect on 3P-MACE	Effect on Stroke
Glucagon-like Peptide 1 Receptor Agonists (GLP1-Ra)	• RCTs show a benefit of subcutaneous liraglutide, dulaglutide, semaglutide, and efpeglenatide [29–33] and non-inferiority for lixisenatide, exenatide, and oral semaglutide [34–36].	• Some evidence of a benefit in RCTs where it was evaluated as a secondary outcome [30,32]. • Several metanalyses support a stroke risk reduction [37,39,40], particularly on isquemic stroke. No effect on hemorrhagic stroke was seen [41].
Sodium–glucose cotransporter type 2 inhibitors (SGLT2i)	• Demonstrated effectiveness in reducing the incidence of hospitalizations for HF and the 3P-MACE composite in CVOTs, although mostly limited to patients with established CVD [56]. • Observational studies have demonstrated the benefit of SGLT2i in both primary and secondary prevention of 3P-MACE events [57].	• In CVOTs, no statistically significant difference was observed regarding stroke [60–63]. Metanalyses also suggest neutrality [37,40,67]. • Data from observational studies do not support a difference in the risk of stroke compared with GLP1-Ra [74]. • May be beneficial in stroke prevention in specific populations, such as those with HF with reduced ejection fraction [56], atrial fibrillation [75], and more severe chronic kidney disease [76].
Dipeptidyl Peptidase 4 Inhibitors (DPP4is)	• Neutral results in CVOTs [81,82].	• Neutral results in CVOTs [83,84].
Tirzepatide	• Non-inferiority vs. glargine [86]. • CVOT is ongoing [87].	• CVOT is ongoing [87] and may provide data.
Finerenone	• Benefit in 3P-MACE [89,90].	• Not shown to specifically prevent stroke in CVOTs [89,90].

CVD—cardiovascular disease; CVOTs—cardiovascular outcome trials; DPP4is—Dipeptidyl peptidase 4 inhibitors; GLP1-Ra—Glucagon-like peptide 1 receptor agonists; HF—heart failure; MACE—major adverse cardiovascular events; RCTs—randomized controlled trials; SGLT2i—Sodium–glucose cotransporter type 2 inhibitors.

5. What about "Older" Pharmacological Options?

CVOTs only became mandatory from 2008 onwards, so for drugs approved before this year, there are not as much solid data regarding cardiovascular outcomes. Still, other types of analyses are available that provide some information.

Metformin is an older drug of established relevance in the treatment of T2DM. There are data suggesting cardiovascular benefits of this drug. In the UKPDS, the metformin arm had a 30% lower risk of cardiovascular complications compared with the diet group, [18] which was also seen in the 10-year follow-up after the trial [91]. A 2017 metanalysis documented the benefit of metformin on all cardiovascular endpoints except stroke, but without reaching statistical significance [92]. In 2019, Han et al. and later Zhang et al. published metanalyses that demonstrated reduced cardiovascular risk with metformin [93,94]. Regarding stroke, there are data suggesting a beneficial effect of metformin, particularly if there is a sustained use pre-event that is maintained afterward [95]. Taking metformin prior to stroke seems to be associated with lower stroke severity and better functional outcomes in patients with small-vessel disease [96].

Within the group of drugs approved prior to the need for CVOTs, glitazones have received the most attention in the context of stroke and are recommended in current guidelines [25,52]. In experimental models, treatment with peroxisome proliferator-activated receptor gamma (PPARγ) agonists improved insulin sensitivity and inhibited the development of atherosclerosis [27]. Additionally, treatment with pioglitazone reduced the area of post-stroke hemorrhagic transformation [97]. In clinical studies, most evidence is of the prevention of recurrent stroke. In the PROactive study, pioglitazone reduced the risk of recurrent stroke by 24% (HR = 0.53, 95% CI = 0.34–0.85; p = 0.0085), but not of the first stroke [98]. In the Insulin Resistance Intervention after Stroke (IRIS) trial, pioglitazone was effective in the secondary prevention of ischemic stroke in patients without DM with insulin resistance [99]. In a Korean publication, a benefit was reported in preventing the first stroke event (odds ratio 0.69, 95% CI (0.60–0.80)), with the greatest benefit in patients with hypertension, obesity, smoking, and a sedentary lifestyle [100].

Sulphonylureas stimulate insulin secretion by closing potassium channels in pancreatic beta-cells independently of plasma glucose levels. The cardiovascular safety of sulfonylureas is controversial. Two metanalyses showed a significantly higher risk of stroke for SUs than for comparator drugs in patients with T2DM [101,102]. In a subsequent population-based cohort study with almost 100,000 patients with T2DM, sulphonylureas use was associated with higher risks of stroke, cardiovascular mortality, and all-cause mortality compared with metformin [103]. A more recent retrospective study with a comparable size demonstrated similar findings [104]. These results suggest that sulfonylureas should be considered carefully or even avoided in patients with high cardiovascular risk.

6. Clinical Implications of Current Data

As previously mentioned, since 2022, the ADA and EASD consensus, and also the current ADA Standards of Care, propose that GLP1-Ra and/or SGLT2i be included in people with T2DM and established or high risk for CVD, HF, and/or CKD to reduce the cardiovascular risk [25,52]. However, given that there is evidence suggesting a greater benefit of GLP1-Ra in atherosclerotic disease and stroke, currently, several authors propose the preferential use of this pharmacological group in patients with a previous history of stroke [49,58]. Pioglitazone is also a drug to be considered by the ADA and the EASD after the previously mentioned drugs in patients with established atherosclerotic CVD [25,52]. Given the relatively frequent coexistence of HF in these patients, it is necessary to take into account HF when considering initiating glitazones and, more recently, the doubt that has also been raised regarding the safety of GLP1-Ra in patients with HF-rEF [53]. Considering all the above-mentioned data, in patients with a history of atherosclerotic disease and/or ischemic stroke, especially without HF, a logical order of introduction of drugs could be GLP1-Ra, followed by SGLT2i, and later pioglitazone. However, in patients with stroke and a history of HF-rEF, advanced CKD, and/or hemorrhagic stroke, the evidence for selection is not as strong and a SGLT2i will often be placed as a first option.

As for the primary prevention of stroke, besides the importance of adequate glycemic control, the specific targeting of obesity, CKD, and other CV risk factors may also influence antidiabetic drug choices. The discussion of the influence of different pharmacological classes on CVD and CKD has been explored in previous sections of this text. As for targeting obesity, both GLP1-Ra and SGLT2i have a beneficial effect on weight, but the

GLP1-Ra may be associated with a greater reduction, particularly semaglutide. Tirzepatide is also associated with an important weight reduction [52].

Figure 1 provides a summary of the proposed recommendations for stroke prevention in type 2 diabetic patients based on current data.

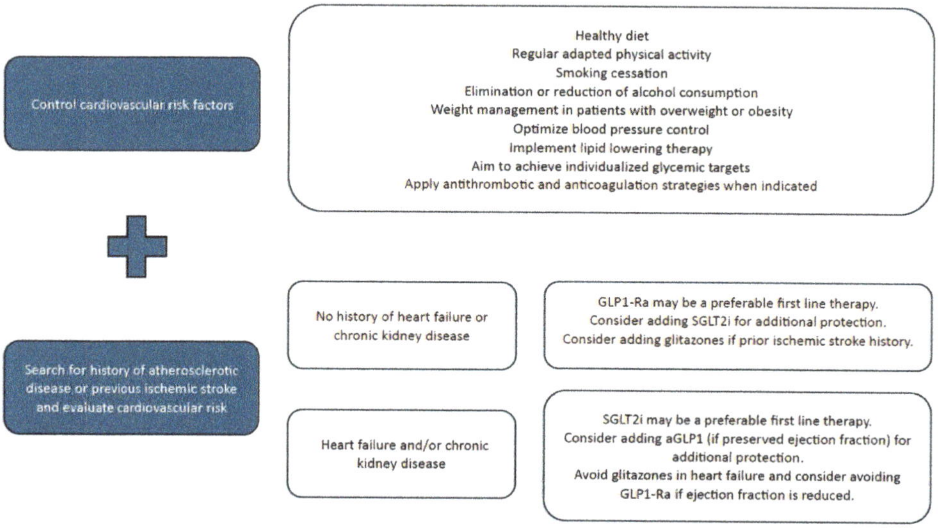

Figure 1. Summary of proposed recommendations for stroke prevention in type 2 diabetic patients. GLP1-Ra—Glucagon-like peptide 1 receptor agonists; SGLT2i—Sodium–glucose cotransporter type 2 inhibitors.

7. Conclusions

In recent decades, CVOTs have brought important data on the role of drugs designed to treat DM in the prevention of cardiovascular events. There is still much to learn, however, on the specific role of these drugs in stroke prevention. Nevertheless, data suggest that GLP1-Ra has a particularly beneficial effect on ischemic stroke. As for hemorrhagic stroke, the available information is less clear, but SGLT2is may be particularly beneficial.

8. Future Perspectives

In recent years, the algorithm of treatment of T2DM has suffered tremendous alterations and currently is not exclusively focused on glycemic control, but also on other goals, such as cardiorenal risk and weight management. Nevertheless, there is still much that can be perfected regarding individual goal definition and treatment personalization.

In the near future, studies on newer pharmacological classes are also expected to emerge and to add useful information. The above-mentioned SURPASS-CVOT is a double-blind, active-controlled CV outcomes trial which is evaluating the cardiovascular safety and efficacy of tirzepatide vs. dulaglutide. As in previous trials, the MACE composite is the primary outcome and data on stroke may be available as a secondary outcome [81]. Most patients with diabetes will be at risk for different types of cardiovascular events (myocardial infarction, ischemic stroke, hemorrhagic stroke, peripheral artery disease, . . .) and will also have several risk factors that may limit the utilization of specific drug classes. As such, it is paramount to stimulate stakeholders to evaluate the effect on each of the macrovascular complications in a detailed manner, for instance, having specific trials with stroke as a primary outcome. In the era of personalized medicine, the exponential increase in knowledge regarding new therapies will hopefully allow clinicians to further take into account the individual characteristics of each patient in the selection of the most adequate treatment combination.

Author Contributions: I.H.V. and T.S.C. made a similar contribution to this article and share first authorship. Conceptualization and methodology, I.H.V. and T.S.C.; writing—original draft preparation, I.H.V. and T.S.C.; review and editing, I.H.V., T.S.C., J.S., L.G. and I.P.; supervision J.S., L.G. and I.P. All authors have read and agreed to the published version of the manuscript.

Funding: This research received no external funding.

Conflicts of Interest: The authors have no conflicts of interest to declare.

References

1. Wafa, H.A.; Wolfe, C.D.A.; Emmett, E.; Roth, G.A.; Johnson, C.O.; Wang, Y. Burden of Stroke in Europe: Thirty-Year Projections of Incidence, Prevalence, Deaths, and Disability-Adjusted Life Years. *Stroke* **2020**, *51*, 2418–2427. [CrossRef] [PubMed]
2. Duration of Diabetes and Risk of Ischemic Stroke | Stroke [Internet]. Available online: https://www.ahajournals.org/doi/10.1161/strokeaha.111.641381 (accessed on 23 March 2024).
3. Williams, D.M.; Atkinson, M.; Evans, M. Stroke Prevention and Treatment in People with Type 2 Diabetes: Is There a Role for GLP-1 (Glucagon-Like Peptide-1) Analogues? *Stroke* **2023**, *54*, 1441–1451. [CrossRef] [PubMed]
4. Fuentes, B. Antidiabetic drugs for stroke prevention in patients with type-2 diabetes. The neurologist's point of view. *Med. Clin.* **2018**, *150*, 275–281. [CrossRef] [PubMed]
5. Caturano, A.; Galiero, R.; Pafundi, P.C. Atrial Fibrillation and Stroke. A Review on the Use of Vitamin K Antagonists and Novel Oral Anticoagulants. *Med. Kaunas Lith.* **2019**, *55*, 617. [CrossRef] [PubMed]
6. Zhang, Z.; Yan, J.; Shi, H. Hyperglycemia as a Risk Factor of Ischemic Stroke. *J. Drug Metab. Toxicol.* **2013**, *4*, 153. [PubMed]
7. Allen, C.L.; Bayraktutan, U. Oxidative stress and its role in the pathogenesis of ischaemic stroke. *Int. J. Stroke Off. J. Int. Stroke Soc.* **2009**, *4*, 461–470. [CrossRef] [PubMed]
8. Caturano, A.; D'Angelo, M.; Mormone, A.; Russo, V.; Mollica, M.P.; Salvatore, T.; Galiero, R.; Rinaldi, L.; Vetrano, E.; Marfella, R.; et al. Oxidative Stress in Type 2 Diabetes: Impacts from Pathogenesis to Lifestyle Modifications. *Curr. Issues Mol. Biol.* **2023**, *45*, 6651–6666. [CrossRef] [PubMed]
9. Salvatore, T.; Galiero, R.; Caturano, A.; Vetrano, E.; Loffredo, G.; Rinaldi, L.; Catalini, C.; Gjeloshi, K.; Albanese, G.; Di Martino, A.; et al. Coronary Microvascular Dysfunction in Diabetes Mellitus: Pathogenetic Mechanisms and Potential Therapeutic Options. *Biomedicines* **2022**, *10*, 2274. [CrossRef] [PubMed]
10. Kamboj, S.S.; Sandhir, R. Protective effect of N-acetylcysteine supplementation on mitochondrial oxidative stress and mitochondrial enzymes in cerebral cortex of streptozotocin-treated diabetic rats. *Mitochondrion* **2011**, *11*, 214–222. [CrossRef] [PubMed]
11. ACCORD Study Group; Cushman, W.C.; Evans, G.W.; Byington, R.P.; Goff, D.C.; Grimm, R.H.; Cutler, J.A.; Simons-Morton, D.G.; Basile, J.N.; Corson, M.A.; et al. Effects of intensive blood-pressure control in type 2 diabetes mellitus. *N. Engl. J. Med.* **2010**, *362*, 1575–1585.
12. Visseren, F.L.J.; Mach, F.; Smulders, Y.M.; Carballo, D.; Koskinas, K.C.; Bäck, M.; Benetos, A.; Biffi, A.; Boavida, J.-M.; Capodanno, D.; et al. 2021 ESC Guidelines on cardiovascular disease prevention in clinical practice. *Eur. Heart J.* **2021**, *42*, 3227–3337. [CrossRef] [PubMed]
13. ElSayed, N.A.; Aleppo, G.; Aroda, V.R.; Bannuru, R.R.; Brown, F.M.; Bruemmer, D.; Collins, B.S.; Das, S.R.; Hilliard, M.E.; Isaacs, D.; et al. 10. Cardiovascular Disease and Risk Management: Standards of Care in Diabetes—2023. *Diabetes Care* **2023**, *46*, S158–S190. [CrossRef]
14. Meschia, J.F.; Bushnell, C.; Boden-Albala, B.; Braun, L.T.; Bravata, D.M.; Chaturvedi, S.; Creager, M.A.; Eckel, R.H.; Elkind, M.S.V.; Fornage, M.; et al. Guidelines for the primary prevention of stroke: A statement for healthcare professionals from the American Heart Association/American Stroke Association. *Stroke* **2014**, *45*, 3754–3832. [CrossRef]
15. Kleindorfer, D.O.; Towfighi, A.; Chaturvedi, S.; Cockroft, K.M.; Gutierrez, J.; Lombardi-Hill, D.; Kamel, H.; Kernan, W.N.; Kittner, S.J.; Leira, E.C.; et al. 2021 Guideline for the Prevention of Stroke in Patients with Stroke and Transient Ischemic Attack: A Guideline from the American Heart Association/American Stroke Association. *Stroke* **2021**, *52*, e364–e467. [CrossRef]
16. Aboyans, V.; Ricco, J.-B.; Bartelink, M.-L.E.L.; Björck, M.; Brodmann, M.; Cohnert, T.; Collet, J.-P.; Czerny, M.; De Carlo, M.; Debus, S.; et al. 2017 ESC Guidelines on the Diagnosis and Treatment of Peripheral Arterial Diseases, in collaboration with the European Society for Vascular Surgery (ESVS): Document covering atherosclerotic disease of extracranial carotid and vertebral, mesenteric, renal, upper and lower extremity arteriesEndorsed by: The European Stroke Organization (ESO)The Task Force for the Diagnosis and Treatment of Peripheral Arterial Diseases of the European Society of Cardiology (ESC) and of the European Society for Vascular Surgery (ESVS). *Eur. Heart J.* **2018**, *39*, 763–816. [PubMed]
17. UK Prospective Diabetes Study (UKPDS) Group. Intensive blood-glucose control with sulphonylureas or insulin compared with conventional treatment and risk of complications in patients with type 2 diabetes (UKPDS 33). *Lancet* **1998**, *352*, 837–853. [CrossRef]
18. UK Prospective Diabetes Study (UKPDS) Group. Effect of intensive blood-glucose control with metformin on complications in overweight patients with type 2 diabetes (UKPDS 34). *Lancet* **1998**, *352*, 854–865. [CrossRef]
19. Skyler, J.S.; Bergenstal, R.; Bonow, R.O.; Buse, J.; Deedwania, P.; Gale, E.A.M.; Howard, B.V.; Kirkman, M.S.; Kosiborod, M.; Reaven, P.; et al. Intensive glycemic control and the prevention of cardiovascular events: Implications of the ACCORD,

ADVANCE, and VA Diabetes Trials: A position statement of the American Diabetes Association and a Scientific Statement of the American College of Cardiology Foundation and the American Heart Association. *J. Am. Coll. Cardiol.* **2009**, *53*, 298–304. [PubMed]
20. Lee, A.K.; Warren, B.; Lee, C.J.; McEvoy, J.W.; Matsushita, K.; Huang, E.S.; Sharrett, A.R.; Coresh, J.; Selvin, E. The Association of Severe Hypoglycemia with Incident Cardiovascular Events and Mortality in Adults with Type 2 Diabetes. *Diabetes Care* **2018**, *41*, 104–111. [CrossRef] [PubMed]
21. Control Group; Turnbull, F.M.; Abraira, C.; Anderson, R.J.; Byington, R.P.; Chalmers, J.P.; Duckworth, W.C.; Evans, G.W.; Gerstein, H.C.; Holman, R.R.; et al. Intensive glucose control and macrovascular outcomes in type 2 diabetes. *Diabetologia* **2009**, *52*, 2288–2298. [CrossRef]
22. American Diabetes Association. Standards of Medical Care in Diabetes-2017 Abridged for Primary Care Providers. *Clin. Diabetes Publ. Am. Diabetes Assoc.* **2017**, *35*, 5–26.
23. Davies, M.J.; D'Alessio, D.A.; Fradkin, J.; Kernan, W.N.; Mathieu, C.; Mingrone, G.; Rossing, P.; Tsapas, A.; Wexler, D.J.; Buse, J.B. Management of Hyperglycemia in Type 2 Diabetes, 2018. A Consensus Report by the American Diabetes Association (ADA) and the European Association for the Study of Diabetes (EASD). *Diabetes Care* **2018**, *41*, 2669–2701. [CrossRef] [PubMed]
24. Novel Antidiabetic Drugs and Risk of Cardiovascular Events in Patients without Baseline Metformin Use: A Meta-Analysis—PubMed. Available online: https://pubmed.ncbi.nlm.nih.gov/33606884/ (accessed on 18 June 2023).
25. Davies, M.J.; Aroda, V.R.; Collins, B.S.; Gabbay, R.A.; Green, J.; Maruthur, N.M.; Rosas, S.E.; Del Prato, S.; Mathieu, C.; Mingrone, G.; et al. Management of Hyperglycemia in Type 2 Diabetes, 2022. A Consensus Report by the American Diabetes Association (ADA) and the European Association for the Study of Diabetes (EASD). *Diabetes Care* **2022**, *45*, 2753–2786. [CrossRef] [PubMed]
26. Sharma, A.; Pagidipati, N.J.; Califf, R.M.; McGuire, D.K.; Green, J.B.; Demets, D.; George, J.T.; Gerstein, H.C.; Hobbs, T.; Holman, R.R.; et al. Impact of Regulatory Guidance on Evaluating Cardiovascular Risk of New Glucose-Lowering Therapies to Treat Type 2 Diabetes Mellitus: Lessons Learned and Future Directions. *Circulation* **2020**, *141*, 843–862. [CrossRef] [PubMed]
27. Lee, S.E.; Nam, H.; Choi, H.S.; Kim, H.; Kyoung, D.-S.; Kim, K.-A. Comparative Effects of Sodium-Glucose Cotransporter 2 Inhibitor and Thiazolidinedione Treatment on Risk of Stroke among Patients with Type 2 Diabetes Mellitus. *Diabetes Metab. J.* **2022**, *46*, 567–577. [CrossRef] [PubMed]
28. Drucker, D.J.; Nauck, M.A. The incretin system: Glucagon-like peptide-1 receptor agonists and dipeptidyl peptidase-4 inhibitors in type 2 diabetes. *Lancet* **2006**, *368*, 1696–1705. [CrossRef] [PubMed]
29. Marso, S.P.; Daniels, G.H.; Brown-Frandsen, K.; Kristensen, P.; Mann, J.F.E.; Nauck, M.A.; Nissen, S.E.; Pocock, S.; Poulter, N.R.; Ravn, L.S.; et al. Liraglutide and Cardiovascular Outcomes in Type 2 Diabetes. *N. Engl. J. Med.* **2016**, *375*, 311–322. [CrossRef] [PubMed]
30. Marso, S.P.; Bain, S.C.; Consoli, A.; Eliaschewitz, F.G.; Jódar, E.; Leiter, L.A.; Lingvay, I.; Rosenstock, J.; Seufert, J.; Warren, M.L.; et al. Semaglutide and Cardiovascular Outcomes in Patients with Type 2 Diabetes. *N. Engl. J. Med.* **2016**, *375*, 1834–1844. [CrossRef]
31. Hernandez, A.F.; Green, J.B.; Janmohamed, S.; D'Agostino, R.B.; Granger, C.B.; Jones, N.P.; Leiter, L.A.; Rosenberg, A.E.; Sigmon, K.N.; Somerville, M.C.; et al. Albiglutide and cardiovascular outcomes in patients with type 2 diabetes and cardiovascular disease (Harmony Outcomes): A double-blind, randomised placebo-controlled trial. *Lancet* **2018**, *392*, 1519–1529. [CrossRef]
32. Gerstein, H.C.; Colhoun, H.M.; Dagenais, G.R.; Diaz, R.; Lakshmanan, M.; Pais, P.; Probstfield, J.; Riesmeyer, J.S.; Riddle, M.C.; Rydén, L.; et al. Dulaglutide and cardiovascular outcomes in type 2 diabetes (REWIND): A double-blind, randomised placebo-controlled trial. *Lancet* **2019**, *394*, 121–130. [CrossRef]
33. Gerstein, H.C.; Sattar, N.; Rosenstock, J.; Ramasundarahettige, C.; Pratley, R.; Lopes, R.D.; Lam, C.S.P.; Khurmi, N.S.; Heenan, L.; Del Prato, S.; et al. Cardiovascular and Renal Outcomes with Efpeglenatide in Type 2 Diabetes. *N. Engl. J. Med.* **2021**, *385*, 896–907. [CrossRef] [PubMed]
34. Pfeffer, M.A.; Claggett, B.; Diaz, R.; Dickstein, K.; Gerstein, H.C.; Køber, L.V.; Lawson, F.C.; Ping, L.; Wei, X.; Lewis, E.F.; et al. Lixisenatide in Patients with Type 2 Diabetes and Acute Coronary Syndrome. *N. Engl. J. Med.* **2015**, *373*, 2247–2257. [CrossRef] [PubMed]
35. Holman, R.R.; Bethel, M.A.; Mentz, R.J.; Thompson, V.P.; Lokhnygina, Y.; Buse, J.B.; Chan, J.C.; Choi, J.; Gustavson, S.M.; Iqbal, N.; et al. Effects of Once-Weekly Exenatide on Cardiovascular Outcomes in Type 2 Diabetes. *N. Engl. J. Med.* **2017**, *377*, 1228–1239. [CrossRef] [PubMed]
36. Husain, M.; Birkenfeld, A.L.; Donsmark, M.; Dungan, K.; Eliaschewitz, F.G.; Franco, D.R.; Jeppesen, O.K.; Lingvay, I.; Mosenzon, O.; Pedersen, S.D.; et al. Oral Semaglutide and Cardiovascular Outcomes in Patients with Type 2 Diabetes. *N. Engl. J. Med.* **2019**, *381*, 841–851. [CrossRef] [PubMed]
37. Fei, Y.; Tsoi, M.-F.; Cheung, B.M.Y. Cardiovascular outcomes in trials of new antidiabetic drug classes: A network meta-analysis. *Cardiovasc. Diabetol.* **2019**, *18*, 112. [CrossRef] [PubMed]
38. Malhotra, K.; Katsanos, A.H.; Lambadiari, V.; Goyal, N.; Palaiodimou, L.; Kosmidou, M.; Krogias, C.; Alexandrov, A.V.; Tsivgoulis, G. GLP-1 receptor agonists in diabetes for stroke prevention: A systematic review and meta-analysis. *J. Neurol.* **2020**, *267*, 2117–2122. [CrossRef] [PubMed]
39. Grewal, S.; Zaman, N.; Borgatta, L.; Nudy, M.; Foy, A.J.; Peterson, B. Usefulness of Glucagon-Like Peptide-1 Receptor Agonists to Reduce Adverse Cardiovascular Disease Events in Patients with Type 2 Diabetes Mellitus. *Am. J. Cardiol.* **2021**, *154*, 48–53. [CrossRef] [PubMed]

40. Palmer, S.C.; Tendal, B.; Mustafa, R.A.; Vandvik, P.O.; Li, S.; Hao, Q.; Tunnicliffe, D.; Ruospo, M.; Natale, P.; Saglimbene, V.; et al. Sodium-glucose cotransporter protein-2 (SGLT-2) inhibitors and glucagon-like peptide-1 (GLP-1) receptor agonists for type 2 diabetes: Systematic review and network meta-analysis of randomised controlled trials. *BMJ* **2021**, *372*, m4573. [CrossRef] [PubMed]
41. Wei, J.; Yang, B.; Wang, R.; Ye, H.; Wang, Y.; Wang, L.; Zhang, X. Risk of stroke and retinopathy during GLP-1 receptor agonist cardiovascular outcome trials: An eight RCTs meta-analysis. *Front. Endocrinol.* **2022**, *13*, 1007980. [CrossRef]
42. Yang, Y.-S.; Chen, H.-H.; Huang, C.-N.; Hsu, C.Y.; Hu, K.-C.; Kao, C.-H. GLP-1RAs for Ischemic Stroke Prevention in Patients with Type 2 Diabetes without Established Atherosclerotic Cardiovascular Disease. *Diabetes Care* **2022**, *45*, 1184–1192. [CrossRef]
43. Strain, W.D.; Frenkel, O.; James, M.A.; Leiter, L.A.; Rasmussen, S.; Rothwell, P.M.; Sejersten Ripa, M.; Truelsen, T.C.; Husain, M. Effects of Semaglutide on Stroke Subtypes in Type 2 Diabetes: Post Hoc Analysis of the Randomized SUSTAIN 6 and PIONEER 6. *Stroke* **2022**, *53*, 2749–2757. [CrossRef]
44. Vergès, B.; Aboyans, V.; Angoulvant, D.; Boutouyrie, P.; Cariou, B.; Hyafil, F.; Mohammedi, K.; Amarenco, P. Protection against stroke with glucagon-like peptide-1 receptor agonists: A comprehensive review of potential mechanisms. *Cardiovasc. Diabetol.* **2022**, *21*, 242. [CrossRef]
45. Arakawa, M.; Mita, T.; Azuma, K.; Ebato, C.; Goto, H.; Nomiyama, T.; Fujitani, Y.; Hirose, T.; Kawamori, R.; Watada, H. Inhibition of monocyte adhesion to endothelial cells and attenuation of atherosclerotic lesion by a glucagon-like peptide-1 receptor agonist, exendin-4. *Diabetes* **2010**, *59*, 1030–1037. [CrossRef]
46. Gaspari, T.; Welungoda, I.; Widdop, R.E.; Simpson, R.W.; Dear, A.E. The GLP-1 receptor agonist liraglutide inhibits progression of vascular disease via effects on atherogenesis, plaque stability and endothelial function in an ApoE$^{-/-}$ mouse model. *Diab. Vasc. Dis. Res.* **2013**, *10*, 353–360. [CrossRef] [PubMed]
47. Rizzo, M.; Rizvi, A.A.; Patti, A.M.; Nikolic, D.; Giglio, R.V.; Castellino, G.; Li Volti, G.; Caprio, M.; Montalto, G.; Provenzano, V.; et al. Liraglutide improves metabolic parameters and carotid intima-media thickness in diabetic patients with the metabolic syndrome: An 18-month prospective study. *Cardiovasc. Diabetol.* **2016**, *15*, 162. [CrossRef]
48. Hogan, A.E.; Gaoatswe, G.; Lynch, L.; Corrigan, M.A.; Woods, C.; O'Connell, J.; O'Shea, D. Glucagon-like peptide 1 analogue therapy directly modulates innate immune-mediated inflammation in individuals with type 2 diabetes mellitus. *Diabetologia* **2014**, *57*, 781–784. [CrossRef] [PubMed]
49. Albert, S.G.; Shrestha, E.; Ahir, V. Stroke Prevention by Antihyperglycemic Drugs in Type 2 Diabetes Mellitus. *Endocr. Pract.* **2024**, *30*, 246–252. [CrossRef]
50. Rodriguez-Valadez, J.M.; Tahsin, M.; Masharani, U.; Park, M.; Hunink, M.G.M.; Yeboah, J.; Li, L.; Weber, E.; Berkalieva, A.; Avezaat, L.; et al. Potential Mediators for Treatment Effects of Novel Diabetes Medications on Cardiovascular and Renal Outcomes: A Meta-Regression Analysis. *J. Am. Heart Assoc.* **2024**, *13*, e032463. [CrossRef] [PubMed]
51. Filippatos, T.D.; Panagiotopoulou, T.V.; Elisaf, M.S. Adverse Effects of GLP-1 Receptor Agonists. *Rev. Diabet. Stud. RDS* **2014**, *11*, 202–230. [CrossRef]
52. American Diabetes Association Professional Practice Committee 9. Pharmacologic Approaches to Glycemic Treatment: Standards of Care in Diabetes-2024. *Diabetes Care* **2024**, *47*, S158–S178. [CrossRef]
53. Neves, J.S.; Packer, M.; Ferreira, J.P. Increased Risk of Heart Failure Hospitalization with GLP-1 Receptor Agonists in Patients with Reduced Ejection Fraction: A Meta-Analysis of the EXSCEL and FIGHT Trials. *J. Card. Fail.* **2023**, *29*, 1107–1109. [CrossRef] [PubMed]
54. Cowie, M.R.; Fisher, M. SGLT2 inhibitors: Mechanisms of cardiovascular benefit beyond glycaemic control. *Nat. Rev. Cardiol.* **2020**, *17*, 761–772. [CrossRef] [PubMed]
55. Salvatore, T.; Galiero, R.; Caturano, A.; Rinaldi, L.; Di Martino, A.; Albanese, G.; Di Salvo, J.; Epifani, R.; Marfella, R.; Docimo, G.; et al. An Overview of the Cardiorenal Protective Mechanisms of SGLT2 Inhibitors. *Int. J. Mol. Sci.* **2022**, *23*, 3651. [CrossRef] [PubMed]
56. Gonzalez, J.; Bates, B.A.; Setoguchi, S.; Gerhard, T.; Dave, C.V. Cardiovascular outcomes with SGLT2 inhibitors versus DPP4 inhibitors and GLP-1 receptor agonists in patients with heart failure with reduced and preserved ejection fraction. *Cardiovasc. Diabetol.* **2023**, *22*, 54. [CrossRef]
57. Seo, B.; Su, J.; Song, Y. Exploring heterogeneities of cardiovascular efficacy and effectiveness of SGLT2 inhibitors in patients with type 2 diabetes: An umbrella review of evidence from randomized clinical trials versus real-world observational studies. *Eur. J. Clin. Pharmacol.* **2022**, *78*, 1205–1216. [CrossRef] [PubMed]
58. Jha, K.K.; Adhikari, R.; Tasdighi, E.; Osuji, N.; Rajan, T.; Blaha, M.J. Transitioning to GLP-1 RAs and SGLT2 Inhibitors as the First Choice for Managing Cardiometabolic Risk in Type 2 Diabetes. *Curr. Atheroscler. Rep.* **2022**, *24*, 925–937. [CrossRef] [PubMed]
59. Hsieh, C.-Y.; Sung, S.-F. From Kidney Protection to Stroke Prevention: The Potential Role of Sodium Glucose Cotransporter-2 Inhibitors. *Int. J. Mol. Sci.* **2022**, *24*, 351. [CrossRef] [PubMed]
60. Fitchett, D.; Inzucchi, S.E.; Cannon, C.P.; McGuire, D.K.; Scirica, B.M.; Johansen, O.E.; Sambevski, S.; Kaspers, S.; Pfarr, E.; George, J.T.; et al. Empagliflozin Reduced Mortality and Hospitalization for Heart Failure Across the Spectrum of Cardiovascular Risk in the EMPA-REG OUTCOME Trial. *Circulation* **2019**, *139*, 1384–1395. [CrossRef]
61. Neal, B.; Perkovic, V.; Mahaffey, K.W.; de Zeeuw, D.; Fulcher, G.; Erondu, N.; Shaw, W.; Law, G.; Desai, M.; Matthews, D.R.; et al. Canagliflozin and Cardiovascular and Renal Events in Type 2 Diabetes. *N. Engl. J. Med.* **2017**, *377*, 644–657. [CrossRef] [PubMed]
62. Wiviott, S.D.; Raz, I.; Bonaca, M.P.; Mosenzon, O.; Kato, E.T.; Cahn, A.; Silverman, M.G.; Zelniker, T.A.; Kuder, J.F.; Murphy, S.A.; et al. Dapagliflozin and Cardiovascular Outcomes in Type 2 Diabetes. *N. Engl. J. Med.* **2019**, *380*, 347–357. [CrossRef]

biomedicines

MDPI

Review

Advances in Pharmacological Approaches for Managing Hypercholesterolemia: A Comprehensive Overview of Novel Treatments

Andrea Mormone [1,†], Giovanni Tortorella [1,†], Francesca Esposito [1,†], Alfredo Caturano [1,2], Aldo Marrone [1], Domenico Cozzolino [1], Raffaele Galiero [1], Raffaele Marfella [1], Ferdinando Carlo Sasso [1] and Luca Rinaldi [3,*]

1 Department of Advanced Medical and Surgical Sciences, "Luigi Vanvitelli" University of Campania, 80131 Naples, Italy; andrea.mormone@studenti.unicampania.it (A.M.); giovanni.tortorella@studenti.unicampania.it (G.T.); francesca.esposito4@studenti.unicampania.it (F.E.); alfredo.caturano@unicampania.it (A.C.); aldo.marrone@unicampania.it (A.M.); domenico.cozzolino@unicampania.it (D.C.); raffaele.galiero@unicampania.it (R.G.); raffaele.marfella@unicampania.it (R.M.); ferdinandocarlo.sasso@unicampania.it (F.C.S.)

2 Department of Experimental Medicine, "Luigi Vanvitelli" University of Campania, 80131 Naples, Italy

3 Department of Medicine and Health Sciences "Vincenzo Tiberio", Università degli Studi del Molise, 86100 Campobasso, Italy

* Correspondence: luca.rinaldi@unicampania.it

† These authors contributed equally to this work.

Abstract: Hypercholesterolemia plays a crucial role in the formation of lipid plaques, particularly with elevated low-density lipoprotein (LDL-C) levels, which are linked to increased risks of cardiovascular disease, cerebrovascular disease, and peripheral arterial disease. Controlling blood cholesterol values, specifically reducing LDL-C, is widely recognized as a key modifiable risk factor for decreasing the morbidity and mortality associated with cardiovascular diseases. Historically, statins, by inhibiting the enzyme β-hydroxy β-methylglutaryl-coenzyme A (HMG)-CoA reductase, have been among the most effective drugs. However, newer non-statin agents have since been introduced into hypercholesterolemia therapy, providing a viable alternative with a favorable cost–benefit ratio. This paper aims to delve into the latest therapies, shedding light on their mechanisms of action and therapeutic benefits.

Keywords: hypercholesterolemia; cardiovascular disease; atherosclerosis; statins; lipid-lowering drugs

1. Introduction

Atherosclerosis is a chronic inflammatory disease that affects the endothelium of large and medium arteries, resulting in the formation of lipid plaques through interactions with other risk factors. Well-recognized contributors to atherosclerosis include hypercholesterolemia, arterial hypertension, diabetes mellitus, obesity, cigarette smoking, and numerous others [1–5]. Our research group conducted a clinical trial, wherein it was reported that the number of risk factors not at target is significantly associated with an increased cardiovascular risk. This investigation emphasizes the paramount significance of addressing a comprehensive array of risk factors to mitigate cardiovascular events [4]. Lipids constitute a pivotal modifiable risk factor for atherosclerotic disease (ASD). The early stages of atherogenesis involve the accumulation and retention of apolipoprotein B (apoB)-containing lipoproteins, particularly low-density lipoproteins (LDL), within arterial intima [6]. Elevated low-density lipoprotein (LDL-C) levels are associated with an increased risk of cardiovascular disease (CAD), cerebrovascular disease, and peripheral arterial disease (PAD) [7–9]. Efficient control of blood cholesterol, especially the reduction in LDL-C, stands as a reliable and achievable modifiable risk factor, significantly reducing the morbidity and mortality associated with cardiovascular disease (CVD) [10,11]. Evidence underscores that the extent and duration of LDL exposure determine the risk of ASD and its complications, underlining the urgency of identifying and treating elevated LDL-C levels [12].

Lovastatin, the first statin, was discovered in the 1970s, but it was only commercially available from 1987, gaining increasing notoriety since 1997 due to the demonstration, in the historic Scandinavian Simvastatin Survival Study, that statins can reduce the risk of cardiovascular disease (CVD) (HR 0.70, 95% CI 0.58, 0.85) [13]. Subsequently, various statin compounds with varying potency in reducing LDL-C levels have been marketed [14]. Statins reduce LDL-C levels by inhibiting the enzyme β-hydroxy β-methylglutaryl-coenzyme A (HMG)-CoA reductase in the cholesterol synthesis pathway, leading to an increased expression of hepatic LDL receptors and, therefore, to a greater absorption of LDL-C from the circulation, reducing its plasma levels [15,16]. Since the 1960s, pharmaceutical companies have started developing non-statin drugs with the sole aim of reducing cholesterol levels, including fibric acid derivatives (e.g., clofibrate, fenofibrate, gemfibrozil), niacins, and bile acid sequestrants/resins (e.g., cholestyramine, colesevelam). Fibrates, agonists of peroxisome proliferator-activated receptor alpha (PPAR-alpha), reduce blood triglyceride levels, increase high-density lipoprotein cholesterol (HDL-C) values, and minimally reduce LDL-C levels [17]. Niacins modulate lipolysis in adipose tissues but have limited tolerability and several side effects [18]. Bile acid resins bind bile acids in the intestine, limiting their reabsorption, eliminating the complex with the feces. Reduced tolerability and dosage formulations limit their use [19]. Another key non-statin therapy is ezetimibe, a well-tolerated drug with modest cardiovascular (CV) risk reduction [20,21]. Ezetimibe selectively inhibits cholesterol absorption by binding to the sterol transporter Niemann–Pick C1-Like 1 (NPC1L1; SLC65A2) in the small intestine, decreasing cholesterol release into the mesenteric veins and increasing its clearance in the blood [22].

Statins, supported by numerous randomized clinical trials, have been the first-line therapy in the primary and secondary prevention of ASD [23,24]. In 2015, the Food and Drug Administration (FDA) approved alirocumab and evolocumab, monoclonal antibodies against proprotein convertase subtilisin/kexin type 9 (PCSK9), representing the most advanced approach for PCSK9 inhibition. PCSK9 is a hepatic secretory protein that negatively regulates the LDL receptor (LDL-R) by binding to its extracellular domain, mediating its internalization and degradation. This process increases the circulating levels of LDL-C and prevents its absorption [25,26]. Monoclonal antibodies (e.g., evolocumab, bococizumab, alirocumab) work synergistically with statins, reducing LDL-C levels by approximately 60% and lowering cardiovascular event incidence [27–29].

In 2013, the primary objective of the American College of Cardiology (ACC) and American Heart Association (AHA) guidelines for hypercholesterolemia treatment shifted to identifying and managing ASD risk rather than treating lipid values alone [30]. Minimal guidance on non-statin therapies was provided, recommending their use in high-risk patients with an unsatisfactory statin response or statin intolerance [30]. In 2016, the ACC designated ezetimibe as the non-statin therapy of choice for clinically stable ASD patients not reaching their LDL-C target values [17]. PCSK9 inhibitors and bile acid sequestrants/resins are considered alternatives to ezetimibe, while niacin is not recommended due to a lack of evidence for its benefit [17].

The 2019 European Society of Cardiology (ESC) and European Atherosclerosis Society (EAS) guidelines updated their recommendations for primary prevention with statin therapy, modifying the 2016 guidelines [31,32]. The general therapeutic approach involves assessing total cardiovascular risk, establishing objectives based on risk, involving the patient in CV risk management decisions, and increasing statin dosage before exploring additional interventions to achieve the selected goal (e.g., ezetimibe or PCSK9 inhibitors) [31]. The purpose of this review is to outline all the available therapies for hypercholesterolemia and their impact on the prevention of overall cardiovascular risk.

Data Collection

A literature review was conducted, updated on 30 December 2023, using PubMed/MEDLINE, Scopus, and Web of Science. We employed a combination of the following keywords: (1) "hypercholesterolemia" OR "low-density lipoprotein" AND "high-density lipoprotein cholesterol" OR "atherosclerotic cardiovascular disease" OR "Diabetes" OR "lipidic plaque" OR "Metabolic Syndrome" OR "Statins" AND "non-statin therapies." Additionally, a manual search for additional publications, both in clinical and pre-clinical studies, was carried out to include any potentially missed through electronic searches. Duplicate records were excluded, along with articles that were not available in English or were deemed ineligible by automation tools (Figure 1).

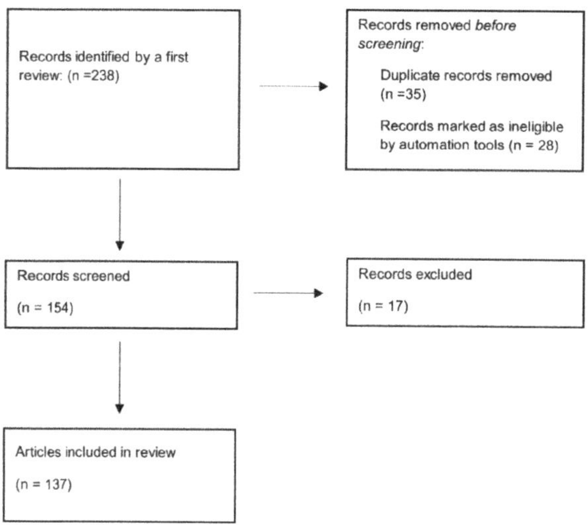

Figure 1. Flow chart.

2. Currently Available Drugs

2.1. Mipomersen

Mipomersen is a second-generation drug designed to reduce the levels of LDL-C by inhibiting the synthesis of apolipoprotein B-100 (apoB). The U.S. Food and Drug Administration has approved mipomersen as third-line therapy for patients with homozygous familial hypercholesterolemia (HoFH) [33,34]. It functions as an antisense oligonucleotide, binding complementarily to human apo-B 100 messenger RNA (mRNA) [35]. This binding triggers the recruitment of a specific catalytic enzyme (Rnase H1), leading to the degradation of the apo-B RNA complex [36]. By reducing the cytoplasmic apo-B 100 mRNA concentration, mipomersen plays a role in lowering the final production of LDL-C.

Administered subcutaneously once a week in a preformulated syringe with 200 mg/mL, mipomersen exhibits good absorption and distribution throughout the human body. It undergoes metabolism not by cytochrome P450 in the liver but by endonucleases in the tissues, with its metabolites ultimately eliminated in the urine. Common adverse events include injection-site reactions (erythema, pruritus, pain), and a flu-like syndrome is reported in about 30% of cases. Clinical trials have indicated the potential for hepatotoxicity; thus, constant monitoring of serum alanine aminotransferase (ALT), aspartate transaminase (AST), total bilirubin, and alkaline phosphatase is crucial during treatment [37,38]. Mipomersen should be discontinued if hepatic cytolysis index levels exceed three times the normal range in the serum or if liver toxicity becomes clinically significant [39]. Contraindications for mipomersen include hypersensitivity/allergic reactions and moderate or severe hepatic impairment (Child–Pugh B or C). In patients with HF and affected by documented atherosclerotic cardiovascular disease (ASCVD), mipomersen significantly reduced apolipoprotein B by 26.3%, total cholesterol by 19.4%, and lipoprotein(a) by 21.1% compared to the placebo (all $p < 0.001$). These reductions contribute to the improvement of atherosclerotic disease [40].

2.2. Lomitapide

Lomitapide is a novel drug designed to lower the cholesterol concentration in the blood. It is indicated for the treatment of patients with HoFH who have an inadequate response to PCSK9 inhibitors. Additionally, it is prescribed for patients with ASCVD whose LDL-C levels exceed 190 mg/dL and do not respond to statin treatment. It has proven effective in reducing cholesterol levels in patients with HoFH, showing reductions in LDL-C and apoB of up to 51% and 56%, respectively. However, there is still a lack of evidence regarding the overall improvement in survival in patients with ASCVD [41–46]. In contrast to the three main classes of cholesterol-lowering drugs (statins, ezetimibe, and bile acid sequestrants), lomitapide acts independently of the expression of LDLR. It achieves this by inhibiting the microsomal triglyceride transfer protein (MTP) in the endoplasmic reticulum lumen, effectively binding to and deactivating MTP. MTP is crucial in cholesterol synthesis as it transports lipid molecules (triglycerides, phospholipids, and cholesterol esters) to apoB-lipoproteins in the endoplasmic reticulum, facilitating the formation of very-low-density lipoprotein (VLDL), low-density lipoprotein (LDL), and chylomicrons [47].

Lomitapide is taken orally on an empty stomach, preferably at least 2 h after meals to mitigate the risk of gastrointestinal side effects. The initial dose is 5 mg per day, gradually increasing over 2–4 weeks to a maximum dose of 60 mg per day if well tolerated. The primary side effects include nausea, vomiting, diarrhea, abdominal pain, and potential liver toxicity. While lomitapide may elevate transaminases, clinically significant elevations in alkaline phosphatase, total bilirubin, or the international normalized ratio (INR) are rare [48,49]. Monitoring liver and renal function tests before initiating treatment and at least monthly during the first year is recommended. Contraindications include pregnancy, liver impairment (Child–Pugh B or C) or unknown increased levels of transaminases [50], and hypersensitivity to the active principle.

2.3. Inclisiran

Inclisiran, a novel drug approved for hypercholesterolemia treatment, acts by inhibiting PCSK9 protein translation in hepatocytes [51]. PCSK9, produced in the liver, is involved in the degradation process of LDL-R on the cell membrane. Inclisiran, a small interfering ribonucleic acid molecule (siRNA), interacts with the RNA-induced silencing complex (RISC), cleaving PCSK9 mRNA, preventing translation of the target protein [52]. The reduction in PCSK9 increases LDL-R availability on the membrane, leading to a greater uptake of circulating LDL and a reduction in serum LDL-C.

The regimen, based on the ORION-1 study's results, involves administering a dose of 284 mg with one subcutaneous injection on day 1, another on day 90, and then one administration every 6 months [53]. The results from the ORION-1 study with a 300 mg dose showed an average reduction of 52.6% (48% to 71%) in LDL-C levels at day 180, with a mean reduction of 47.2% at day 240 after receiving the two doses. In these studies, a reduction in PCSK9 levels by an average of 69.1 ± 12.1% at day 180 and at day 240 of 40% was observed. A one-year follow-up of the ORION-1 participants showed an LDL-C reduction of 31.4% at 360 days, signifying a sustained but waning effect over time [54].

The inclisiran phase 3 trials, particularly ORION-9, evaluated the efficacy of inclisiran in patients with HoFH already treated with the maximum dose of statin and ezetimibe with a baseline level of LDL-C more than 100 mg/dL; it showed an average reduction of 47.9% (95% CI −53% to −42.73 $p < 0.001$) compared to a placebo [55]. ORION-10 and -11 evaluated the efficacy of inclisiran in patients with ASCVD or ASCVD equivalent risk and LDL levels of more than 70 mg/dL; in this study, it was seen how inclisiran is able to lead to an average reduction of 52.3% (−52.3% (95% CI −55.7 to −48.8%; $p < 0.001$), thus proving effective in improving ASCVD [56].

Regarding the impact of inclisiran in cardiovascular outcomes trials, the results are still ongoing; however, a recently published pooled patient-level analysis of ORION-9, -10, and -11 showed that the occurrence episodes of major adverse cardiovascular events (MACE) (131 vs. 172 events; hazard ratio (HR) 0.75, 95% CI 0.60–0.94), fatal/non-fatal MI (33 vs. 41 events; HR 0.81, 95% CI 0.51–1.29), and fatal/non-fatal stroke (13 vs. 15 events; HR 0.80, 95% CI 0.39–1.67) were all lower in the group of patients treated with inclisiran [57]. This is indicated in the treatment of hypercholesterolemia in patients with HeFH or ASCVD already treated with the maximum dose of statins and ezetimibe that require further lowering of LDL-C [58]. Off-label, it could be useful also in patients with contraindication or intolerance to statin treatment.

Safety and side-effects were evaluated in all of these three clinical trials; the most common side effects are injection site reactions (5% in the inclisiran vs. 0.7% in the placebo group; risk ratio 7.54), bronchitis (4.3% for inclisiran vs. 2.7% placebo; risk ratio 1.55), hypertension (5.7% for inclisiran vs. 5.7% for placebo), arthralgia (5.0% for inclisiran vs. 4.0% for placebo), back pain (4.5% for inclisiran vs. 4.2% for placebo), urinary tract infection (4.4% for inclisiran vs. 3.6% for placebo), and an increase in serum creatine phosphokinase (2.3% in inclisiran vs. 3.2% in placebo) [59]. Longer-term information about safety and tolerability is not currently available; however, recently published data from the ORION-4 study showed good results [60]. The safety data of inclisiran in patients with CKD, severe hepatic dysfunctions, and pregnancy are not yet available; however, data suggest that it could be considered safe in patients with CKD [61].

2.4. Bempedoic Acid

The need for increasingly stringent targets in controlling LDL-C values for preventing cardiovascular risk, coupled with the not-very-strict adherence to statin treatment [62], has spurred growing interest in developing new oral drugs for cholesterol therapy. Bempedoic acid (formerly ETC1002), a long-chain tetramethyl-substituted keto diacid, is a molecule first studied in 2003 that belongs to the family of so-called "fraudulent fatty acids", along with fibrates, ω-3 fatty acids, and pantethine [63]. This acid inhibits ATP citrate lyase (ACLY), a cytosolic enzyme involved in lipid and glycide metabolism and synthesis. Specifically, ACLY plays a role in the complex reaction transforming citrate into acetyl-coA, a fundamental precursor for HMG-coA synthesis, an essential substrate for cholesterol production [64]. Blocking this enzyme increases LDL-R on the membrane, resulting in reduced circulating LDL, lipid reduction, decreased hepatic steatosis, and increased weight loss [65,66].

Bempedoic acid exhibits good absorption after oral administration, with excellent gastrointestinal tolerability and bioavailability. It is strongly bound to plasma proteins, possesses a half-life of about 21 h, and is primarily metabolized by the liver through hepatic glucuronidation [67]. Metabolism by cytochrome P-450 is minimal, avoiding significant drug interactions and allowing administration in patients with mild–moderate renal impairment [68]. Currently available commercially in 180 mg tablets [69], it is also available in a fixed combination with 10 mg of ezetimibe [70]. Indications include treating adult patients with hypercholesterolemia (familial and non-familial) and mixed dyslipidemia in addition to statins if the target is unattainable with the maximum tolerated dose of statins and ezetimibe or when statins are not tolerated or contraindicated.

The tolerability and safety profile were addressed naïvely the CLEAR program, comprising four phase 3 trials: (1) CLEAR Tranquility (in statin-intolerant patients) [71]; (2) CLEAR Harmony (patients with LDL-C $\geq$ 70 mg/dL despite maximally tolerated statin therapy) [72]; (3) CLEAR Wisdom (patients with ASCVD, HeFH, or both, on optimal statin treatment) [73]; and (4) CLEAR Serenity (statin-intolerant patients with ASCVD and inadequately controlled LDL-C) [74]. Despite the excellent results of bempedoic acid in the CLEAR studies in terms of LDL-C reduction (18% in combination with statin and 24%

when administered in patients intolerant to statins or contraindicated) [75], a challenge arises from the reported meta-analyses, as the trials lasted a maximum of 52 weeks [76]. An open-label extension emerged to extend the drug evaluation period. This work indicates that the safety and efficacy results (a stable reduction of about 14% in LDL-C) persist for 2.5 years in patients with hypercholesterolemia and ASCVD and/or HeFH. This trial demonstrated that bempedoic acid effectively reduces LDL compared to a placebo, leading to improved global outcomes and long-term cardiovascular outcomes for patients with established ASCVD or those at high risk [76].

Regarding adverse reactions, bempedoic acid proves to be a safe drug. Notably, significant hepatic or muscular cytolysis occurs in only 2.8% compared with a placebo. Compared to statins, muscle damage is minimal because the enzyme it acts upon is predominantly concentrated in hepatocytes rather than muscle cells [75]. Severe complications, such as Achilles tendon rupture, have only been observed in patients with other associated risk factors [77]. The sole drug-related adverse effect is increased uric acid (mean rise is 0.7 mg/dL, 95% CI, 0.5–0.9 mg/dL) with a higher rate of gout flare (OR = 3.2; 95% CI, 0.12–8.2), primarily due to renal organic anion transporter 2 inhibition [78]. Therefore, evaluating uric acid before treatment and monitoring during treatment is recommended [79].

2.5. Pelacarsen

Pelacarsen is a new type of antisense oligonucleotide drug involved in reducing the level of Lp(a) by inhibiting the translation of mRNA of the Lp(a) gene in hepatocytes [80]. Lp(a), a lipoprotein similar to LDL in which ApoB is linked to Apo(a) [81,82], appears to be involved in the development of ASCVD. Although there is not yet a precise analysis of the role of Lp(a) in ASCVD due to a lack of FDA-approved pharmacological therapies, it should be considered an independent risk factor with values in the blood above 30 mg/dL to 50 mg/dL [83–87]. Lp(a) seems to exert this negative action in the development of atherosclerotic disease through three different ways: firstly, it carries out proinflammatory activity due to its high content of oxidized phospholipids; then, it has a prothrombotic effect due to the plasminogen-like protease domain on Apo(a), with a possible role also as an antifibrinolytic agent; finally, it has proatherogenic activity for the LDL-like moiety [88,89].

The first randomized trial to evaluate the use of a specific drug that acts on reducing Lp(a) levels was the IONIS-APO(a)Rx phase 2 trial. This work has shown that this new drug is able to reduce Lp(a) levels by between 67% and 72%; moreover, a simultaneous reduction was also noted in the overall levels of LDL-C, Apo(a), and ApoB, which finally leads to a reduction in the inflammatory activity of monocytes associated with oxidized phospholipids. The IONIS-APO[a]-LRX phase $\frac{1}{2}$a trial showed how the conjugation of IONIS-APO(a)Rx with the GalNAc3 complex, mediating hepatocyte delivery via asialoglycoprotein [73], improves the potency of the drug by about 30 times, with an average reduction in Lp(a) blood levels of about 92.4%, also reducing the dose and without particular side effects. The AKCEA-APO(a)-LRx phase 2 trial, in which 286 patients with cardiovascular maladaptive disease and Lp(a) levels greater than 60 mg/dL were recruited, showed a dose-dependent reduction in patients treated with APO(a)-LRx compared to a placebo [88]. In particular, it has been seen how a dose of 20 mg per week is able to lead to an average reduction in Lp(a) blood levels of about 92% in the absence of serious adverse reactions such as flu-like syndrome, liver impairment, kidney damage, or thrombocytopenia. Finally, Lp(a) HORIZON, a phase 3 randomized controlled trial that started in 2019 and will probably end in 2024, aims to study the occurrence of major cardiovascular events as the primary outcome in a cohort of 8323 patients with blood levels of LPA greater than 70 mg/dl and randomly treated with pelacarsen or a placebo.

3. Novel Therapeutic Options That Are Not on the Market Yet

3.1. Olpasiran

Olpasiran is new si-RNA drug involved in the synthesis of Lp(a); in particular, it acts by inhibiting the translation of Lp(a) m-RNA. In preclinical studies in transgenic mice, olpasiran has been shown to lead to a dose-dependent decrease in serum Lp(a). In a phase 1 study, however, it showed an ability to reduce serum Lp(a) in a percentage between 72 and 97. The phase 2 OCEAN(a)-DOSE study demonstrated, in a cohort of patients randomly treated with 225 mg of olpasiran every 12 weeks or a placebo, a reduction in Lp(a) compared to low values of approximately 90% in the absence of significant adverse reactions [90].

3.2. ANGPTL3

Lipoprotein lipase (LPL) is a member of the lipase family situated on the luminal surface of capillaries that catabolizes plasma triglycerides of lipoproteins like chylomicrons and VLDL [91]. Its deficiency leads to severe hypertriglyceridemia [83,92] and a reduction in HDL-C [93], thereby increasing the risk of ischemic heart disease [94]. Angiopoietin-like proteins (ANGPTLs) are a family of proteins able to induce the posttranslational regulation of LPL, determining its inhibition [94]. Koishi R. [95] et al. investigated the role of angiopoietin-like protein 3 (ANGPTL3), a member of the vascular endothelial growth factor (VEGF) family expressed and secreted by the liver. Treating mice with this protein determined an increase in total cholesterol, triglycerides, and non-esterified fatty acids one day after injection, peaking after four days, suggesting an important potential role of ANGPTL3 in elevating serum lipids. This effect seems to be determined by an LDL-R-independent mechanism. Adam et al. [96] studied the inhibition process mediated by ANGPTL3 on LPL and endothelial lipase. A fully human monoclonal antibody, evinacumab, capable of inactivating ANGPTL3 in LDL-R-deficient mice, lowered the levels of triglyceride and cholesterol by derepressing LPL and EL, determining VLDL remodeling, resulting in the formation of lipid-depleted remnants, which were removed from circulation. This ended in a reduction in LDL-C in serum. EL, in the absence of LDL-R, seems to be the key to this process because the inhibition of this protein leads to an increase in LDL-C. In the ELIPSE HoFH [97] trial, the effect on LDL-C reduction in patients with homozygous familial hypercholesterolemia (HoFH) taking evinacumab versus a placebo was compared. At week 24, the patients in the evinacumab group registered a reduction of 47.1% in LDL-C, while in the placebo group, there was a 1.9% increase. The monoclonal antibody was well tolerated, and the most common adverse events were nasopharyngitis, influenza-like illness, dizziness, rhinorrhea, and nausea. In null–null homozygotes patients, there was a complete absence of LDL-R expression. Statins and PCSK9 inhibitors have a low-to-zero effect on cholesterol reduction, and evinacumab, approved by FDA for the treatment of HoFH, is already an important choice for them. Rosenson et al. [98], in a randomized double-blind phase 2 trial, examined 272 patients with refractory hypercholesterolemia, meaning patients with heterozygous familiar hypercholesterolemia or non-heterozygous familiar hypercholesterolemia with atherosclerotic cardiovascular disease; these patients were non-responders to other lipid-lowering therapies. The trial was designed in groups with different dosages of subcutaneous evinacumab (450 mg, 300 mg every week or every 2 weeks, or placebo) or intravenous evinacumab (15 mg/kg every 4 weeks, 5 mg/kg every 4 weeks, or placebo every 4 weeks). The reduction in LDL was observed from week 2 to week 16, and it was similar in the subcutaneous and the intravenous group, demonstrating the possibility of this human monoclonal antibody for lowering cholesterol not only in HoFH patients but also in every patient with refractory hypercholesterolemia. Other options in development for the inhibition of ANGPTL3 are targeting its RNA. Vupanorsen (AKCEA-ANGPTL3-L) is an antisense oligonucleotide that targets ANGPTL3 mRNA [99]. It showed promising results in lowering triglycerides and LDL, but recently, considering the insufficient results and adverse reactions, the development program was discontinued [100]. Another example is the investigational RNAi ARO-ANG3 trial, which has now completed its second phase; the key findings were a mean reduction in ANGPTL3 of up to 82%, LDL-C of up to 48.1%, and ApoB of up to 39.2% in patients with HoFH [101]. No serious adverse reactions were identified.

3.3. CETP

Cholesteryl ester transfer protein (CETP) is a hydrophobic glycoprotein produced in the liver and adipose tissue that catalyzes the transfer of cholesteryl esters from HDL to triglyceride-rich lipoproteins (LDL, VLDL) [102]. Patients with a CETP deficiency have increased HDL-C [103], which has a beneficial cardiovascular role, as HDL particles are considered to have anti-inflammatory, anti-oxidative, anti-apoptotic, and anti-thrombotic roles, along with a reduction in non-HDL cholesterol [104,105]. This evidence has led to an increasing interest in the inhibition of CETP to reduce the impact of cholesterol on the cardiovascular system; following this idea, several drugs have been developed.

Hovingh G.K. [106] et al. conducted a randomized, double-blind phase 2 study on obitracepib (TA-8995), a CETP inhibitor, with the conclusion that 10 mg of this drug alone reduced LDL-C by up to 45.3% and by up to 68% in patients receiving obitracepib plus 20 mg of atorvastatin; HDL-C increased by up to 179% in the 10 mg obitracepib group. A similar result was achieved in another randomized, double-blind, placebo-controlled trial by Nicholls et al. [107]; in a group of 120 patients with a background of high-intensity statin medication, the add-on treatment with 10 mg of obitracepib significantly reduced LDL, Lp(a), and ApoB and increased HDL-C. The most common adverse reactions were nausea and headache.

The effect of this drug seems very promising for reducing cardiovascular deaths; several studies are evaluating this subject: PREVAIL [108] is a placebo-controlled, double-blind, randomized phase 3 study consisting of 9000 patients that has been focusing on the effect of 10 mg of obitracepib on patients with a history of ASCVD not controlled by traditional lipid-lowering therapies; REVEAL [109] is another randomized phase 3 trial with almost 30,000 patients with previous cardiovascular disease already taking a statin; they also received placebo or another CETP inhibitor, anacetrapib. The study has already demonstrated a significant reduction in the primary endpoint of coronary death and myocardial infarction or coronary revascularization. No severe side effects were highlighted [110]. At the conclusion of these two trials, we will have novel information on the potential use of these medications. CETP inhibitors could represent another choice of therapy for several patients with a high cardiovascular risk who are intolerant to statins or that may need a more impactful reduction in cholesterol not achieved with other therapies.

Figure 2 illustrates a visual representation of the mechanisms of the drugs listed above.

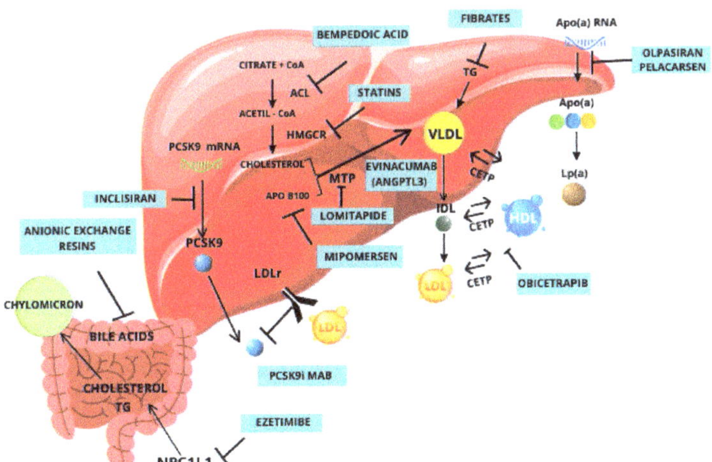

Figure 2. The mechanisms of the main cholesterol-lowering drugs.

3.4. HMG-CoA Reductase Degrader

The introduction of statins to the market has changed cholesterol-lowering therapies; these drugs are still the most commonly prescribed thanks to their low cost and great benefits. Statins bind to and inhibit the catalytic domain of their target, the 3-hydroxy-3-methylglutaryl–coenzyme A reductase (HMGCR) [111], stopping the conversion of HMG-CoA to mevalonate, a key reaction for cholesterol synthesis. Mevalonate derivatives are known to control HMGCR levels through a multivalent feedback mechanism, and in the absence of serum cholesterol, there is a higher activity of HMGCR [112]. Statins, by blocking this reductase, induce a compensatory increase in HMGCR [113] that can paradoxically reduce the effect of the drug in lowering cholesterol. Jiang et al. [114] identified a specific HMGCR degrader, Cmpd81; LDL mice treated with Cmdp81 alone or lovastatin and Cmpd81 showed a decrease in VLDL and LDL in their liver cells and fewer atherosclerotic plaques. No effects on body weight, food intake, nor cardiovascular toxicity were associated with Cmdp81 during the study. This is a promising new approach for reducing cholesterol alone or in a synergistic way in patients already in treatment with statins.

3.5. ASGR1

The asialoglycoprotein receptor (ASGPR) was discovered in the mid-1960s by Ashwell, Morell, and colleagues [115,116] in their studies of the uptake of serum glycoproteins by hepatocytes. It is mainly expressed in the liver, where it is responsible for the endocytosis and degradation of desialylated glycoproteins with terminal galactose (Gal) or N-acetylgalactosamine (GalNAc) residues, making its most interesting role the removal of desialylated forms of glycoproteins from circulation [117]. ASGPR consists of two subunits: ASGR1 and ASGR2 [118]; the first and major one has been investigated for its potential role in regulating serum cholesterol.

Nioi et al. [119] discovered that two loss-of-function variants in ASGR1, del12 and p.W158X, are associated with a non-HDL-C reduction, an increase in levels of alkaline phosphatase and vitamin B12, and a reduced risk of coronary artery diseases. Wang et al. [120] revealed that the inhibition of ASGR1 in mice determined the impossibility to internalize asialoglycoproteins, activating the enzyme AMPK, and finally increasing LXRα, upregulating the ATP-binding cassette transporter (ABCA1), which delivers cholesterol to HDL, and ABCG5/G8, which expels cholesterol to the bile; AMPK also inhibits the transcription factor SREBP and consequently blocks lipogenesis. ASGR1 mice liver cells displayed lower triglycerides and serum cholesterol compared to wild-type mice and an increase in biliary cholesterol in the gallbladder, posing a potential risk for gallstones.

Inhibition of ASGR1 could represent an interesting future approach to reducing cardiovascular risk by lowering cholesterol through its excretion into the biliary system; the localization of the receptor is mainly in the liver, which could avoid adverse reactions depending on AMPK activation in other organs. Additionally, another advantage is that ASGR1 inhibitors synergize with other cholesterol-lowering drugs like statins and ezetimibe, providing other choices for therapy. The limit of this potential drug is its role in balancing the uptake of glycoproteins that may cause hepatic damage [121], cholelithiasis, and the interaction with platelet function [122].

The first randomized, double-blind, phase 1 trial with 48 participants was conducted in 2017 using a specific ASGR1 inhibitor, the human monoclonal antibody AMG-529 [123,124], to assess the potential risk of this treatment. The antibody showed an acceptable safety profile, and the most common reaction was a headache, with an increase in alkaline phosphatase noted. More studies in the future will clarify the benefits and disadvantages of this ASGR1 inhibition.

3.6. PCSK9 Vaccine

PCSK9 inhibition is considered, since the approval of evolocumab, to be one of the most impactful therapies regarding cholesterol reduction, but due to the elevated cost and frequent administration, in recent years, another idea that has been explored is developing a vaccine capable of inducing an immune response against PCSK9 and therefore blocking its function. Pan et al. [125] designed and injected a PCSK9 vaccine in mice; five PCSK9 epitope peptides were conjugated with Qβ-virus-like-particles (VLP), creating the PCSK9Qβ-003 vaccine. Administering this medication to mice determined a decrease in triglycerides and non-HDL cholesterol after the third dose; the vaccine was able to inhibit LDLR degradation mediated by PCSK9, it synergized with statins, and no significant adverse reactions were found in the mice treated with the vaccine. Another recent randomized, double-blind, placebo-controlled phase 1 study [126,127] is evaluating the effect of VXX-401, a vaccine designed to stimulate the immune response against PCSK9 in humans; it has already been tested in rats, pigs, and monkeys with sufficient results. The 48 participants, naïve to statins and divided into four treatment cohorts, have been receiving a dosage of 100 mcg or 300 mcg of the drug and two placebo groups. At the conclusion of this trial, we will have more information on the effect and safety of this promising PCSK9 inhibitor in humans.

3.7. Additional Emerging Strategies

An oral PCSK9 inhibitor, MK-0616, was the subject of a phase 2, randomized, double-blind, placebo-controlled study [128,129]. The promising drug has the same mechanism as the other PCSK9 inhibitors with the advantage of being administered once a day orally. A total of 381 participants with hypercholesterolemia were divided into four groups receiving a different dosage of MK-0616, and after 8 weeks, they showed a significant reduction in LDL-C (60.9% in the 30 mg group) compared to a placebo; no serious adverse reactions were reported.

Clustered regularly interspaced short palindromic repeats is a DNA base editor that functions without double-strand breaks and determines A->G edits in target DNA; this technology was used to design a specific PCSK9 editor. With a single infusion, it knocked down PCSK9 in almost every hepatocyte in cynomolgus monkeys and lowered LDL-C by up to 60% for a period of 8 months. Similar results were obtained in another study with non-human primates [130]. These promising results have determined the start of a phase 1 single-ascending dose to evaluate the safety of VERVE-101, a CRISPR base-editing drug assembled by a messenger RNA for an adenine base editor and a guide RNA and designed to block PCSK9 in patients with HeFH, atherosclerotic cardiovascular disease, and uncontrolled hypercholesterolemia [131].

A summary of the available and emerging LDL-C-lowering therapies is provided in Table 1.

Table 1. Available and emerging LDL-C-lowering therapies.

Name	Target	Phase	LDL-C Reduction	Adverse Reactions	Mechanism	Clinical Use or Perspectives
Statins [12–16]	HMGCR	Approved	20% to 50%	Rhabdomyolysis	Competitively inhibits HMG-CoA reductase	Primary and secondary prevention of ASCVD Severe hypercholesterolemia
Ezetimibe [20–22]	NPC1L1	Approved	23%	Stomach pain, mucle pain and cramps, asthenia	Inhibits the intestinal absorption of cholesterol by blocking NPC1L1	Add-on to statin therapy or alone for ASCVD and for severe hypercholesterolemia
Mipomersen [35–38]	ApoB100 mRNA	Approved, FDA only	26%	Injection-site reactions, flu-like symptoms, ALT elevations	Anti-sense oligonucleotide that prevents the production of apolipoprotein B	HoFH treatment
Lomitapide [41–50]	MTP	Approved	40% to 50%	Liver toxicity, GI adverse reactions	Blocks MTP protein	HoFH treatment

Table 1. *Cont.*

Name	Target	Phase	LDL-C Reduction	Adverse Reactions	Mechanism	Clinical Use or Perspectives
PCSK9i antibody [27–29]	PCSK9	Approved	47%	Nasopharyngitis, upper respiratory tract infection, back pain, joint pain, flu-like symptoms, injection-site reactions	Inhibits PCSK9, preventing its interaction with cholesterol receptors	HoFH treatment and prevention of ASCVD in association with statins or alone.
Bempedoic acid [62–79]	ACL	Approved	17% to 21%	Hyperuricaemia, pain in arms or legs, anaemia	Blocks adenosine triphosphate citrate lyase	Add-on to statin for HeFH and prevention of ASCVD
Inclisiran [51–61]	PCSK9 mRNA	Approved	50%	Pain and rash at the injection site.	Reduces the production of PCSK9 through gene silencing	Add-on to statin for HeFH and prevention of ASCVD
Evinacumab [101,102]	ANGPTL3	Approved	47%	Nasopharyngitis, influenza-like illness, dizziness, rhinorrhea, nausea.	Stops ANGPTL3 from blocking vascular lipases that break down fats	HoFH treatment
Pelacarsen [80–88]	LPA mRNA	Phase 3	26%	Flu-like syndrome, liver impairment, kidney damage, thrombocytopenia	Blocks translation of mRNA of the LPA gene	Prevention of ASCVD
Olpasiran [90]	Lp(a)	Phase 3	Lp(a) < 90%	Injection-site pain	Small-interfering RNA that prevents the assembly of Lp(a)	Reduction in Lp(a)
Obicetrapib [110]	CETP	Phase 3	45%	Nausea, urinary tract infection, headache	Inhibits CETP, which catalyzes the transfer of cholesteryl esters from HDL to LDL and VLDL	Reduction in LDL and apoB and increase in HDL
HMARO-ANG3 [99]	ANGPTL3 mRNA	Phase 2	44–48%	Headache, respiratory tract infections, local injection-site reactions.	RNAi, which inhibits ANGPTL3	Treatment of dyslipidemias, familiar hypercholesterolemia, and hypertriglyceridemia.
MK-0616 [128,129]	PCSK9	Phase 2	60.9%	Arthralgia, diarrhea, nausea, dyspepsia	Oral PCSK9 inhibitor	Treatment of hypercholesterolemia
PCSK9 vaccine (VXX-401) [126,127]	PCSK9	Phase 1	30–50% *	No damage detected *	Induces immune response against PCSK9, blocking it	Treatment of hypercholesterolemia by inducing antibodies against PCSK9
VERVE-101 [131]	PCSK9 gene	Phase 1	69% *	Elevations in liver function tests *	Inhibits PCSK9 through a CRISPR base-editing technique	Treatment of HeFH, hypercholesterolemia, and ASCVD.
ASGR1i [121–124]	ASGR1	One phase 1 study in 2017		Potential liver toxicity	Increases cholesterol efflux to bile	Treatment of hypercholesterolemia and ASCVD.
HMGCR degrader [114]	HMGCR	No human trial		No damage detected°	Reduces statin-induced HMGCR accumulation	Reduction in cholesterol

ACL: ATP citrate lyase; ANGPTL3: angiopoetin-like 3 protein; CETP: cholesteryl ester transfer protein; FDA: Food and Drug Administration; ASCVD: atherosclerotic cardiovascular disease; HMGCR: 3-hydroxy-3-methylglutaryl–coenzyme A reductase; HoFH: homozygous familial hypercholesterolemia; HeFH: heterozygous familiar hypercholesterolemia; VLDL: very-low-density lipoprotein; LDL-C: low-density lipoprotein; HDL: high-density lipoprotein; LP(a): lipoprotein (a); MTP: microsomal triglyceride transfer protein; NPC1L1: Niemann–Pick-like protein 1C1; PCSK9i: proprotein convertase subtilisin kexin type 9 inhibiting; ASGR1i: asialoglycoprotein receptor inhibitor; ALT: alanine aminotransferase; GI: gastrointestinal; CRISPR: clustered regularly interspaced short palindromic.

4. Conclusions

ASCVD stands out as the most impactful cause of morbidity and mortality globally, particularly among the elderly [132]. In 2019 alone, an estimated 17.9 million deaths were attributed to CVDs, representing 32% of all causes of death during that year [132]. Mitigating ASCVD remains a formidable challenge in modern medicine, which is tightly linked to behavioral risk factors such as tobacco use, an imbalanced and unhealthy diet, and alcohol abuse, exacerbated by insufficient physical activity. While intervening in these factors is crucial, it often proves inadequate in shielding individuals from heart attacks and strokes, the predominant causes of CV death [133–135].

The advent of statins over 30 years ago marked a pivotal breakthrough in LDL-C-lowering drugs, with atorvastatin remaining one of the most widely prescribed medications globally. Unfortunately, its efficacy falls short in individuals intolerant to statins or those failing to achieve LDL targets through statin monotherapy. Over the past two decades, a slew of novel medications aimed at combatting ASCVD have secured approval and entered the market. Noteworthy among them are ezetimibe, targeting intestinal cholesterol absorption and often used in combination with statins; mipomersen and lomitapide, prescribed to reduce LDL-C in patients with HoFH; and evolocumab and alirocumab, potent PCSK9 inhibitors exerting a significant impact on cholesterol levels, which is integral in secondary therapies when statins prove insufficient. Recent additions to this roster include bempedoic acid, which inhibits LDL synthesis in the liver; inclisiran, another formidable PCSK9 inhibitor; and evinacumab, which disrupts ANGPTL3, impeding its ability to decelerate fat-degrading enzymes.

Future prospects in cholesterol-lowering therapies hold promise with the emergence of obicetrapib, a CETP inhibitor, which concurrently lowers LDL-C and elevates HDL-C, either alone or in combination with statins; ARO-ANG3, an RNAi agent akin to evinacumab, which inhibits ANGPTL3; and olpasiran, a small-interfering RNA, and pelacarsen, an antisense oligonucleotide, which prevent the assembly of Lp(a), a recognized cardiovascular risk factor [136] historically unaddressed by specific cholesterol-reducing therapies. Drugs such as PCSK9 inhibitors, mipomersen, and CETP inhibitors are known to lower Lp(a).

Exploring additional avenues, potential medications in development include ASGR1 inhibitors, which enhance cholesterol efflux to bile and consequently reduce serum levels, and HMGCR degraders that optimize statin effects by mitigating compensatory increases in HMGCR. This diverse array of emerging therapies holds the potential to substantially lower serum cholesterol levels, alleviating the burden of cardiovascular diseases.

Author Contributions: Conceptualization, A.M. (Andrea Mormone), G.T., F.E. and L.R.; writing—original draft preparation, A.M. (Andrea Mormone), G.T., F.E., A.C., L.R. and A.M. (Aldo Marrone); writing—review and editing, A.C., D.C., R.G. and A.M. (Aldo Marrone); supervision R.M., F.C.S. and L.R. All authors have read and agreed to the published version of the manuscript.

Funding: The authors received no financial support for the research, authorship, and/or publication of this article.

Institutional Review Board Statement: The authors have reviewed the literature data and have reported results coming from studies approved by local ethics committees.

Informed Consent Statement: Not applicable.

Data Availability Statement: No dataset was generated for the publication of this article.

Conflicts of Interest: The authors declare no conflicts of interest.

References

1. Libby, P.; Sukhova, G.; Lee, R.T.; Liao, J.K. Molecular biology of atherosclerosis. *Int. J. Cardiol.* **1997**, *62*, S23–S29. [CrossRef]
2. Kumric, M.; Borovac, J.A.; Martinovic, D.; Kurir, T.T.; Bozic, J. Circulating Biomarkers Reflecting Destabilization Mechanisms of Coronary Artery Plaques: Are We Looking for the Impossible? *Biomolecules* **2021**, *11*, 881. [CrossRef]
3. Yurdagul, A.; Finney, A.C.; Woolard, M.D.; Orr, A.W. The arterial microenvironment: The where and why of atherosclerosis. *Biochem. J.* **2016**, *473*, 1281–1295. [CrossRef]

4. Sasso, F.C.; Simeon, V.; Galiero, R.; Caturano, A.; De Nicola, L.; Chiodini, P.; Rinaldi, L.; Salvatore, T.; Lettieri, M.; Nevola, R.; et al. The number of risk factors not at target is associated with cardiovascular risk in a type 2 diabetic population with albuminuria in primary cardiovascular prevention. Post-hoc analysis of the NID-2 trial. *Cardiovasc. Diabetol.* **2022**, *21*, 235. [CrossRef]
5. Caturano, A.; D'Angelo, M.; Mormone, A.; Russo, V.; Mollica, M.P.; Salvatore, T.; Galiero, R.; Rinaldi, L.; Vetrano, E.; Marfella, R.; et al. Oxidative Stress in Type 2 Diabetes: Impacts from Pathogenesis to Lifestyle Modifications. *Curr. Issues Mol. Biol.* **2023**, *45*, 6651–6666. [CrossRef]
6. Bore'n, J.; Chapman, M.J.; Krauss, R.M.; Packard, C.J.; Bentzon, J.F.; Binder, C.J.; Daemen, M.J.; Demer, L.L.; Hegele, R.A.; Nicholls, S.J.; et al. Low-density lipoproteins cause atherosclerotic cardiovascular disease: Pathophysiological, genetic, and therapeutic insights: A consensus statement from the European Atherosclerosis Society Consensus Panel. *Eur. Heart J.* **2020**, *41*, 2313–2330. [CrossRef] [PubMed]
7. Mihaylova, B.; Emberson, J.; Blackwell, L.; Keech, A.; Simes, J.; Barnes, E.H.; Voysey, M.; Gray, A.; Collins, R.; Baigent, C.; et al. The effects of lowering LDL cholesterol with statin therapy in people at low risk of vascular disease: Meta-analysis of individual data from 27 randomised trials. *Lancet* **2012**, *380*, 581–590. [PubMed]
8. Roth, G.A.; Mensah, G.A.; Johnson, C.O.; Addolorato, G.; Ammirati, E.; Baddour, L.M.; Barengo, N.C.; Beaton, A.Z.; Benjamin, E.J.; Benziger, C.P.; et al. Global Burden of Cardiovascular Diseases and Risk Factors, 1990–2019: Update From the GBD 2019 Study. *J. Am. Coll. Cardiol.* **2020**, *76*, 2982–3021. [CrossRef] [PubMed]
9. Herrington, W.; Lacey, B.; Sherliker, P.; Armitage, J.; Lewington, S. Epidemiology of Atherosclerosis and the Potential to Reduce the Global Burden of Atherothrombotic Disease. *Circ. Res.* **2016**, *118*, 535–546. [CrossRef] [PubMed]
10. Ward, N.C.; Watts, G.F.; Eckel, R.H. Statin toxicity mechanistic insights and clinical implications. *Circ. Res.* **2019**, *124*, 328–350. [CrossRef] [PubMed]
11. Salvatore, T.; Galiero, R.; Caturano, A.; Vetrano, E.; Loffredo, G.; Rinaldi, L.; Catalini, C.; Gjeloshi, K.; Albanese, G.; Di Martino, A.; et al. Coronary Microvascular Dysfunction in Diabetes Mellitus: Pathogenetic Mechanisms and Potential Therapeutic Options. *Biomedicines* **2022**, *10*, 2274. [CrossRef]
12. Emerging Risk Factors Collaboration; Di Angelantonio, E.; Gao, P.; Pennells, L.; Kaptoge, S.; Caslake, M.; Thompson, A.; Butterworth, A.S.; Sarwar, N.; Wormser, D.; et al. Lipid-related markers and cardiovascular disease prediction. *JAMA* **2012**, *307*, 2499–2506.
13. Scandinavian Simvastatin Survival Study Group. Randomised trial of cholesterol lowering in 4444 patients with coronary heart disease: The Scandinavian Simvastatin Survival Study (4S). *Lancet* **1994**, *344*, 1383–1389.
14. Hajar, R. Statins: Past and present. *Heart Views* **2011**, *12*, 121–127. [CrossRef]
15. Sirtori, C.R. The pharmacology of statins. *Pharm. Res.* **2014**, *88*, 3–11. [CrossRef]
16. Gentile, S.; Turco, S.; Guarino, G.; Sasso, C.F.; Amodio, M.; Magliano, P.; Salvatore, T.; Corigliano, G.; Agrusta, M.; De Simone, G.; et al. Comparative efficacy study of atorvastatin vs simvastatin, pravastatin, lovastatin and placebo in type 2 diabetic patients with hypercholesterolaemia. *Diabetes Obes. Metab.* **2000**, *2*, 355–362. [CrossRef] [PubMed]
17. Naeem, F.; McKay, G.; Fisher, M. Cardiovascular outcomes trials with non-statin lipid-lowering drugs in diabetes. *Br. J. Diabetes* **2018**, *18*, 5. [CrossRef]
18. Habibe, M.N.; Kellar, J.Z. Niacin Toxicity. In *StatPearls*; StatPearls Publishing: Treasure Island, FL, USA, 2023.
19. Lloyd-Jones, D.M.; Morris, P.B.; Ballantyne, C.M.; Birtcher, K.K.; Daly, D.D., Jr.; De Palma, S.M.; Minissian, M.B.; Orringer, C.E.; Smith, S.C., Jr. ACC expert consensus decision pathway on the role of non-statin therapies for ldl-cholesterol lowering in the management of atherosclerotic cardiovascular disease risk: A report of the American college of cardiology task force on clinical expert consensus documents. *J. Am. Coll. Cardiol.* **2016**, *68*, 92–125. [PubMed]
20. Baigent, C.; Landray, M.J.; Reith, C.; Emberson, J.; Wheeler, D.C.; Tomson, C.; Wanner, C.; Krane, V.; Cass, A.; Craig, J.; et al. The effects of lowering LDL cholesterol with simvastatin plus ezetimibe in patients with chronic kidney disease (Study of Heart and Renal Protection): A randomised placebo-controlled trial. *Lancet* **2011**, *377*, 2181–2192. [CrossRef] [PubMed]
21. Rossebo, A.B.; Pedersen, T.R.; Boman, K.; Brudi, P.; Chambers, J.B.; Egstrup, K.; Gerdts, E.; Gohlke-Bärwolf, C.; Holme, I.; Kesäniemi, Y.A.; et al. Intensive lipid lowering with simvastatin and ezetimibe in aortic stenosis. *N. Engl. J. Med.* **2008**, *359*, 1343–1356. [CrossRef] [PubMed]
22. Kosoglou, T.; Statkevich, P.; Johnson-Levonas, A.O.; Paolini, J.F.; Bergman, A.J.; Alton, K.B. Ezetimibe: A review of its metabolism, pharmacokinetics and drug interactions. *Clin. Pharmacokinet.* **2005**, *44*, 467–494. [CrossRef] [PubMed]
23. Shapiro, M.D.; Fazio, S. From Lipids to Inflammation: New Approaches to Reducing Atherosclerotic Risk. *Circ. Res.* **2016**, *118*, 732–749. [CrossRef] [PubMed]
24. Grundy, S.M.; Stone, N.J.; Bailey, A.L.; Beam, C.; Birtcher, K.K.; Blumenthal, R.S.; Braun, L.T.; de Ferranti, S.; Faiella-Tommasino, J.; Forman, D.E.; et al. AHA/ACC/AACVPR/AAPA/ABC/ACPM/ADA/AGS/APhA/ASPC/NLA/PCNA Guideline on the Management of Blood Cholesterol: A Report of the American College of Cardiology/American Heart Association Task Force on Clinical Practice Guidelines. *Circulation* **2019**, *139*, e1082–e1143. [PubMed]
25. Qian, Y.W.; Schmidt, R.J.; Zhang, Y.; Chu, S.; Lin, A.; Wang, H.; Wang, X.; Beyer, T.P.; Bensch, W.R.; Li, W.; et al. Secreted PCSK9 downregulates low density lipoprotein receptor through receptor-mediated endocytosis. *J. Lipid Res.* **2007**, *48*, 1488–1498. [CrossRef] [PubMed]
26. Kwon, H.J.; Lagace, T.A.; McNutt, M.C.; Horton, J.D.; Deisenhofer, J. Molecular basis for LDL receptor recognition by PCSK9. *Proc. Natl. Acad. Sci. USA* **2008**, *105*, 1820–1825. [CrossRef]

27. Ballantyne, C.M.; Neutel, J.; Cropp, A.; Duggan, W.; Wang, E.Q.; Plowchalk, D.; Sweeney, K.; Kaila, N.; Vincent, J.; Bays, H. Results of bococizumab, a monoclonal antibody against proprotein convertase subtilisin/kexin type 9, from a randomized, placebo-controlled, dose-ranging study in statin-treated subjects with hypercholesterolemia. *Am. J. Cardiol.* **2015**, *115*, 1212–1221. [CrossRef]
28. Robinson, J.G.; Farnier, M.; Krempf, M.; Bergeron, J.; Luc, G.; Averna, M.; Stroes, E.S.; Langslet, G.; Raal, F.J.; El Shahawy, M.; et al. Efficacy and safety of alirocumab in reducing lipids and cardiovascular events. *N. Engl. J. Med.* **2015**, *372*, 1489–1499. [CrossRef]
29. Sabatine, M.S.; Giugliano, R.P.; Wiviott, S.D.; Raal, F.J.; Blom, D.J.; Robinson, J.; Ballantyne, C.M.; Somaratne, R.; Legg, J.; Wasserman, S.M.; et al. Efficacy and safety of evolocumab in reducing lipids and cardiovascular events. *N. Engl. J. Med.* **2015**, *372*, 1500–1509. [CrossRef]
30. Stone, N.J.; Robinson, J.G.; Lichtenstein, A.H.; Bairey Merz, C.N.; Blum, C.B.; Eckel, R.H.; Goldberg, A.C.; Gordon, D.; Levy, D.; Lloyd-Jones, D.M.; et al. 2013 ACC/AHA guideline on the treatment of blood cholesterol to reduce atherosclerotic cardiovascular risk in adults: A report of the American College of Cardiology/American Heart Association Task Force on Practice Guidelines. *Circulation* **2014**, *129*, S1–S45. [CrossRef]
31. Mach, F.; Baigent, C.; Catapano, A.L.; Koskinas, K.C.; Casula, M.; Badimon, L.; Chapman, M.J.; De Backer, G.G.; Delgado, V.; Ference, B.A.; et al. 2019 ESC/EAS Guidelines for the management of dyslipidaemias: Lipid modification to reduce cardiovascular risk. *Eur. Heart J.* **2020**, *41*, 111–188. [CrossRef]
32. Puri, R.; Mehta, V.; Duell, P.B.; Nair, D.; Mohan, J.C.; Yusuf, J.; Dalal, J.J.; Mishra, S.; Kasliwal, R.R.; Agarwal, R.; et al. Proposed low-density lipoprotein cholesterol goals for secondary prevention and familial hypercholesterolemia in India with focus on PCSK9 inhibitor monoclonal antibodies: Expert consensus statement from Lipid Association of India. *J. Clin. Lipidol.* **2020**, *14*, e1–e13. [CrossRef]
33. Goldberg, A.C. Novel therapies and new targets of treatment for familial hypercholesterolemia. *J. Clin. Lipidol.* **2010**, *4*, 350–356. [CrossRef] [PubMed]
34. Wong, E.; Goldberg, T. Mipomersen (kynamro): A novel antisense oligonucleotide inhibitor for the management of homozygous familial hypercholesterolemia. *Pharm. Ther.* **2014**, *39*, 119–122.
35. Parham, J.S.; Goldberg, A.C. Mipomersen and its use in familial hypercholesterolemia. *Expert Opin. Pharmacother.* **2019**, *20*, 127–131. [CrossRef] [PubMed]
36. Crooke, S.T.; Geary, R.S. Clinical pharmacological properties of mipomersen (Kynamro), a second generation antisense inhibitor of apolipoprotein B. *Br. J. Clin. Pharmacol.* **2013**, *76*, 269–276. [CrossRef]
37. McGowan, M.P.; Tardif, J.C.; Ceska, R.; Burgess, L.J.; Soran, H.; Gouni-Berthold, I.; Wagener, G.; Chasan-Taber, S. Randomized, placebo-controlled trial of mipomersen in patients with severe hypercholesterolemia receiving maximally tolerated lipid-lowering therapy. *PLoS ONE* **2012**, *7*, e49006. [CrossRef]
38. Chambergo-Michilot, D.; Alur, A.; Kulkarni, S.; Agarwala, A. Mipomersen in Familial Hypercholesterolemia: An Update on Health-Related Quality of Life and Patient-Reported Outcomes. *Vasc. Health Risk Manag.* **2022**, *18*, 73–80. [CrossRef]
39. Astaneh, B.; Makhdami, N.; Astaneh, V.; Guyatt, G. The Effect of Mipomersen in the Management of Patients with Familial Hypercholesterolemia: A Systematic Review and Meta-Analysis of Clinical Trials. *J. Cardiovasc. Dev. Dis.* **2021**, *8*, 82. [CrossRef] [PubMed]
40. Stein, E.A.; Dufour, R.; Gagne, C.; Gaudet, D.; East, C.; Donovan, J.M.; Chin, W.; Tribble, D.L.; McGowan, M. Apolipoprotein B synthesis inhibition with mipomersen in heterozygous familial hypercholesterolemia: Results of a randomized, double-blind, placebo-controlled trial to assess efficacy and safety as add-on therapy in patients with coronary artery disease. *Circulation* **2012**, *126*, 2283–2292. [CrossRef] [PubMed]
41. Jellinger, P.S. Impact of new lipid management guidelines on the treatment of extreme and very high-risk patients: AACE/ACE and AHA/ACC guidelines. *J. Diabetes* **2020**, *12*, 105–109. [CrossRef]
42. Jellinger, P.S.; Handelsman, Y.; Rosenblit, P.D.; Bloomgarden, Z.T.; Fonseca, V.A.; Garber, A.J.; Grunberger, G.; Guerin, C.K.; Bell, D.S.H.; Mechanick, J.I.; et al. American association of clinical endocrinologists and american college of endocrinology guidelines for management of dyslipidemia and prevention of cardiovascular disease—Executive summarycomplete Appendix to Guidelines. *Endocr. Pract.* **2017**, *23*, 479–497. [CrossRef]
43. Lloyd-Jones, D.M.; Morris, P.B.; Ballantyne, C.M.; Birtcher, K.K.; Daly, D.D.; DePalma, S.M.; Minissian, M.B.; Orringer, C.E.; Smith, S.C. 2017 Focused Update of the 2016 ACC Expert Consensus Decision Pathway on the Role of Non-Statin Therapies for LDL-Cholesterol Lowering in the Management of Atherosclerotic Cardiovascular Disease Risk: A Report of the American College of Cardiology Task Force on Expert Consensus Decision Pathways. *J. Am. Coll. Cardiol.* **2017**, *70*, 1785–1822. [PubMed]
44. Grundy, S.M.; Stone, N.J.; Bailey, A.L.; Beam, C.; Birtcher, K.K.; Blumenthal, R.S.; Braun, L.T.; de Ferranti, S.; Faiella-Tommasino, J.; Forman, D.E.; et al. 2018 AHA/ACC/AACVPR/AAPA/ABC/ACPM/ADA/AGS/APhA/ASPC/NLA/PCNA Guideline on the Management of Blood Cholesterol: A Report of the American College of Cardiology/American Heart Association Task Force on Clinical Practice Guidelines. *J. Am. Coll. Cardiol.* **2019**, *73*, e285–e350. [CrossRef] [PubMed]
45. Samaha, F.F.; McKenney, J.; Bloedon, L.T.; Sasiela, W.J.; Rader, D.J. Inhibition of microsomal triglyceride transfer protein alone or with ezetimibe in patients with moderate hypercholesterolemia. *Nat. Clin. Pract. Cardiovasc. Med.* **2008**, *5*, 497–505. [CrossRef] [PubMed]
46. Andrus, B.; Lacaille, D. 2013 ACC/AHA guideline on the assessment of cardiovascular risk. *J. Am. Coll. Cardiol.* **2014**, *63*, 2886. [CrossRef] [PubMed]

47. Ajufo, E.; Rader, D.J. New Therapeutic Approaches for Familial Hypercholesterolemia. *Annu. Rev. Med.* **2018**, *69*, 113–131. [CrossRef]
48. Cuchel, M.; Bloedon, L.T.; Szapary, P.O.; Kolansky, D.M.; Wolfe, M.L.; Sarkis, A.; Millar, J.S.; Ikewaki, K.; Siegelman, E.S.; Gregg, R.E.; et al. Inhibition of microsomal triglyceride transfer protein in familial hypercholesterolemia. *N. Engl. J. Med.* **2007**, *356*, 148–156. [CrossRef] [PubMed]
49. Cuchel, M.; Meagher, E.A.; du Toit Theron, H.; Blom, D.J.; Marais, A.D.; Hegele, R.A.; Averna, M.R.; Sirtori, C.R.; Shah, P.K.; Gaudet, D.; et al. Efficacy and safety of a microsomal triglyceride transfer protein inhibitor in patients with homozygous familial hypercholesterolaemia: A single-arm, open-label, phase 3 study. *Lancet* **2013**, *381*, 40–46. [CrossRef] [PubMed]
50. Crismaru, I.; Pantea Stoian, A.; Bratu, O.G.; Gaman, M.A.; Stanescu, A.M.A.; Bacalbasa, N.; Diaconu, C.C. Low-density lipoprotein cholesterol lowering treatment: The current approach. *Lipids Health Dis.* **2020**, *19*, 85. [CrossRef]
51. Soffer, D.; Stoekenbroek, R.; Plakogiannis, R. Small interfering ribonucleic acid for cholesterol lowering—Inclisiran: Inclisiran for cholesterol lowering. *J. Clin. Lipidol.* **2022**, *16*, 574–582. [CrossRef]
52. Alshaer, W.; Zureigat, H.; Al Karaki, A.; Al-Kadash, A.; Gharaibeh, L.; Hatmal, M.M.; Aljabali, A.A.A.; Awidi, A. siRNA: Mechanism of action, challenges, and therapeutic approaches. *Eur. J. Pharmacol.* **2021**, *905*, 174178. [CrossRef] [PubMed]
53. Ray, K.K.; Landmesser, U.; Leiter, L.A.; Kallend, D.; Dufour, R.; Karakas, M.; Hall, T.; Troquay, R.P.; Turner, T.; Visseren, F.L.; et al. Inclisiran in patients at high cardiovascular risk with elevated LDL cholesterol. *N. Engl. J. Med.* **2017**, *376*, 1430–1440. [CrossRef] [PubMed]
54. Ray, K.K.; Stoekenbroek, R.M.; Kallend, D.; Nishikido, T.; Leiter, L.A.; Landmesser, U.; Wright, R.S.; Wijngaard, P.L.J.; Kastelein, J.J.P. Effect of 1 or 2 doses of inclisiran on low-density lipoprotein cholesterol levels: One-year follow-up of the ORION-1 randomized clinical trial. *JAMA Cardiol.* **2019**, *4*, 1067–1075. [CrossRef] [PubMed]
55. Raal, F.J.; Kallend, D.; Ray, K.K.; Turner, T.; Koenig, W.; Wright, R.S.; Wijngaard, P.L.J.; Curcio, D.; Jaros, M.J.; Leiter, L.A.; et al. Inclisiran for the treatment of heterozygous familial hypercholesterolemia. *N. Engl. J. Med.* **2020**, *382*, 1520–1530. [CrossRef] [PubMed]
56. Ray, K.K.; Wright, R.S.; Kallend, D.; Koenig, W.; Leiter, L.A.; Raal, F.J.; Bisch, J.A.; Richardson, T.; Jaros, M.; Wijngaard, P.L.J.; et al. Two phase 3 trials of inclisiran in patients with elevated LDL cholesterol. *N. Engl. J. Med.* **2020**, *382*, 1507–1519. [CrossRef]
57. Ray, K.K.; Raal, F.J.; Kallend, D.G.; Jaros, M.J.; Koenig, W.; Leiter, L.A.; Landmesser, U.; Schwartz, G.G.; Lawrence, D.; Friedman, A.; et al. Inclisiran and cardiovascular events: A patient-level analysis of phase III trials. *Eur. Heart J.* **2023**, *44*, 129–138. [CrossRef]
58. US Food & Drug Administration. Drugs@FDA—Leqvio (Inclisiran). Available online: https://www.accessdata.fda.gov/drugsatfda_docs/nda/2022/214012Orig1s000TOC.cfm (accessed on 27 June 2023).
59. Wright, R.S.; Ray, K.K.; Raal, F.J.; Kallend, D.G.; Jaros, M.; Koenig, W.; Leiter, L.A.; Landmesser, U.; Schwartz, G.G.; Friedman, A.; et al. Pooled patient-level analysis of inclisiran trials in patients with familial hypercholesterolemia or atherosclerosis. *J. Am. Coll. Cardiol.* **2021**, *77*, 1182–1193. [CrossRef]
60. Ray, K.K.; Troquay, R.P.T.; Visseren, F.L.J.; Leiter, L.A.; Scott Wright, R.; Vikarunnessa, S.; Talloczy, Z.; Zang, X.; Maheux, P.; Lesogor, A.; et al. Long-term efficacy and safety of inclisiran in patients with high cardiovascular risk and elevated LDL cholesterol (ORION-3): Results from the 4-year open-label extension of the ORION-1 trial. *Lancet Diabetes Endocrinol.* **2023**, *11*, 109–119. [CrossRef]
61. Wright, R.S.; Collins, M.G.; Stoekenbroek, R.M.; Robson, R.; Wijngaard, P.L.J.; Landmesser, U.; Leiter, L.A.; Kastelein, J.J.P.; Ray, K.K.; Kallend, D. Effects of renal impairment on the pharmacokinetics, efficacy, and safety of inclisiran: An analysis of the ORION-7 and ORION-1 studies. *Mayo Clin. Proc.* **2020**, *95*, 77–89. [CrossRef] [PubMed]
62. Vrablik, M.; Seifert, B.; Parkhomenko, A.; Banach, M.; Jóźwiak, J.J.; Kiss, R.G.; Gaita, D.; Rašlová, K.; Zachlederova, M.; Bray, S.; et al. Lipid-lowering therapy use in primary and secondary care in Central and East ern Europe: DA VINCI observational study. *Atherosclerosis* **2021**, *334*, 66–75. [CrossRef] [PubMed]
63. Sirtori, C.R.; Galli, C.; Franceschini, G. Fraudulent (and non fraudulent) fatty acids for human health. *Eur. J. Clin. Investig.* **1993**, *23*, 686. [CrossRef]
64. Ruscica, M.; Banach, M.; Sahebkar, A.; Corsini, A.; Sirtori, C.R. ETC-1002 (Bempedoic acid) for the management of hyperlipidemia: From preclinical studies to phase 3 trials. *Expert Opin. Pharmacother.* **2019**, *20*, 791–803. [CrossRef]
65. Pinkosky, S.L.; Newton, R.S.; Day, E.A.; Ford, R.J.; Lhotak, S.; Austin, R.C.; Birch, C.M.; Smith, B.K.; Filippov, S.; Groot, P.H.E.; et al. Liver-specific ATP citrate lyase inhibition by bempedoic acid decreases LDL-C and attenuates atherosclerosis. *Nat. Commun.* **2016**, *7*, 13457. [CrossRef]
66. Pinkosky, S.L.; Filippov, S.; Srivastava, R.A.; Hanselman, J.C.; Bradshaw, C.D.; Hurley, T.R.; Cramer, C.T.; Spahr, M.A.; Brant, A.F.; Houghton, J.L.; et al. AMP-activated protein kinase and ATP-citrate lyase are two distinct molecular targets for ETC-1002, a novel small molecule regulator of lipid and carbohydrate metabolism. *J. Lipid. Res.* **2013**, *54*, 134–151. [CrossRef]
67. Ballantyne, C.M.; Bays, H.; Catapano, A.L.; Goldberg, A.; Ray, K.K.; Saseen, J.J. Role of bempedoic acid in clinical practice. *Cardiovasc. Drugs Ther.* **2021**, *35*, 853–864. [CrossRef]
68. Amore, B.M.; Sasiela, W.J.; Ries, D.K.; Tresh, P.; Emery, M.G. Pharma cokinetics of bempedoic acid in patients with renal impairment. *Clin. Transl. Sci.* **2022**, *15*, 789–798. [CrossRef]
69. Nilemdo. Available online: https://www.ema.europa.eu/en/medicines/human/EPAR/nilemdo (accessed on 19 December 2023).
70. Nustendi. Available online: https://www.ema.europa.eu/en/medicines/human/EPAR/nustendi#product-information-section] (accessed on 19 December 2023).

71. Ballantyne, C.M.; Banach, M.; Mancini, G.B.J.; Lepor, N.E.; Hanselman, J.C.; Zhao, X.; Leiter, L.A. Efficacy and safety of bempedoic acid added to ezetimibe in statin-intolerant patients with hypercholesterolemia: A randomized, placebo controlled study. *Atherosclerosis* **2018**, *277*, 195–203. [CrossRef]
72. Ray, K.K.; Bays, H.E.; Catapano, A.L.; Lalwani, N.D.; Bloedon, L.T.; Sterling, L.R.; Robinson, P.L.; Ballantyne, C.M. Safety and efficacy of bempedoic acid to reduce LDL cholesterol. *N. Engl. J. Med.* **2019**, *380*, 1022–1032. [CrossRef] [PubMed]
73. Goldberg, A.C.; Leiter, L.A.; Stroes, E.S.G.; Baum, S.J.; Hanselman, J.C.; Bloedon, L.T.; Lalwani, N.D.; Patel, P.M.; Zhao, X.; Duell, P.B. Effect of bempe doic acid vs placebo added to maximally tolerated statins on low-density lipoprotein cholesterol in patients at high risk for cardiovascular disease: The CLEAR Wisdom Randomized Clini cal Trial. *JAMA* **2019**, *322*, 1780–1788. [CrossRef] [PubMed]
74. Laufs, U.; Banach, M.; Mancini, G.B.J.; Gaudet, D.; Bloedon, L.T.; Sterling, L.R.; Kelly, S.; Stroes, E.S.G. Efficacy and safety of bempedoic acid in patients with hypercholesterolemia and statin intolerance. *J. Am. Heart Assoc.* **2019**, *8*, e011662. [CrossRef] [PubMed]
75. Banach, M.; Duell, P.B.; Gotto, A.M., Jr.; Laufs, U.; Leiter, L.A.; Mancini, G.B.J.; Ray, K.K.; Flaim, J.; Ye, Z.; Catapano, A.L. Association of bempedoic acid administration with atherogenic lipid levels in phase 3 randomized clinical trials of patients with hypercho lesterolemia. *JAMA Cardiol.* **2020**, *5*, 1124–1135. [CrossRef] [PubMed]
76. Ballantyne, C.M.; Banach, M.; Bays, H.E.; Catapano, A.L.; Laufs, U.; Stroes, E.S.G.; Robinson, P.; Lei, L.; Ray, K.K. Long-term safety and efficacy of bempedoic acid in patients with atherosclerotic cardio vascular disease and/or heterozygous familial hypercholesterolemia (from the CLEAR Harmony Open-Label Extension Study). *Am. J. Cardiol.* **2022**, *174*, 1–11. [CrossRef] [PubMed]
77. Bays, H.E.; Banach, M.; Catapano, A.L.; Duell, P.B.; Gotto, A.M., Jr.; Laufs, U.; Leiter, L.A.; Mancini, G.B.J.; Ray, K.K.; Bloedon, L.T.; et al. Bempedoic acid safety analysis: Pooled data from four phase 3 clinical trials. *J. Clin. Lipidol.* **2020**, *14*, 649–659.e646. [CrossRef] [PubMed]
78. Di Minno, A.; Lupoli, R.; Calcaterra, I.; Poggio, P.; Forte, F.; Spadarella, G.; Ambrosino, P.; Iannuzzo, G.; Di Minno, M.N.D. Efficacy and safety of bempedoic acid in patients with hypercholesterolemia: Systematic review and meta-analysis of randomized controlled trials. *J. Am. Heart Assoc.* **2020**, *9*, e016262. [CrossRef]
79. Dehlin, M.; Jacobsson, L.; Roddy, E. Global epidemiology of gout: Prevalence, incidence, treatment patterns and risk factors. *Nat. Rev. Rheumatol.* **2020**, *16*, 380–390. [CrossRef]
80. Crooke, S.T.; Witztum, J.L.; Bennett, C.F.; Baker, B.F. RNA-targeted therapeutics. *Cell Metab.* **2018**, *27*, 714–739. [CrossRef]
81. Berg, K. A new serum type system in man-the Lp system. *Acta Pathol. Microbiol. Scand.* **1963**, *59*, 369–382. [CrossRef]
82. Schmidt, K.; Noureen, A.; Kronenberg, F.; Utermann, G. Structure, function, and genetics of lipoprotein (a). *J. Lipid Res.* **2016**, *57*, 1339–1359. [CrossRef]
83. Khera, A.V.; Everett, B.M.; Caulfield, M.P.; Hantash, F.M.; Wohlgemuth, J.; Ridker, P.M.; Hantash, F.M.; Wohlgemuth, J.; Ridker, P.M.; Mora, S. Lipoprotein(a) concentrations, rosuvastatin therapy, and residual vascular risk: An analysis from the JUPITER Trial (Justification for the Use of Statins in Prevention: An Intervention Trial Evaluating Rosuvastatin). *Circulation* **2014**, *129*, 635–642. [CrossRef]
84. Nordestgaard, B.G.; Chapman, M.J.; Ray, K.; Borén, J.; Andreotti, F.; Watts, G.F.; Ginsberg, H.; Amarenco, P.; Catapano, A.; Descamps, O.S.; et al. Lipoprotein(a) as a cardiovascular risk factor: Current status. *Eur. Heart J.* **2010**, *31*, 2844–2853. [CrossRef]
85. Varvel, S.; McConnell, J.P.; Tsimikas, S. Prevalence of elevated Lp(a) mass levels and patient thresholds in 532 359 patients in the United States. *Arterioscler. Thromb. Vasc. Biol.* **2016**, *36*, 2239–2245. [CrossRef] [PubMed]
86. Capoulade, R.; Chan, K.L.; Yeang, C.; Mathieu, P.; Bossé, Y.; Dumesnil, J.G.; Tam, J.W.; Teo, K.K.; Mahmut, A.; Yang, X.; et al. Oxidized phospholipids, lipoprotein(a), and progression of calcific aortic valve stenosis. *J. Am. Coll. Cardiol.* **2015**, *66*, 1236–1246. [CrossRef] [PubMed]
87. van Buuren, F.; Horstkotte, D.; Knabbe, C.; Hinse, D.; Mellwig, K.P. Incidence of elevated lipoprotein (a) levels in a large cohort of patients with cardiovascular disease. *Clin. Res. Cardiol. Suppl.* **2017**, *12*, 55–59. [CrossRef] [PubMed]
88. Tsimikas, S.; Karwatowska-Prokopczuk, E.; Gouni-Berthold, I.; Tardif, J.C.; Baum, S.J.; Steinhagen-Thiessen, E.; Shapiro, M.D.; Stroes, E.S.; Moriarty, P.M.; Nordestgaard, B.G.; et al. Lipoprotein(a) reduction in persons with cardiovascular disease. *N. Engl. J. Med.* **2020**, *382*, 244–255. [CrossRef] [PubMed]
89. Tsimikas, S. A test in context: Lipoprotein(a): Diagnosis, prognosis, controversies, and emerging therapies. *J. Am. Coll. Cardiol.* **2017**, *69*, 692–711. [CrossRef]
90. O'Donoghue, M.L.; López, J.A.G.; Knusel, B.; Gencer, B.; Wang, H.; Wu, Y.; Kassahun, H.; Sabatine, M.S. Study design and rationale for the Olpasiran trials of Cardiovascular Events And lipoproteiN(a) reduction-DOSE finding study (OCEAN(a)-DOSE). Study design and rationale for the Olpasiran trials of Cardiovascular Events and lipoproteiN(a) reduction-DOSE finding study (OCEAN(a)-DOSE). *Am. Heart J.* **2022**, *251*, 61–69.
91. Tsutsumi, K. Lipoprotein lipase and atherosclerosis. *Curr. Vasc. Pharmacol.* **2003**, *1*, 11–17. [CrossRef]
92. Langlois, S.; Deeb, S.; Brunzell, J.D.; Kastelein, J.J.; Hayden, M.R. A major insertion accounts for a significant proportion of mutations underlying human lipoprotein lipase deficiency. *Proc. Natl. Acad. Sci. USA* **1989**, *86*, 948–952. [CrossRef] [PubMed]
93. Nordestgaard, B.G.; Abildgaard, S.; Wittrup, H.H.; Steffensen, R.; Jensen, G.; Tybjaerg-Hansen, A. Heterozygous lipoprotein lipase deficiency: Frequency in the general population, effect on plasma lipid levels, and risk of ischemic heart disease. *Circulation* **1997**, *96*, 1737–1744. [CrossRef] [PubMed]

94. Kersten, S. New insights into angiopoietin-like proteins in lipid metabolism and cardiovascular disease risk. *Curr. Opin. Lipidol.* **2019**, *30*, 205–211. [CrossRef] [PubMed]
95. Koishi, R.; Ando, Y.; Ono, M.; Shimamura, M.; Yasumo, H.; Fujiwara, T.; Horikoshi, H.; Furukawa, H. Angptl3 regulates lipid metabolism in mice. *Nat. Genet.* **2002**, *30*, 151–157. [CrossRef]
96. Adam, R.C.; Mintah, I.J.; Alexa-Braun, C.A.; Shihanian, L.M.; Lee, J.S.; Banerjee, P.; Hamon, S.C.; Kim, H.I.; Cohen, J.C.; Hobbs, H.H.; et al. Angiopoietin-like protein 3 governs LDL-cholesterol levels through endothelial lipase-dependent VLDL clearance. *J. Lipid Res.* **2020**, *61*, 1271–1286. [CrossRef]
97. Raal, F.J.; Rosenson, R.S.; Reeskamp, L.F.; Hovingh, G.K.; Kastelein, J.J.P.; Rubba, P.; Ali, S.; Banerjee, P.; Chan, K.C.; Gipe, D.A.; et al. ELIPSE HoFH Investigators. Evinacumab for Homozygous Familial Hypercholesterolemia. *N. Engl. J. Med.* **2020**, *383*, 711–720. [CrossRef]
98. Rosenson, R.S.; Burgess, L.J.; Ebenbichler, C.F.; Baum, S.J.; Stroes, E.S.G.; Ali, S.; Khilla, N.; Hamlin, R.; Pordy, R.; Dong, Y.; et al. Evinacumab in Patients with Refractory Hypercholesterolemia. *N. Engl. J. Med.* **2020**, *383*, 2307–2319. [CrossRef]
99. Gaudet, D.; Karwatowska-Prokopczuk, E.; Baum, S.J.; Hurh, E.; Kingsbury, J.; Bartlett, V.J.; Figueroa, A.L.; Piscitelli, P.; Singleton, W.; Witztum, J.L.; et al. Vupanorsen, an N-acetyl galactosamine-conjugated antisense drug to ANGPTL3 mRNA, lowers triglycerides and atherogenic lipoproteins in patients with diabetes, hepatic steatosis, and hypertriglyceridaemia. *Eur. Heart J.* **2020**, *41*, 3936–3945. [CrossRef]
100. Available online: https://www.pfizer.com/news/press-release/press-release-detail/pfizer-and-ionis-announce-discontinuation-vupanorsen (accessed on 19 December 2023).
101. Available online: https://classic.clinicaltrials.gov/ct2/show/NCT05217667 (accessed on 19 December 2023).
102. Hesler, C.B.; Swenson, T.L.; Tall, A.R. Purification and characterization of a human plasma cholesteryl ester transfer protein. *J. Biol. Chem.* **1987**, *262*, 2275–2282. [CrossRef] [PubMed]
103. Inazu, A.; Brow, M.L.; Hesler, C.B.; Agellon, L.B.; Koizumi, J.; Takata, K.; Maruhama, Y.; Mabuchi, H.; Tall, A.R. Increased high-density lipoprotein levels caused by a common cholesteryl-ester transfer protein gene mutation. *N. Engl. J. Med.* **1990**, *323*, 1234–1238. [CrossRef] [PubMed]
104. Tall, A.R.; Rader, D. Trials and Tribulations of CETP Inhibitors. *Circ. Res.* **2018**, *122*, 106–112. [CrossRef] [PubMed]
105. Sasso, F.C.; Pafundi, P.C.; Gelso, A.; Bono, V.; Costagliola, C.; Marfella, R.; Sardu, C.; Rinaldi, L.; Galiero, R.; Acierno, C.; et al. High HDL cholesterol: A risk factor for diabetic retinopathy? Findings from NO BLIND study. *Diabetes Res. Clin. Pract.* **2019**, *150*, 236–244. [CrossRef]
106. Hovingh, G.K.; Kastelein, J.J.; Van Deventer, S.J.; Round, P.; Ford, J.; Saleheen, D.; Rader, D.J.; Brewer, H.B.; Barter, P.J. Cholesterol ester transfer protein inhibition by TA-8995 in patients with mild dyslipidaemia (TULIP): A randomised, double-blind, placebo-controlled phase 2 trial. *Lancet.* **2015**, *386*, 452–460. [CrossRef] [PubMed]
107. Nicholls, S.J.; Ditmarsch, M.; Kastelein, J.J.; Rigby, S.P.; Kling, D.; Curcio, D.L.; Alp, N.J.; Davidson, M.H. Lipid lowering effects of the CETP inhibitor obicetrapib in combination with high-intensity statins: A randomized phase 2 trial. *Nat. Med.* **2022**, *28*, 1672–1678. [CrossRef]
108. Available online: https://classic.clinicaltrials.gov/ct2/show/NCT05202509 (accessed on 19 December 2023).
109. Available online: https://classic.clinicaltrials.gov/ct2/show/NCT01252953 (accessed on 19 December 2023).
110. Bowman, L.; Hopewell, J.C.; Chen, F.; Wallendszus, K.; Stevens, W.; Collins, R.; Wiviott, S.D.; Cannon, C.P.; Braunwald, E.; Sammons, E.; et al. Effects of Anacetrapib in Patients with Atherosclerotic Vascular Disease. *N. Engl. J. Med.* **2017**, *377*, 1217–1227. [CrossRef] [PubMed]
111. Istvan, E.S.; Deisenhofer, J. Structural mechanism for statin inhibition of HMG-CoA reductase. *Science* **2001**, *292*, 1160–1164. [CrossRef] [PubMed]
112. Brown, M.S.; Goldstein, J.L. Multivalent feedback regulation of HMG CoA reductase, a control mechanism coordinating isoprenoid synthesis and cell growth. *J. Lipid Res.* **1980**, *21*, 505–517. [CrossRef] [PubMed]
113. Reihnér, E.; Rudling, M.; Ståhlberg, D.; Berglund, L.; Ewerth, S.; Björkhem, I.; Einarsson, K.; Angelin, B. Influence of pravastatin, a specific inhibitor of HMG-CoA reductase, on hepatic metabolism of cholesterol. *N. Engl. J. Med.* **1990**, *323*, 224–228. [CrossRef] [PubMed]
114. Jiang, S.Y.; Li, H.; Tang, J.J.; Wang, J.; Luo, J.; Liu, B.; Wang, J.K.; Shi, X.J.; Cui, H.W.; Tang, J.; et al. Discovery of a potent HMG-CoA reductase degrader that eliminates statin-induced reductase accumulation and lowers cholesterol. *Nat. Commun.* **2018**, *9*, 5138. [CrossRef] [PubMed]
115. Ashwell, G.; Morell, A.G. The role of surface carbohydrates in the hepatic recognition and transport of circulating glycoproteins. *Adv. Enzymol. Relat. Areas Mol. Biol.* **1974**, *41*, 99–128. [PubMed]
116. Ashwell, G.; Harford, J. Carbohydrate-specific receptors of the liver. *Annu. Rev. Biochem.* **1982**, *51*, 531–554. [CrossRef] [PubMed]
117. Weigel, P.H.; Yik, J.H. Glycans as endocytosis signals: The cases of the asialoglycoprotein and hyaluronan/chondroitin sulfate receptors. *Biochim. Biophys. Acta* **2002**, *1572*, 341–363. [CrossRef]
118. Hoober, J.K. ASGR1 and Its Enigmatic Relative, CLEC10A. *Int. J. Mol. Sci.* **2020**, *21*, 4818. [CrossRef]
119. Nioi, P.; Sigurdsson, A.; Thorleifsson, G.; Helgason, H.; Agustsdottir, A.B.; Norddahl, G.L.; Helgadottir, A.; Magnusdottir, A.; Jonasdottir, A.; Gretarsdottir, S.; et al. Variant ASGR1 Associated with a Reduced Risk of Coronary Artery Disease. *N. Engl. J. Med.* **2016**, *374*, 2131–2141. [CrossRef] [PubMed]

120. Wang, J.Q.; Li, L.L.; Hu, A.; Deng, G.; Wei, J.; Li, Y.F.; Liu, Y.B.; Lu, X.Y.; Qiu, Z.P.; Shi, X.J.; et al. Inhibition of ASGR1 decreases lipid levels by promoting cholesterol excretion. *Nature* **2022**, *608*, 413–420. [CrossRef] [PubMed]
121. Xie, B.; Shi, X.; Li, Y.; Xia, B.; Zhou, J.; Du, M.; Xing, X.; Bai, L.; Liu, E.; Alvarez, F.; et al. Deficiency of ASGR1 in pigs recapitulates reduced risk factor for cardiovascular disease in humans. *PLoS Genet.* **2021**, *17*, e1009891. [CrossRef] [PubMed]
122. Zhao, W.; Xu, S.; Weng, J. ASGR1: An emerging therapeutic target in hypercholesterolemia. *Signal Transduct. Target. Ther.* **2023**, *23*, 43. [CrossRef] [PubMed]
123. Janiszewski, M.; Sohn, W.; Su, C.; Hsu, Y.H.; Finger, E.; Kaufman, A. A randomized, placebo-controlled, double-blind, ascending single-dose, phase 1 study to evaluate the safety, tolerability, pharmacokinetics, and pharmacodynamics of amg 529, a novel anti-asgr1 monoclonal antibody, in healthy subjects. *J. Am. Coll. Cardiol.* **2019**, *73*, 1755. [CrossRef]
124. Available online: https://classic.clinicaltrials.gov/ct2/show/NCT03170193 (accessed on 22 December 2023).
125. Pan, Y.; Zhou, Y.; Wu, H.; Chen, X.; Hu, X.; Zhang, H.; Zhou, Z.; Qiu, Z.; Liao, Y. A Therapeutic Peptide Vaccine Against PCSK9. *Sci. Rep.* **2017**, *7*, 12534. [CrossRef]
126. Available online: https://classic.clinicaltrials.gov/ct2/show/NCT05762276 (accessed on 22 December 2023).
127. Dodart, J.; Boyd, J.; Chirinos-Rojas, C.; Lu, H.; Wang, S.; Ding, S.; Thibodeaux, B.; Vroom, M.; Sahni, J.; Ramos, M.M.; et al. Vxx-401, an investigational pcsk9 vaccine for the prevention of cardiovascular disease. *J. Am. Coll. Cardiol.* **2023**, *81*, 1636. [CrossRef]
128. Available online: https://classic.clinicaltrials.gov/ct2/show/NCT05261126 (accessed on 22 December 2023).
129. Ballantyne, C.M.; Banka, P.; Mendez, G.; Garcia, R.; Rosenstock, J.; Rodgers, A.; Mendizabal, G.; Mitchel, Y.; Catapano, A.L. Phase 2b Randomized Trial of the Oral PCSK9 Inhibitor MK-0616. *J. Am. Coll. Cardiol.* **2023**, *81*, 1553–1564. [CrossRef]
130. Musunuru, K.; Chadwick, A.C.; Mizoguchi, T.; Garcia, S.P.; DeNizio, J.E.; Reiss, C.W.; Wang, K.; Iyer, S.; Dutta, C.; Clendaniel, V.; et al. In vivo CRISPR base editing of PCSK9 durably lowers cholesterol in primates. *Nature* **2021**, *593*, 429–434. [CrossRef]
131. Lee, R.G.; Mazzola, A.M.; Braun, M.C.; Platt, C.; Vafai, S.B.; Kathiresan, S.; Rohde, E.; Bellinger, A.M.; Khera, A.V. Efficacy and Safety of an Investigational Single-Course CRISPR Base-Editing Therapy Targeting PCSK9 in Nonhuman Primate and Mouse Models. *Circulation* **2023**, *147*, 242–253. [CrossRef]
132. GBD 2019 Diseases and Injuries Collaborators. Global burden of 369 diseases and injuries in 204 countries and territories, 1990–2019: A systematic analysis for the Global Burden of Disease Study 2019. *Lancet* **2020**, *396*, 1204–1222. [CrossRef]
133. Available online: https://www.who.int/news-room/fact-sheets/detail/cardiovascular-diseases-(cvds) (accessed on 22 December 2023).
134. Sasso, F.C.; Pafundi, P.C.; Gelso, A.; Bono, V.; Costagliola, C.; Marfella, R.; Sardu, C.; Rinaldi, L.; Galiero, R.; Acierno, C.; et al. Relationship between albuminuric CKD and diabetic retinopathy in a real-world setting of type 2 diabetes: Findings from No blind study. *Nutr. Metab. Cardiovasc. Dis.* **2019**, *29*, 923–930. [CrossRef] [PubMed]
135. Di Francia, R.; Rinaldi, L.; Cillo, M.; Varriale, E.; Facchini, G.; D'Aniello, C.; Marotta, G.; Berretta, M. Antioxidant diet and genotyping as tools for the prevention of liver disease. *Eur. Rev. Med. Pharmacol. Sci.* **2016**, *20*, 5155–5163. [PubMed]
136. Nordestgaard, B.G.; Langsted, A. Lipoprotein (a) as a cause of cardiovascular disease: Insights from epidemiology, genetics, and biology. *J. Lipid. Res.* **2016**, *57*, 1953–1975. [CrossRef] [PubMed]

biomedicines

MDPI

Review

Novel Insights into the Cardioprotective Effects of the Peptides of the Counter-Regulatory Renin–Angiotensin System

Janette Alejandra Gamiño-Gutiérrez [1], Ivana María Terán-Hernández [2], Jairo Castellar-Lopez [3], Wendy Villamizar-Villamizar [2], Estefanie Osorio-Llanes [3], Mariali Palacios-Cruz [4], Wendy Rosales [3], Aileen Y. Chang [5], Luis Antonio Díaz-Ariza [2], María Clara Ospino [2] and Evelyn Mendoza-Torres [2,*]

1 School of Medicine, University of Guadalajara, Guadalajara 44360, Mexico; janettea-gaminog@unilibre.edu.co

2 Grupo de Investigación Avanzada en Biomedicina, Faculty of Health Sciences, Universidad Libre Seccional Barranquilla, Barranquilla 081001, Colombia; ivanam-teranh@unilibre.edu.co (I.M.T.-H.); wendyp-villamizarv@unilibre.edu.co (W.V.-V.); luis-diazariza@unilibre.edu.co (L.A.D.-A.); mariac-ospinog@unilibre.edu.co (M.C.O.)

3 Grupo de Investigación Avanzada en Biomedicina, Faculty of Exact and Natural Sciences, Universidad Libre Seccional Barranquilla, Barranquilla 081001, Colombia; jairoa-castellarl@unilibre.edu.co (J.C.-L.); estefanie-osoriol@unilibre.edu.co (E.O.-L.); wendyd.rosalesr@unilibre.edu.co (W.R.)

4 Faculty of Medicine, Universidad Veracruzana, Veracruz 91090, Mexico; zs19009332@estudiantes.uv.mx

5 School of Medicine and Health Sciences, The George Washington University, Washington, DC 20052, USA; chang@email.gwu.edu

* Correspondence: evelyn.mendozat@unilibre.edu.co

Abstract: Currently, cardiovascular diseases are a major contributor to morbidity and mortality worldwide, having a significant negative impact on both the economy and public health. The renin–angiotensin system contributes to a high spectrum of cardiovascular disorders and is essential for maintaining normal cardiovascular homeostasis. Overactivation of the classical renin–angiotensin system is one of the most important pathophysiological mechanisms in the progression of cardiovascular diseases. The counter-regulatory renin–angiotensin system is an alternate pathway which favors the synthesis of different peptides, including Angiotensin-(1-7), Angiotensin-(1-9), and Alamandine. These peptides, via the angiotensin type 2 receptor (AT2R), MasR, and MrgD, initiate multiple downstream signaling pathways that culminate in the activation of various cardioprotective mechanisms, such as decreased cardiac fibrosis, decreased myocardial hypertrophy, vasodilation, decreased blood pressure, natriuresis, and nitric oxide synthesis. These cardioprotective effects position them as therapeutic alternatives for reducing the progression of cardiovascular diseases. This review aims to show the latest findings on the cardioprotective effects of the main peptides of the counter-regulatory renin–angiotensin system.

Keywords: cardiovascular diseases; heart failure; renin–angiotensin system; angiotensin-(1-7); angiotensin-(1-9); alamandine

1. Introduction

Acute myocardial infarction (AMI), atherosclerosis, heart failure, valvular diseases, cardiac rhythm disorders, cerebrovascular disease, venous thromboembolism, pulmonary thromboembolism, arterial hypertension, and peripheral arterial disease are just a few of the pathologies that fall under the umbrella term of cardiovascular diseases (CVDs) [1,2]. It is essential to maximize our understanding of CVDs because they are all major global causes of morbidity and mortality and have a significant effect on public health and the economy [3]. According to estimates, 17.9 million people worldwide die from CVDs each year, making them the leading cause of death [4–6].

According to the American Heart Association, there are around 2380 deaths caused by CVD every day and one person dies from one of these conditions in the US every 36 s [6].

In Mexico, the statistics presented by the National Institute of Statistics and Geography show that from January to August 2020, 141,873 people died from CVD, a number that even exceeded deaths from COVID-19 [7]. Over time, and with the exponential growth of scientific advances, the pathophysiological mechanisms involved in the progression of CVD have been determined [8]. In Colombia, the vital statistics registered by the National Administrative Department of Statistics show that during 2021, 55,717 people died from CVD, and of these deaths, 47,621 were due to AMI, 4589 to primary hypertension, and 3507 to hypertensive heart disease with heart failure [9].

Under physiological conditions, the renin-angiotensin system (RAS) [10] participates in the regulation of cardiac output, vasoconstriction, hydroelectrolytic balance, cell growth, and the integrity of the vascular wall. However, under pathological conditions, the over-activation of this system promotes the development of acute or chronic CVD through mechanisms of proliferation, remodeling, and inflammation [11,12]. The RAS is a pathway mediated by multiple enzymatic reactions that produce a wide variety of peptides. This system starts with the renin produced in the juxtaglomerular cells of the kidney, which then cleaves angiotensinogen from the liver [13] to form angiotensin I (Ang I). Later, angiotensin converting enzyme (ACE) cleaves Ang I to convert it into angiotensin II (Ang II), which can bind to the angiotensin type II receptor (AT1R) to favor increases in total peripheral resistance (TPR), the production of aldosterone, and peripheral vasoconstriction which increases arterial pressure [14]. It was previously believed that the product of the system, Ang II, was the main and only functional peptide and primary ligand of the AT1R and that its binding primarily regulates blood pressure control [15].

Currently, it has been described that the RAS is more complex and that the products generated in the pathway are potentially functional since its target receptors determine different effects that are important objects of study for a better understanding of the system, its role as a pathophysiological determinant of CVD, and its importance as a future target and therapeutic resource [10].

Angiotensin-(1-7) (Ang-[1-7]), angiotensin-(1-9) (Ang-[1-9]), and alamandine are three peptides of the counter-regulatory RAS that have shown cardioprotective effects [12,16,17]. Ang-(1-7), Ang-(1-9), and alamandine bind to the Mas receptor (MasR), AT2R, and MrgD, respectively, promoting ligand/receptor binding and antagonizing the effects of Ang II, including vasodilator, antihypertensive, and antifibrotic effects [18–20]. The objective of this review is to present the latest evidence supporting the cardioprotective effects of Ang-(1-9), Ang-(1-7), and alamandine.

2. Cardiovascular Diseases

CVDs are the leading cause of death, disability, and medical spending globally [21,22]. The American Heart Association reports that coronary heart disease (CHD) is by far the main cause of death (41.3%), followed by stroke (17.2%), high blood pressure (HBP) (11.7%), heart failure (HF) (9.9%), diseases of the arteries (2.8%), and other minor CVD causes combined (17.3%) (Figure 1) [23].

2.1. *Coronary Heart Disease (CHD)*

Coronary heart disease occurs when there is an imbalance between the supply and demand of cardiac tissue. The demand corresponds directly to the amount of blood supply required by the myocardium, while the supply refers to the amount of blood that perfuses this tissue [24]. Coronary blood flow can be reduced by the presence of atheromatous plaques or by different degrees of vasoconstriction present in the coronary arteries [25]. Coronary heart disease thus influences the development of different heart diseases.

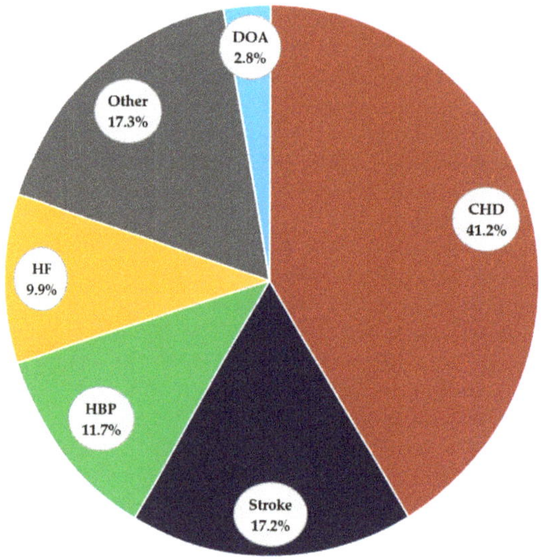

Figure 1. Causes of CVD death. CVD: cardiovascular disease, CHD: coronary heart disease, Other: other minor CVDs combined, HBP: high blood pressure, HF: heart failure, and DOA: diseases of the arteries.

The main cause of CHD is AMI, which is defined according to the fourth universal definition as the presence of cardiomyocyte necrosis in a clinical context consistent with acute myocardial ischemia, detected by a rise or fall of hs-cTn (high-sensitivity cardiac troponin) values with at least one value above the 99th percentile [26,27], with symptoms of myocardial ischemia (chest pain radiating from the left arm to the neck, dyspnea, sweating, nausea, vomiting, abnormal heartbeats, anxiety, fatigue, and weakness, among others [28,29]), changes in the electrocardiogram (ECG), image of evident myocardial damage, or the finding of coronary thrombus at autopsy.

During AMI, the hypoxic environment generated by the absence of irrigation causes ionic and metabolic alterations in the tissue, causing the subsequent necrosis of cardiomyocytes [27,30]. After ischemia, and secondary to the release of mediators, the inflammatory phase is established in the injury area [31]. Once completed, the proliferation phase begins which is characterized by an increase in the population of myofibroblasts with the subsequent production of fibers and contractile proteins that contribute to the process of remodeling and repair of the injured myocardium [32,33].

2.2. Stroke

Stroke is caused by a decrease in cerebral flow that causes neuronal injury. Each year, 795,000 individuals in the United States experience a stroke, of which 87% (690,000) are ischemic and 185,000 are recurrent [34]. There are three main causes of stroke. The first one is the presence of atheromatous plaques in the cerebral vasculature. The second cause is cerebral infarction of cardiogenic origin, and the final cause is the presence of lacunar infarcts due to injury of small vessels [35]. There are different pathophysiological mechanisms including a decrease in flow conditions, a lower supply of glucose to the tissue, alteration in the synthesis of ATP, the development of edema, inflammation, and neuronal death, thus contributing to the development of neurological deficits [36].

2.3. High Blood Pressure (HBP)

There are multiple pathophysiological mechanisms that cause the development of arterial hypertension. These include mechanisms involving the RAS, natriuretic peptides, factors of the vascular endothelium, and the central nervous system [37]. High blood pressure is one of the main risk factors that contributes to the development of cardiovascular disease [38]. The primary cardiovascular disease associated with high blood pressure is acute myocardial infarction [39]. There is a strong association between hypertension and the development of heart failure, secondary to cardiac remodeling, diastolic dysfunction, and alterations in the ejection fraction [40].

2.4. Heart Failure (HF)

Heart failure (HF) is often caused by a structural or functional cardiac disorder, such as AMI, which is the leading cause of HF in the world, that leads to a reduction in heart rate and that causes an alteration in cardiac output. Patients with HF report orthopnea, paroxysmal nocturnal dyspnea, and edema of the lower extremities. On physical examination, it is common to find elevated jugular venous pressure and pulmonary congestion [41–44].

Heart failure in patients hospitalized for AMI has a frequency of presentation ranging from 14% to 36% [45]. In fact, it is mandatory to perform the Killip–Kimbal classification according to the presence of signs of HF in patients with AMI [46]. As previously mentioned, after an AMI there is a remodeling process in the cardiac tissue [47,48]. HF after AMI is a consequence of cardiomyocyte death, the formation of scars by fibroblasts that repair the necrotic area, and adaptive effects that are activated to maintain adequate hemodynamic function [49–51].

The most common cause of HF in the world is related to an AMI. After the initial insult, an inflammatory phase occurs; then, a repair and proliferation phase with subsequent myocardial remodeling, which may result in mechanical, electrical, or hemodynamic alterations, which leads to deterioration in the patient's quality of life, increased prescriptions of medications, and more admissions to hospitalization. This may explain the great economic and social impact that AMI has on the population.

2.5. Other CVDs

There are other minor CVDs that are worth mentioning in this review. These can appear as a direct complication of major cardiovascular disease [23].

Heart rhythm disorders are a common condition. It is known that the main risk factor for developing atrial fibrillation is the presence of high blood pressure. There are other situations such as AMI that are directly associated with the appearance of rhythm disorders such as ventricular arrhythmias [52].

Valvular diseases are similarly correlated with high blood pressure. According to the American Heart Association, patients with high blood pressure have an odds ratio (OR) of 1.71 (95% CI) of developing aortic stenosis [23,53]. Similarly, high blood pressure correlates with the development of peripheral arterial disease (OR 1.47 CI 95%) and is considered one of the main preventable risk factors [23].

3. Renin–Angiotensin System (RAS)

The RAS has been studied for a long time, due to its fundamental role in regulating the functioning of the cardiovascular system [54]. The role of the classical RAS in the regulation of renal and cardiovascular physiology has been widely studied, which has also led to the identification of its implications in the pathological context. However, recently new components have been identified that constitute a noncanonical and counter-regulatory RAS that antagonizes the deleterious effects of the classical RAS. Further research is needed to determine therapeutic targets in the counter-regulatory RAS.

3.1. Classical RAS

The classical RAS begins with the production of pre-prorenin in the juxtaglomerular cells of the kidney, which is cleaved to form prorenin prior to becoming active renin. Renin is released into the systemic circulation under specific stimuli, such as low systemic blood pressure, situations of hypovolemia of any etiology, and decreased sodium or sympathetic stimulation [54].

rats prone to stroke. These effects are mediated by the AT2R [69]. This peptide can increase the plasma fibrinogen level, increasing the generation of fibrin, similarly to Ang II [71].

Ang-(1-9) has a protective effect on the heart and blood vessels against I/R injury, which could have promising results as a therapeutic target for the induction of reverse ventricular remodeling in patients with heart failure and coronary artery disease.

3.2.3. Alamandine

Alamandine is a recently identified heptapeptide that is a product of the decarboxylation of Ang-(1-7) [72]. This peptide is structurally similar to Ang-(1-7) and differs in a single N-terminal alanine residue [73] instead of an aspartate residue [74,75]. Alamandine shows an affinity for MrgD, a member of the Mas-related G protein-coupled receptor (MRGPR) family. The MrgD receptor has 42% sequence similarity and 20% identity within the seven-transmembrane domain of the AT1R receptor [76]. Lautner et al. used almandine labeled with fluorescein to test its specific binding to MrgD in Chinese hamster ovary (CHO) cells transfected and not transfected with MrgD. Specific union with MrgD and almandine was determined [77].

The alamandine/MrgD complex initiates a downstream signaling pathway that significantly reduces the levels of TNF-α, IL-1β, IL-6, and NO [78]. Alamandine has several physiological effects that are similar to those of Ang-(1-7), including vasodilation, antifibrosis, and blood pressure lowering. Its actions are independent of the recognized vasodilator receptors of the RAS and MasR receptors, according to current research [73,74].

4. Cardioprotective Effects of the Peptides of the Counter-Regulatory RAS

4.1. Cardioprotective Effects of Ang-(1-7)

As previously stated, Ang-(1-7) acts via MasR [79], a G protein-coupled receptor (Figure 2). After binding of Ang-(1-7) to MasR, multiple signaling pathways are activated that generate cardioprotective effects and attenuate the effects induced by Ang II [79,80]. Figure 3 shows the signaling and cardiac effects of Ang-(1-7).

Ang-(1-7) promotes vasodilation via the activation of the MasR through the NO–soluble guanylyl cyclase pathway, opposing the effects produced by Ang II [81]. Carver et al. demonstrated that Ang-(1-7) increases DUSP1 (dual-specificity phosphatase 1), to reduce MAP kinase/Smad/CTGF signaling and consequently decrease fibrosis in resistance arterioles [82]. Wang LP et al. (2016) showed for the first time that the ACE2–Ang-(1-7)–MasR axis significantly prevented cardiac fibrosis in murine models by inhibiting the effect on KCa3.1 channels through the ERK1/2 pathway [83]. In hypertensive two-kidney rats trained with a single clip, administration of Ang-(1-7) decreased fibrosis and was accompanied by upregulation of MasR and phosphorylation of eNOS [2,84].

The regulation of several extracellular matrix proteins may also play a role in the antiproliferative and antifibrotic action of MasR activation in the heart [85]. Ang-(1-7) decreased TGF-β1 mRNA levels in cultured cardiac fibroblasts [86], reduced plasma TGF-β1 levels in a rat model of myocardial infarction [87], and increased vascular remodeling [88]. Oral treatment with the nonpeptide Ang-(1-7) analog, AV0991, reduces cardiac remodeling in hypertensive rats [89]. In cardiac fibroblasts, Ang-(1-7) reduced DNA, protein, and collagen synthesis after stimulation with serum and endothelin-1 [90].

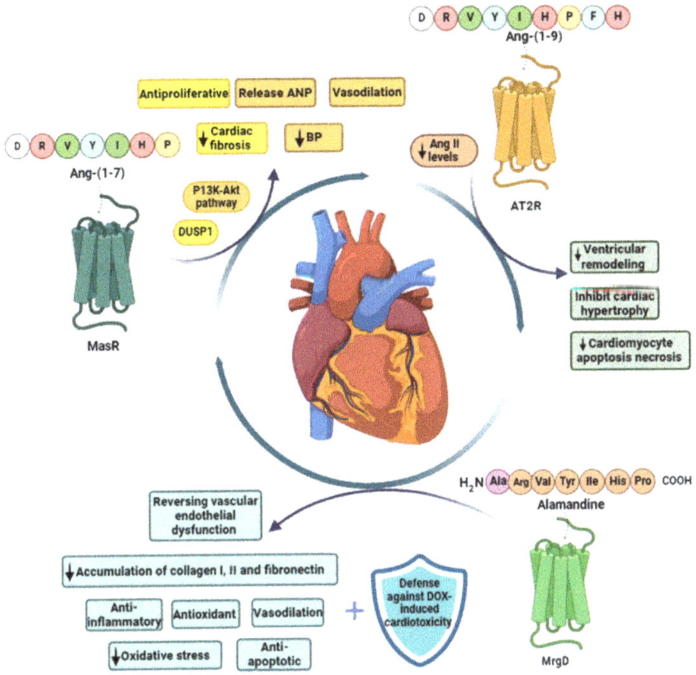

Figure 3. Cardioprotective effects of Ang-(1-9), Ang-(1-7), and alamandine. AT2R: angiotensin II type 2 receptor, Ang II: angiotensin II, BP: blood pressure, MasR: Mas receptor, and ANP: atrial natriuretic peptide. ↑: increase; ↓: decrease.

Recently, it has been shown that a formulation including Ang-(1-7) in hydroxypropyl β-cyclodextrin produced an improvement in diastolic and systolic functions and reduced the expression of fibrosis scar markers (TGF-β and type I collagen) in a rat model of myocardial infarction induced by left coronary artery occlusion [91]. In endothelial cells, Ang-(1-7) was discovered to be an antisenescence peptide that functions independently of the RAS by concurrently activating klotho and Nrf2/HO-1. Therefore, avoiding endothelial cell senescence and its associated vascular problems may be possible with the use of Ang-(1-7) mimetic drugs [92]. Ang-(1-7) enhanced collagen deposition in vivo. Ang-(1-7) decreased the expressions of collagen type I and α-SMA and increased the expressions of ACE2 and MasR in silicotic rat lung tissue and fibroblasts stimulated by Ang II. Ang-(1-7) exerted a protective effect on Ang II-induced myofibroblast differentiation and silicotic fibrosis by regulating the ACE2–Ang-(1-7)–MasR axis [93]. Chronic infusion of Ang-(1-7) into the brain modulates inflammatory mediators, RAS components, and iNOS in the hypothalamus, suggesting a possible additional antihypertensive mechanism of Ang-(1-7) in the central nervous system [94]. Stoyell-Conti et al. compared HR in a saline-infused control group versus a group administered Ang-(1-7) as well as iodine Ang-(1-7). Ang-(1-7) and iodoAng-(1-7) prevented the increase in HR in the saline group during the protocol. The iodoAng-(1-7) group had a lower heart rate than the saline group [95]. Ang-(1-7) could be a recurrent additive in heart surgery and cardioprotection strategies.

The cardioprotective effects of Ang-(1-7) are explained by multiple pathways, one of which is the PI3K–Akt signaling pathway that can induce ANP secretion and vascular regulation mediated by IGF-1 and VEGF; it also decreases microvascular fibrosis through the DUSP1 pathway and its effects on TGF-β1 by reducing ventricular remodeling [91–95].

4.2. Cardioprotective Effects of Ang-(1-9)

Ang-(1-9) exerts cardioprotective effects via AT2R, a G protein-coupled receptor [79] (Figure 2). Ang-(1-9) is a relatively more stable intermediate than Ang-(1-7) in terms of ACE2 regulation and is also thought to reduce Ang II levels because it competes with Ang I at the active site of ACE, increases Ang-(1-7), and stimulates bradykinin release from endothelial cells [79]. Ang-(1-9) can inhibit cardiac hypertrophy after myocardial infarction, attenuates cardiac fibrosis in stroke-prone spontaneously hypertensive rats and prevents cardiomyocyte hypertrophy by regulating mitochondrial dynamics [17,96,97]. Furthermore, this peptide also prevents vascular remodeling by a Foxo1-dependent mechanism [98] and decreases cardiomyocyte death during simulated I/R [99]. These findings show the potential of Ang-(1-9) to improve recovery of the cardiac function after AMI or cardiac surgeries in which the use of cardioplegia is necessary [100,101]. Both Ang-(1-9) and Ang-(1-7) may prevent cardiomyocyte hypertrophy and pathological ventricular remodeling [101–103].

When Ang I was injected into the pulmonary and renal arteries of dogs, it was discovered that leucine quickly began to manifest. This discovery provided the first proof for this peptide. The authors suggested that a carboxypeptidase was involved in the catalysis of Ang I to form a compound known at the time as des-Leu10 Ang I [104] now known as Ang-(1-9). Initially, it was thought that this peptide lacked biological activity and only indirect action was attributed to it due to its ability to compete with Ang I for the active sites of ACE, generating high levels of Ang-(1-7) and decreasing the Ang II [105]. However, in recent years, evidence of a direct effect of Ang-(1-9) on the cardiovascular system has increased [106].

Sotomayor Flores-C et al. confirmed that changes in mitochondrial dynamics and Ca^{2+} handling are related to the development and progression of pathological cardiac hypertrophy. They also showed for the first time that Ang-(1-9) controls this mitochondrial process in a model of neonatal rat cardiomyocytes, upregulating miR-129-3p and inhibiting protein kinase A inhibitor (PKIA). Ang-(1-9) also inhibits mitochondrial fission, a crucial process underlying its pro-hypertrophic actions, as previously mentioned [97]. This has been very beneficial for research because, at the cellular level, cardiac hypertrophy is associated with metabolic changes that are specifically linked to the alteration of mitochondrial function and morphology, because this mitochondrial function supports the modulation of intracellular Ca^{2+} signaling, which in turn affects changes in gene and protein expression, among other processes, and helps to satisfy the high demands of energy. The importance of this organelle in preserving good cardiac function is highlighted by the fact that approximately 70% of ATP synthesis takes place in the mitochondrial matrix, highlighting its prominent involvement in the heart [97]. Norambuena-Soto et al. also conducted a study to evaluate the anti-vascular-remodeling effects of Ang-(1-9), giving special focus to the control of the vascular smooth muscle cell phenotype. Through this research, they showed that Ang-(1-9) decreased blood pressure and aortic thickness in spontaneously hypertensive rats and that the same thickness reduction was associated with decreased smooth muscle cell proliferation. In addition, Ang-(1-9) treatment inhibited migration and decreased the effects induced by platelet-derived growth factor-BB [98]. Mendoza Torres et al. showed that Ang-(1-9) limited reperfusion-induced cell death via an AT2R and Akt dependent mechanism [99]. Figure 3 shows the signaling and cardiac effects of Ang-(1-9).

Protein kinase B (Akt) is a crucial component of the cell cycle process. It has been linked to cancer, cell growth, inactivity, and aging [107]. Activation of PI3K further phosphorylates and activates Akt, which localizes to the cell membrane and once activated serves a variety of functions, including activation of cAMP-response element-binding protein, inhibition of p27, localization of protein O in the cytoplasm, and the activation of phosphatidylinositol 3-phosphate, among others [107]. The PI3K/Akt signal transduction pathway, which involves the activation of PI3K, results in the binding of Akt to the cell membrane with the aid of phosphoinositide-dependent kinase. However, Akt is activated because of threonine and serine phosphorylation, which also mediates other enzymatic biological effects such as those related to cell growth, apoptosis suppression, cell migration, vesicle transport, and transformation cell malignancy [107]. Recent research on the signaling pathways that are activated by the counter-regulatory RAS has highlighted it as a potential therapeutic target for the management of CVD [17]. Ang-(1-9) has been linked to the PI3K/Akt signaling system; evidence suggests that it can stimulate ANP secretion activating the endothelial PI3K–Akt–NO synthase pathway [17]. The interaction of Ang-(1-9) with AT2R may activate Akt signaling pathway leading to natriuresis and NO production, which promotes vasodilatory effects and lowers blood pressure [17]. Mendoza Torres et al. showed that Ang-(1-9) decreases apoptosis and necrosis in neonatal rat cardiomyocytes subjected to simulated I/R and improves left ventricular function and decreases infarct size in isolated rat hearts through an AT2R and Akt-dependent mechanism [99]. The PI3K–Akt signaling pathway associated with insulin-like growth factor (IGF-1) is considered one of the key molecular mechanisms responsible for exercise-induced cardiac growth and protection, considering it to be the primary signaling pathway in the physiological onset of cardiac hypertrophy [108]. Activation of this signaling cascade has also been shown to protect the heart in mouse models of cardiac injury and cardiovascular disease, whereas reduced IGF1–PI3K–Akt signaling is detrimental to cardiac function and accelerates disease progression [17]. Another important function that has been associated with Akt is in the process of angiogenesis through the regulation of the NO signaling pathway. The PI3K/Akt pathway releases a group of angiogenic factors including vascular endothelial growth factor (VEGF) [81]. Receptor 2 for VEGF has a central role in angiogenesis which, in turn, is required for endothelial cell migration and enables the formation of capillary-like structures through a PI3K/Akt-dependent manner. NO is released from the endothelium and represents the main mediator of smooth muscle tone causing vasodilation through endothelial-type nitric oxide synthase activity [81]. For all the above, the important role that PI3K/Akt signaling pathway plays as a regulatory mechanism in physiological processes and the disadvantages that its deregulation entails are made evident. Furthermore, the evidence that demonstrates the influence of Ang-(1-9) on the regulation of Akt promotes the development of studies to explore other effects that this peptide may exert through the PI3K/Akt signaling pathway.

The mechanisms by which Ang-(1-9) exerts its beneficial effects on the heart are explained by the regulation of intracellular calcium and the inhibition of mitochondrial fission, crucial processes in cardiomyocyte hypertrophy.

4.3. Cardioprotective Effects of Alamandine

Alamandine is an endogenous ligand of MrgD [72,79]. This has been supported by a study in Wistar rats treated with isoproterenol, where oral administration of alamandine contained in 2-hydroxypropyl-cyclodextrin reduced the accumulation of collagen I and III, as well as fibronectin, in cardiac tissue of rats treated with isoproterenol [77,109]. In another study conducted in male C57BL/6J mice, which were divided into three groups, namely, (1) Simulated surgery, (2) Operated, and (3) Operated + treated with alamandine-HPβCD (2-hydroxypropyl-β-cyclodextrin, 30 μg/kg/day, via probe), administration of alamandine for 14 days decreased arterial remodeling, resulting in a reduction in the thickness of the middle layer of the ascending aorta, along with an attenuation of fibrosis at this same level and reduction in the vascular expression of proinflammatory genes (CCL2, TNF-α, IL-1β) [110]. Lautner et al. demonstrated that alamandine prevented the development of cardiomyocyte hypertrophy and the evolution to cardiac fibrosis and decreased molecules that are activated during cardiac remodeling [77]. Treatment with alamandine, 20 min before ischemia, reduced the infarct size, apoptotic proteins, and LDH levels in isolated rat hearts subjected to global ischemia for 20 min and 50 min of reperfusion [77].

On the other hand, alamandine exerts antioxidant, anti-inflammatory, and antiapoptotic effects, and is a cardioprotective alternative against doxorubicin (DOX)-induced cardiotoxicity [110]. Hekmat et al. discovered that the administration of alamandine restored the alterations induced by DOX in the cardiac muscle as well as at the level of vascular congestion, relieving effects such as cardiac contractility, decreased systolic and diastolic blood pressure, and increased left ventricular end-diastolic pressure. Alamandine also decreased oxidative stress and inflammatory cytokines [110,111]. Furthermore, alamandine counteracted the hypertrophic effects generated by Ang II in isolated ventricular cardiomyocytes from C57BL/6 mice through activation of the AMPK/NO signaling pathway via MrgD [75]. In a mouse model of heart failure induced by myocardial infarction, alamandine was administered via intraperitoneal injection for two weeks, resulting in a reduction in fibrosis, oxidative stress, apoptosis biomarkers, and cardiac dysfunction [112].

The N-terminal Asp/Ala amino acid is the only difference between alamandine and Ang-(1-7). This could account for the striking similarity of most of the biological impacts examined. Alamandine can cause endothelium-dependent vasodilation in the aortic rings of mice and rats as has been demonstrated with Ang-(1-7) [113]. Additionally, alamandine microinjections generated cardiovascular effects comparable to those of Ang-(1-7): elevated blood pressure in the rostral ventrolateral medulla oblongata and lowered blood pressure in the caudal ventrolateral medulla oblongata [77]. Although alamandine and Ang-(1-7) have comparable actions, their respective receptors are different [114]. In addition to the cardioprotective effects, alamandine exerted protective effects at the renal level against I/R injury. In fact, alamandine improved renal function, and attenuated inflammation and apoptosis,and decreased serum levels of creatinine, blood cystatin C, and blood urea nitrogen, as well as oxidative stress [114]. Figure 3 shows the impact of alamandine on cell signaling in cardiovascular signaling.

Alamandine is a molecule similar to Ang-(1-7) that appears to prevent the development of myocardial hypertrophy and fibrosis, in addition to having anti-inflammatory and antioxidant effects. It has become an important focus in the understanding of the cardioprotective and reno-protective mechanisms of the alternative pathways of the RAS. Preclinical studies with almandine for damage reduction and myocardial fibrosis have shown promising results, which opens the door for clinical studies to corroborate these effects in humans.

Table 1 summarizes the main cardioprotective effects of Ang-(1-7), Ang-(1-9), and alamandine.

Table 1. Main cardioprotective effects of the peptides of the counter-regulatory RAS.

Peptide	Cardioprotective Effects
Angiotensin-(1-9)	Prevention of cardiac hypertrophy in myocardial infarcted rats [102].
	Attenuation of cardiac fibrosis in stroke-prone spontaneously hypertensive rats [96].
	Cardioprotection against I/R injury via AT2R/Akt pathway in neonatal rat cardiomyocytes and isolated rat hearts [99].
	Prevention of cardiomyocyte hypertrophy by regulating mitochondrial dynamics in neonatal rat cardiomyocytes [97].
Angiotensin-(1-7)	Promotion of vasodilation via the activation of the MasR and NO–soluble guanylyl cyclase pathway in spontaneously hypertensive rats [81].
	Decreasing fibrosis in resistant arterioles via DUSP1/MAP kinase/Smad/CTGF signaling in rats with Ang II-induced hypertension [82].
	Reduction in cardiac fibrosis by inhibiting effect on KCa3.1 channels through ERK1/2 pathway, decreasing TGF-β1, and reducing collagen synthesis in mice treated with Ang II via osmotic mini-pumps [83].
Alamandine	Reduction in the accumulation of collagen and fibronectin in cardiac tissue of rats treated with isoproterenol [77,109].
	Reduction in the vascular expression of proinflammatory genes (CCL2, TNF-α, and IL-1β) in rats treated with doxorubicin [110].
	Prevention of Ang II-induced hypertrophy through AMPK/NO via the MrgD in neonatal rat cardiomyocytes [75].

5. Clinical Trials with the Peptides of the Counter-Regulatory RAS

In the race to make the leap from the bench to the bedside, Ang-(1-7) has certain advantage over Ang-(1-9), and alamandine. This may be due to the fact that the functional role of Ang-(1-7) in the antagonism of the effects of Ang II was known before the discovery of ACE2 [115] and initially Ang-(1-9) was thought to be biologically inactive, operating indirectly by competing with Ang I for the ACE and leading to reduction in Ang II levels while increasing those of Ang-(1-7) [105,116]. It took several years for evidence to appear showing that Ang-(1-9) exerts direct cardiovascular effects through AT2R [96,102,117]. Furthermore, the low plasma levels for Ang-(1-9), ranging from 5 to 50 fmol/mL [118,119], raise suspicions of its low half-life which is up to now still unknown. However, clinical trials listed on www.clinicaltrials.gov explore the safety of other alternatives for AT2R agonists, such as LP2 and C21 and recombinant ACE2 (rACE2), but no clinical trials have been found that study the direct effects of Ang-(1-9) or a more stable pharmacological alternative of this peptide. The safety and tolerability of rACE2, GSK2586881 from GlaxoSmithKline, and APN01 from Apeiron Biologics, have been evaluated in two double-blind, placebo-controlled dose-escalation phase 1 clinical trials. rACE2 was shown to be safe and well tolerated [120,121].

On the other hand, there is a phase 1, open-label, single-center clinical trial that evaluated the effects of C21 on forearm blood flow in healthy male subjects by use of strain-gauge venous occlusion plethysmography but the results have not yet been published [122]. To date, there are no clinical trials related to alamandine due to its recent discovery and the lack of greater preclinical evidence to continue the evaluation of its effects in patients [111].

Due to the cardioprotective effects demonstrated in preclinical models, Ang-(1-7) has become a therapeutic target for reducing cardiovascular risk, especially in scenarios of heart failure and ischemic heart disease. This has motivated the conduct of clinical trials aimed at demonstrating its beneficial effects on the cardiovascular system. While most of these trials are still ongoing, it is expected that the results will shed light on a new therapeutic arsenal that can help decrease the overall burden of cardiovascular disease.

A total of 24 interventional clinical trials with Ang-(1-7) were found in the literature, of which 8 correspond to the evaluation of its cardiovascular benefits; Four clinical trials are in the recruitment phase (phase 1 and 2), two in active status, one in completed status and one was in withdrawn status due to discontinuation of the drug for intervention.

Considering that aging is one of the risk factors for the development of cardiovascular diseases, there is a study (NCT05301192, recruitment status phase 1) that seeks to demonstrate the effect of Ang-(1-7) on sympathetic nervous system activity to restore β2 vascular adrenergic receptor signaling, which may help reduce cardiovascular risk during aging. Participants in this clinical trial will receive Ang-(1-7) intravenously for 110 min, administered in escalating doses of 2 ng/kg/min, 4 ng/kg/min, and 8 ng/kg/min (each of these doses will be infused for 10 min). After the dose escalation, Ang-(1-7) will be administered at 8 ng/kg/min for an additional 80 min. Blood and endothelial cell samples are taken before and after each infusion to measure endothelial function [123].

Another clinical trial (NCT03604289, recruitment status early phase 1) aims to assess the effect of Ang-(1-7) in patients with obesity and hypertension, intending to demonstrate whether there is an improvement in cardiovascular health in this group of patients [124].

Another clinical trial (NCT03240068, active status) aims to determine the cardiovascular effects of Ang-(1-7) in patients with peripheral artery disease (men or women between 21 and 80 years old) through acute intravenous infusions (five escalating doses of 10 min each: 1, 2, 4, 8, and 12 ng/kg/min). They will evaluate whether Ang-(1-7) leads to improvements in lower limb blood flow and reduces systemic inflammatory action in participants [125].

An open multicenter clinical trial is currently being conducted, in phase 2 recruitment (NCT06013839), that evaluates its usefulness and effectiveness in patients with cardiomyopathy related to Duchenne muscular dystrophy. In this study, the change in ejection fraction will be evaluated at 6 and 12 months in patients who received an Ang-(1-7) regimen at a dose of 0.5 mg/kg/day for 6 months [126].

In the context of strokes, a double-blind, randomized, placebo-controlled, hybrid decentralized study (NCT06135103; recruitment status phase 2) aims to evaluate the safety and efficacy of daily subcutaneous injection of Ang-(1-7) in post-ischemic stroke patients to improve their motor and sensory functions as measured with the Fugl-Meyer Assessment of Upper Extremity (FMA-UE). Subjects will receive either Ang-(1-7) 0.5 mg/kg or a placebo for 12 weeks started 6 to 24 months post ischemic stroke, and they will have a 12-week follow up visit after treatment has ended [127].

Likewise, a study carried out in 2022 evaluated the cardioprotective effects of counterregulatory peptides in diabetic patients through endomyocardial biopsies. The study reported that patients with poor metabolic control presented non-enzymatic glycation of four lysine residues of the ACE2 receptor (GlycACE2). An interesting finding was an inverse relationship between the presence of GlycACE2 and Ang-(1-7), Ang-(1-9), and MasR levels (Ang 1-7: $R = -0.844$, $p < 0.001$; Ang 1-9: $R = -0.762$, $p < 0.001$; MasR: $R = -0.613$, $p < 0.001$) [128]. The clinical impact of this discovery lies in highlighting the importance of the achievement of tight glycemic control which normalizes the antiremodeling effects of RAS-inhibition.

On the other hand, there is a clinical trial (NCT04401423, completed, phase 2) whose purpose is to identify the preventive effect of Ang-(1-7) against acute kidney injury, as well as the deterioration of multiorgan failure resulting from COVID-19 in severely affected patients. Participants will be exposed to a 3 h dose of TXA127 intravenously at 0.5 mg/kg per day for 10 consecutive days or until medical discharge. This trial demonstrated safe administration in critically ill COVID-19 patients. Additionally, it would be interesting and beneficial to document the effect of TXA127 in patients who have previously suffered acute myocardial infarction [129]. Interest in the effects of Ang-(1-7) is growing, so there are several ongoing clinical trials to evaluate its effects in different scenarios. To date, the results obtained in the different clinical trials show a promising future and a paradigm shift in the treatment of cardiovascular diseases, pointing to Ang-(1-7) and the MasR axis as new therapeutic targets for the reduction in the burden of cardiovascular morbidity and mortality.

6. Perspectives and Conclusions

It is important to investigate the new therapeutic strategies for the treatment of cardiovascular diseases, one of the main causes of death worldwide. Starting from the understanding of the overactivation of the classical RAS as a pathophysiological determinant in their progression is essential.

This review of the literature shows that the counter-regulatory RAS mainly ends with the synthesis of Ang-(1-7), Ang-(1-9), and alamandine. After binding to their specific receptors, these peptides activate multiple signaling pathways and cause beneficial effects on the cardiovascular system. Multiple studies have sought to analyze in vivo and in vitro the level of protection conferred by peptides of the counter-regulatory RAS; even though the evidence is convincing, there is still a long way to go. There are still several challenges such as improving techniques for its rapid detection in patient plasma and thus knowing the physiological levels and variations that can occur in a pathological context. These data are important for establishing doses for clinical trials. On the other hand, the short half-life of RAS counter-regulatory peptides has encouraged the development of a new field of research and innovation that consists of the development of more stable forms of these peptides or mimetic peptides. With respect to Ang-(1-9), a molecule was published in a patent application and consists in a peptidomimetic synthesized with D amino acids by inverting the original sequence of Ang-(1-9) (retro-enantio Ang-[1-9]) which retains the antihypertensive and cardioprotective activities of Ang-(1-9) [130]. By expanding knowledge about these peptides and innovating in forms of administration, we will move closer to novel therapies for use in clinical practice.

Author Contributions: Conceptualization, E.M.-T. and J.A.G.-G.; methodology, E.M.-T.; investigation, J.A.G.-G., I.M.T.H., J.C.-L., W.V.-V., E.O.-L., L.A.D.-A. and M.C.O.; writing—original draft preparation,

J.A.G.-G., I.M.T.H., J.C.-L., W.V.-V., E.O.-L., L.A.D.-A., M.P.-C. and M.C.O.; writing—review and editing, E.M.-T., J.A.G.-G., L.A.D.-A., M.C.O., W.R. and A.Y.C.; visualization, L.A.D.-A. and M.P.-C.; supervision, E.M.-T.; project administration, W.R.; funding acquisition, E.M.-T. and W.R. All authors have read and agreed to the published version of the manuscript.

Funding: This research was funded by MINCIENCIAS-Colombia, grant number 120884468190 and the APC was funded by Universidad Libre Seccional Barranquilla, Colombia.

Institutional Review Board Statement: Not applicable.

Informed Consent Statement: Not applicable.

Data Availability Statement: Not applicable.

Conflicts of Interest: The authors declare no conflicts of interest.

References

1. Mensah, G.A.; Roth, G.A.; Fuster, V. The Global Burden of Cardiovascular Diseases and Risk Factors. *J. Am. Coll. Cardiol.* **2019**, *74*, 2529–2532. [CrossRef] [PubMed]
2. Shufelt, C.L.; Pacheco, C.; Tweet, M.S.; Miller, V.M. Sex-Specific Physiology and Cardiovascular Disease. *Adv. Exp. Med. Biol.* **2018**, *1065*, 433–454. [PubMed]
3. Gheorghe, A.; Griffiths, U.; Murphy, A.; Legido-Quigley, H.; Lamptey, P.; Perel, P. The Economic Burden of Cardiovascular Disease and Hypertension in Low- and Middle-Income Countries: A Systematic Review. *BMC Public Health* **2018**, *18*, 975. [CrossRef] [PubMed]
4. Kraus, W.E.; Powell, K.E.; Haskell, W.L.; Janz, K.F.; Campbell, W.W.; Jakicic, J.M.; Troiano, R.P.; Sprow, K.; Torres, A.; Piercy, K.L.; et al. Physical Activity, All-Cause and Cardiovascular Mortality, and Cardiovascular Disease. *Med. Sci. Sport. Exerc.* **2019**, *51*, 1270–1281. [CrossRef] [PubMed]
5. Liu, S.; Li, Y.; Zeng, X.; Wang, H.; Yin, P.; Wang, L.; Liu, Y.; Liu, J.; Qi, J.; Ran, S.; et al. Burden of Cardiovascular Diseases in China, 1990–2016. *JAMA Cardiol.* **2019**, *4*, 342–352. [CrossRef] [PubMed]
6. Cardiovascular Diseases. Available online: https://www.who.int/health-topics/cardiovascular-diseases/ (accessed on 8 July 2023).
7. Defunciones Registradas en México 2020. Available online: https://www.inegi.org.mx/contenidos/saladeprensa/boletines/2021/EstSociodemo/DefuncionesRegistradas2020_Pre_07.pdf (accessed on 28 July 2023).
8. Te Riet, L.; Van Esch, J.H.; Roks, A.J.; van den Meiracker, A.H.; Danser, A.H. Hypertension: Renin-angiotensin-aldosterone system alterations. *Circ. Res.* **2015**, *116*, 960–975. [CrossRef]
9. Defunciones Fetales y No Fetales—Dane. Available online: https://www.dane.gov.co/files/investigaciones/poblacion/bt_estadisticasvitales_defunciones_Itrim_2022pr.pdf (accessed on 25 July 2023).
10. Miller, A.J.; Arnold, A.C. The Renin–Angiotensin System in Cardiovascular Autonomic Control: Recent Developments and Clinical Implications. *Clin. Auton. Res.* **2018**, *29*, 231–243. [CrossRef]
11. Forrester, S.J.; Booz, G.W.; Sigmund, C.D.; Coffman, T.M.; Kawai, T.; Rizzo, V.; Scalia, R.; Eguchi, S. Angiotensin II Signal Transduction: An Update on Mechanisms of Physiology and Pathophysiology. *Physiol. Rev.* **2018**, *98*, 1627–1738. [CrossRef]
12. Santos, R.A.; Oudit, G.Y.; Verano-Braga, T.; Canta, G.; Steckelings, U.M.; Bader, M. The Renin-Angiotensin System: Going beyond the Classical Paradigms. *Am. J. Physiol. Heart Circ. Physiol.* **2019**, *316*, 958–970. [CrossRef]
13. Yang, T.; Xu, C. Physiology and Pathophysiology of the Intrarenal Renin-Angiotensin System: An Update. *J. Am. Soc. Nephrol.* **2017**, *28*, 1040–1049. [CrossRef]
14. Chaszczewska-Markowska, M.; Sagan, M.; Bogunia-Kubik, K. The Renin-Angiotensin-Aldosterone System (RAAS)—Physiology and Molecular Mechanisms of Functioning. *Postep. Hyg. Med. Dosw. (Online)* **2016**, *70*, 917–927. [CrossRef] [PubMed]
15. Nishiyama, A.; Kobori, H. Independent Regulation of Renin–Angiotensin–Aldosterone System in the Kidney. *Clin. Exp. Nephrol.* **2018**, *22*, 1231–1239. [CrossRef]
16. Bitker, L.; Burrell, L.M. Classic and Nonclassic Renin-Angiotensin Systems in the Critically Ill. *Crit. Care Clin.* **2019**, *35*, 213–227. [CrossRef] [PubMed]
17. Ocaranza, M.P.; Riquelme, J.A.; García, L.; Jalil, J.E.; Chiong, M.; Santos, R.A.; Lavandero, S. Counter-Regulatory Renin–Angiotensin System in Cardiovascular Disease. *Nat. Rev. Cardiol.* **2019**, *17*, 116–129. [CrossRef] [PubMed]
18. Li, X.C.; Zhang, J.; Zhuo, J.L. The Vasoprotective Axes of the Renin-Angiotensin System: Physiological Relevance and Therapeutic Implications in Cardiovascular, Hypertensive and Kidney Diseases. *Pharmacol. Res.* **2017**, *125*, 21–38. [CrossRef]
19. Karnik, S.S.; Singh, K.D.; Tirupula, K.; Unal, H. Significance of Angiotensin 1–7 Coupling with MAS1 Receptor and Other GPCRs to the Renin-angiotensin System: IUPHAR Review 22. *Br. J. Pharmacol.* **2017**, *174*, 737–753. [CrossRef]
20. Kangussu, L.M.; Guimaraes, P.S.; Nadu, A.P.; Melo, M.B.; Santos, R.A.S.; Campagnole-Santos, M.J. Activation of Angiotensin-(1–7)/Mas Axis in the Brain Lowers Blood Pressure and Attenuates Cardiac Remodeling in Hypertensive Transgenic (MREN2)27 Rats. *Neuropharmacology* **2015**, *97*, 58–66. [CrossRef]

21. Roth, G.A.; Mensah, G.A.; Johnson, C.O.; Addolorato, G.; Ammirati, E.; Baddour, L.M.; Barengo, N.C.; Beaton, A.Z.; Benjamin, E.J.; Benziger, C.P.; et al. Global Burden of Cardiovascular Diseases and Risk Factors, 1990–2019. *J. Am. Coll. Cardiol.* **2020**, *76*, 2982–3021. [CrossRef]
22. Aguiar, J.E. Preventing Premature Mortality from Cardiovascular Disease: A Prime Goal. *Rev. Port. Cardiol.* **2020**, *39*, 35–36. [CrossRef]
23. Tsao, C.; Aday, A. Correction to: Heart Disease and Stroke Statistics—2022 Update: A Report from the American Heart Association. *Circulation* **2022**, *146*, 141.
24. Medina-Leyte, D.J.; Zepeda-García, O.; Domínguez-Pérez, M.; González-Garrido, A.; Villarreal-Molina, T.; Jacobo-Albavera, L. Endothelial Dysfunction, Inflammation and Coronary Artery Disease: Potential Biomarkers and Promising Therapeutical Approaches. *Int. J. Mol. Sci.* **2021**, *22*, 3850. [CrossRef] [PubMed]
25. Taqueti, V.R.; Di Carli, M.F. Coronary Microvascular Disease Pathogenic Mechanisms and Therapeutic Options: JACC State-of-the-Art Review. *J. Am. Coll. Cardiol.* **2018**, *72*, 2625–2641. [CrossRef] [PubMed]
26. Thygesen, K. Consenso ESC 2018 Sobre la Cuarta Definición Universal del Infarto. *Rev. Esp. Cardiol.* **2019**, *72*, 72.
27. Frangogiannis, N.G. Pathophysiology of Myocardial Infarction. *Compr. Physiol.* **2015**, *5*, 1841–1875. [PubMed]
28. Lu, L.; Liu, M.; Sun, R.; Zheng, Y.; Zhang, P. Myocardial Infarction: Symptoms and Treatments. *Cell Biochem. Biophys.* **2015**, *72*, 865–867. [CrossRef] [PubMed]
29. Ferry, A.V.; Anand, A.; Strachan, F.E.; Mooney, L.; Stewart, S.D.; Marshall, L. Presenting Symptoms in Men and Women Diagnosed with Myocardial Infarction Using Sex-Specific Criteria. *J. Am. Heart Assoc.* **2019**, *8*, e012307. [CrossRef] [PubMed]
30. Hausenloy, D.J.; Chilian, W.; Crea, F.; Davidson, S.M.; Ferdinandy, P.; Garcia-Dorado, D.; van Royen, N.; Schulz, R.; Heusch, G. The Coronary Circulation in Acute Myocardial Ischaemia/Reperfusion Injury: A Target for Cardioprotection. *Cardiovasc. Res.* **2019**, *115*, 1143–1155. [CrossRef]
31. Ong, S.B.; Hernández-Reséndiz, S.; Crespo-Avilan, G.E.; Mukhametshina, R.T.; Kwek, X.Y.; Cabrera-Fuentes, H.A.; Hausenloy, D.J. Inflammation Following Acute Myocardial Infarction: Multiple Players, Dynamic Roles, and Novel Therapeutic Opportunities. *Pharmacol. Ther.* **2018**, *186*, 73–87. [CrossRef]
32. Prabhu, S.D.; Frangogiannis, N.G. The Biological Basis for Cardiac Repair after Myocardial Infarction: From Inflammation to Fibrosis: From Inflammation to Fibrosis. *Circ. Res.* **2016**, *119*, 91–112. [CrossRef]
33. Hao, K.; Lei, W.; Wu, H.; Wu, J.; Yang, Z.; Yan, S.; Lu, X.A.; Li, J.; Xia, X.; Han, X.; et al. Lncrna-Safe Contributes to Cardiac Fibrosis through Safe-Sfrp2-HuR Complex in Mouse Myocardial Infarction. *Theranostics* **2019**, *9*, 7282–7297. [CrossRef]
34. Kleindorfer, D.O.; Towfighi, A.; Chaturvedi, S.; Cockroft, K.M.; Gutierrez, J.; Lombardi-Hill, D.; Kamel, H.; Kernan, W.N.; Kittner, S.J.; Leira, E.C.; et al. 2021 Guideline for the Prevention of Stroke in Patients with Stroke and Transient Ischemic Attack: A Guideline from the American Heart Association/American Stroke Association. *Stroke* **2021**, *52*, e364–e467. [CrossRef] [PubMed]
35. Zhao, Y.; Zhang, X.; Chen, X.; Wei, Y. Neuronal injuries in cerebral infarction and ischemic stroke: From mechanisms to treatment (Review). *Int. J. Mol. Med.* **2022**, *49*, 15. [CrossRef] [PubMed]
36. Qin, C.; Yang, S.; Chu, Y.H.; Zhang, H.; Pang, X.W.; Chen, L.; Zhou, L.Q.; Chen, M.; Tian, D.S.; Wang, W. Signaling pathways involved in ischemic stroke: Molecular mechanisms and therapeutic interventions. *Signal Transduct. Target. Ther.* **2022**, *7*, 215. [CrossRef] [PubMed]
37. Oparil, S.; Acelajado, M.C.; Bakris, G.L.; Berlowitz, D.R.; Cífková, R.; Dominiczak, A.F.; Grassi, G.; Jordan, J.; Poulter, N.R.; Rodgers, A.; et al. Hypertension. *Nat. Rev. Dis. Prim.* **2018**, *4*, 18014. [CrossRef] [PubMed]
38. Fuchs, F.D.; Whelton, P.K. High Blood Pressure and Cardiovascular Disease. *Hypertension* **2020**, *75*, 285–292. [CrossRef] [PubMed]
39. Al Ghorani, H.; Götzinger, F.; Böhm, M.; Mahfoud, F. Arterial hypertension—Clinical trials update 2021. *Nutr. Metab. Cardiovasc. Dis.* **2022**, *32*, 21–31. [CrossRef]
40. Messerli, F.H.; Rimoldi, S.F.; Bangalore, S. The Transition from Hypertension to Heart Failure: Contemporary Update. *JACC Heart Fail.* **2017**, *5*, 543–551. [CrossRef]
41. Jugdutt, B.I. Aging and Heart Failure: Changing Demographics and Implications for Therapy in the Elderly. *Heart Fail. Rev.* **2010**, *15*, 401–405. [CrossRef]
42. Arrigo, M.; Jessup, M.; Mullens, W.; Reza, N.; Shah, A.M.; Sliwa, K. Acute Heart Failure. *Nat. Rev. Dis. Prim.* **2020**, *6*, 16. [CrossRef]
43. Kurmani, S.; Squire, I. Acute Heart Failure: Definition, Classification and Epidemiology. *Curr. Heart Fail. Rep.* **2017**, *14*, 385–392. [CrossRef]
44. Long, B.; Koyfman, A.; Gottlieb, M. Diagnosis of Acute Heart Failure in the Emergency Department: An Evidence-Based Review. *West. J. Emerg. Med.* **2019**, *20*, 875–884. [CrossRef] [PubMed]
45. Bahit, M.C.; Kochar, A.; Granger, C.B. Post-Myocardial Infarction Heart Failure. *JACC Heart Fail.* **2018**, *6*, 179–186. [CrossRef] [PubMed]
46. Zhang, Q.; Zhou, L.; Cai, H.L.; Lu, H.H. Relationship of the ORBIT and HAS-BLED Scores with Killip Class 3-4 in Patients with ST-Segment Elevation Myocardial Infarction. *Medicine* **2019**, *98*, e14578. [CrossRef] [PubMed]
47. Curley, D.; Lavin Plaza, B.; Shah, A.M.; Botnar, R.M. Molecular Imaging of Cardiac Remodelling after Myocardial Infarction. *Basic Res. Cardiol.* **2018**, *113*, 10. [CrossRef] [PubMed]
48. Peet, C.; Ivetic, A.; Bromage, D.I.; Shah, A.M. Cardiac Monocytes and Macrophages after Myocardial Infarction. *Cardiovasc. Res.* **2020**, *116*, 1101–1112. [CrossRef]

49. Gabriel-Costa, D. The Pathophysiology of Myocardial Infarction-Induced Heart Failure. *Pathophysiology* **2018**, *25*, 277–284. [CrossRef]
50. Jenča, D.; Melenovský, V.; Stehlik, J.; Staněk, V.; Kettner, J.; Kautzner, J.; Adámková, V.; Wohlfahrt, P. Heart Failure after Myocardial Infarction: Incidence and Predictors. *ESC Heart Fail.* **2021**, *8*, 222–237. [CrossRef]
51. Bostan, M.M.; Stătescu, C.; Anghel, L.; Șerban, I.L.; Cojocaru, E.; Sascău, R. Post-Myocardial Infarction Ventricular Remodeling Biomarkers—The Key Link between Pathophysiology and Clinic. *Biomolecules* **2020**, *10*, 1587. [CrossRef]
52. Frampton, J.; Ortengren, A.R.; Zeitler, E.P. Arrhythmias after Acute Myocardial Infarction. *Yale J. Biol. Med.* **2023**, *96*, 83–94. [CrossRef]
53. Liakos, C.I.; Grassos, C.A.; Papadopoulos, D.P.; Dimitriadis, K.S.; Tsioufis, C.P.; Tousoulis, D. Arterial hypertension and aortic valve stenosis: Shedding light on a common "liaison". *Hell. J. Cardiol.* **2017**, *58*, 261–266. [CrossRef]
54. Morales Olivas, F.J.; Estañ Yago, L. Conceptos Nuevos Sobre el Sistema Renina Angiotensina. *Hipertens. Riesgo Vasc.* **2010**, *27*, 211–217. [CrossRef]
55. Ames, M.K.; Atkins, C.E.; Pitt, B. The Renin-Angiotensin-Aldosterone System and Its Suppression. *J. Vet. Intern. Med.* **2019**, *33*, 363–382. [CrossRef] [PubMed]
56. Bruce, E.B.; de Kloet, A.D. The Intricacies of the Renin-Angiotensin-System in Metabolic Regulation. *Physiol. Behav.* **2017**, *178*, 157–165. [CrossRef] [PubMed]
57. Cohen, J.B.; Hanff, T.C.; Bress, A.P.; South, A.M. Relationship between ACE2 and Other Components of the Renin-Angiotensin System. *Curr. Hypertens. Rep.* **2020**, *22*, 44. [CrossRef] [PubMed]
58. Lelis, D.F.; Freitas, D.F.; Machado, A.S.; Crespo, T.S.; Santos, S.H.S. Angiotensin-(1-7), Adipokines and Inflammation. *Metabolism* **2019**, *95*, 36–45. [CrossRef]
59. Santos, R.A.; Simoes e Silva, A.C.; Maric, C.; Silva, D.M.; Machado, R.P.; de Buhr, I.; Heringer-Walther, S.; Pinheiro, S.V.; Lopes, M.T.; Bader, M.; et al. Angiotensin-(1-7) is an endogenous ligand for the G protein-coupled receptor Mas. *Proc. Natl. Acad. Sci. USA* **2003**, *100*, 8258–8263. [CrossRef] [PubMed]
60. Yamamoto, K.; Takeshita, H.; Rakugi, H. ACE2, Angiotensin 1-7 and Skeletal Muscle: Review in the Era of COVID-19. *Clin. Sci.* **2020**, *134*, 3047–3062. [CrossRef]
61. Santos, R.A.S.; Sampaio, W.O.; Alzamora, A.C.; Motta-Santos, D.; Alenina, N.; Bader, M. The ACE2/Angiotensin-(1-7)/MAS Axis of the Renin-Angiotensin System: Focus on Angiotensin-(1-7). *Physiol. Rev.* **2018**, *98*, 505–553. [CrossRef]
62. Medina, D.; Arnold, A.C. Angiotensin-(1-7): Translational Avenues in Cardiovascular Control. *Am. J. Hypertens.* **2019**, *32*, 1133–1142. [CrossRef]
63. Freitas, R.A.; Junior, R.R.P.; Justina, V.D.; Bressan, A.F.M.; Bomfim, G.F.; Carneiro, F.S.; Giachini, F.R.; Lima, V.V. Angiotensin (1-7)-Attenuated Vasoconstriction is Associated with the Interleukin-10 Signaling Pathway. *Life Sci.* **2020**, *262*, 118552. [CrossRef]
64. Miller, A.J.; Bingaman, S.S.; Mehay, D.; Medina, D.; Arnold, A.C. Angiotensin-(1-7) Improves Integrated Cardiometabolic Function in Aged Mice. *Int. J. Mol. Sci.* **2020**, *21*, 5131. [CrossRef] [PubMed]
65. Kittana, N. Angiotensin-Converting Enzyme 2-Angiotensin 1-7/1-9 System: Novel Promising Targets for Heart Failure Treatment. *Fundam. Clin. Pharmacol.* **2018**, *32*, 14–25. [CrossRef] [PubMed]
66. McKinney, C.A.; Fattah, C.; Loughrey, C.M.; Milligan, G.; Nicklin, S.A. Angiotensin-(1-7) and Angiotensin-(1-9): Function in Cardiac and Vascular Remodelling. *Clin. Sci.* **2014**, *126*, 815–827. [CrossRef] [PubMed]
67. Varagic, J.; Ahmad, S.; Nagata, S.; Ferrario, C.M. ACE2: Angiotensin II/Angiotensin-(1-7) Balance in Cardiac and Renal Injury. *Curr. Hypertens. Rep.* **2014**, *16*, 420. [CrossRef]
68. Higuchi, S.; Ohtsu, H.; Suzuki, H.; Shirai, H.; Frank, G.D.; Eguchi, S. Angiotensin II Signal Transduction through the AT1 Receptor: Novel Insights into Mechanisms and Pathophysiology. *Clin. Sci.* **2007**, *112*, 417–428. [CrossRef] [PubMed]
69. Gonzalez, L.; Novoa, U.; Moya, J.; Gabrielli, L.; Jalil, J.E.; García, L.; Chiong, M.; Lavandero, S.; Ocaranza, M.P. Angiotensin-(1-9) Reduces Cardiovascular and Renal Inflammation in Experimental Renin-Independent Hypertension. *Biochem. Pharmacol.* **2018**, *156*, 357–370. [CrossRef] [PubMed]
70. Flores-Muñoz, M.; Smith, N.J.; Haggerty, C.; Milligan, G.; Nicklin, S.A. Angiotensin1-9 antagonises pro-hypertrophic signalling in cardiomyocytes via the angiotensin type 2 receptor. *J. Physiol.* **2011**, *589*, 939–951. [CrossRef]
71. Kramkowski, K.; Mogielnicki, A.; Leszczynska, A.; Buczko, W. Angiotensin-(1-9), the Product of Angiotensin I Conversion in Platelets, Enhances Arterial Thrombosis in Rats. *J. Physiol. Pharmacol.* **2010**, *61*, 317–324.
72. Schleifenbaum, J. Alamandine and its Receptor MrgD Pair up to Join the Protective Arm of the Renin-Angiotensin System. *Front. Med.* **2019**, *6*, 107. [CrossRef]
73. Park, B.M.; Phuong, H.T.A.; Yu, L.; Kim, S.H. Alamandine Protects the Heart against Reperfusion Injury via the MrgD Receptor. *Circ. J.* **2018**, *82*, 2584–2593. [CrossRef]
74. Jesus, I.C.G.; Mesquita, T.R.R.; Monteiro, A.L.L.; Parreira, A.B.; Santos, A.K.; Coelho, E.L.X.; Silva, M.M.; Souza, L.A.C.; Campagnole-Santos, M.J.; Santos, R.S.; et al. Alamandine Enhances Cardiomyocyte Contractility in Hypertensive Rats through a Nitric Oxide-Dependent Activation of Camkii. *Am. J. Physiol. Cell* **2020**, *318*, 740–750. [CrossRef]
75. Jesus, I.C.G.; Scalzo, S.; Alves, F.; Marques, K.; Rocha-Resende, C.; Bader, M.; Santos, R.A.S.; Guatimosim, S. Alamandine Acts via MrgD to Induce AMPK/NO Activation against ANG II Hypertrophy in Cardiomyocytes. *Am. J. Physiol. Cell Physiol.* **2018**, *314*, 702–711. [CrossRef] [PubMed]

76. Qaradakhi, T.; Matsoukas, M.T.; Hayes, A.; Rybalka, E.; Caprnda, M.; Rimarova, K.; Sepsi, M.; Büsselberg, D.; Kruzliak, P.; Matsoukas, J.; et al. Alamandine Reverses Hyperhomocysteinemia-Induced Vascular Dysfunction via PKA-Dependent Mechanisms. *Cardiovasc. Ther.* **2017**, *35*, e12306. [CrossRef] [PubMed]
77. Lautner, R.Q.; Villela, D.C.; Fraga-Silva, R.A.; Silva, N.; Verano-Braga, T.; Costa-Fraga, F. Discovery and Characterization of Alamandine: A Novel Component of the Renin-Angiotensin System. *Circ. Res.* **2013**, *112*, 1104–1111. [CrossRef] [PubMed]
78. Song, X.D.; Feng, J.P.; Yang, R.X. Alamandine Protects Rat from Myocardial Ischemia-Reperfusion Injury by Activating JNK and Inhibiting NF-κB. *Eur. Rev. Med. Pharmacol. Sci.* **2019**, *23*, 6718–6726.
79. Mendoza-Torres, E.; Oyarzún, A.; Mondaca-Ruff, D.; Azocar, A.; Castro, P.F.; Jalil, J.E.; Chiong, M.; Lavandero, S.; Ocaranza, M.P. ACE2 and Vasoactive Peptides: Novel Players in Cardiovascular/Renal Remodeling and Hypertension. *Ther. Adv. Cardiovasc. Dis.* **2015**, *9*, 217–237. [CrossRef] [PubMed]
80. Samakova, A.; Gazova, A.; Sabova, N.; Valaskova, S.; Jurikova, M.; Kyselovic, J. The PI3k/Akt Pathway is Associated with Angiogenesis, Oxidative Stress and Survival of Mesenchymal Stem Cells in Pathophysiologic Condition in Ischemia. *Physiol. Res.* **2019**, *68*, 131–138. [CrossRef]
81. Zhang, F.; Tang, H.; Sun, S.; Luo, Y.; Ren, X.; Chen, A. Angiotensin-(1-7) induced vascular relaxation in spontaneously hypertensive rats. *Nitric Oxide* **2019**, *88*, 1–9. [CrossRef]
82. Carver, K.A.; Smith, T.L.; Gallagher, P.E.; Tallant, E.A. Angiotensin-(1-7) Prevents Angiotensin II-Induced Fibrosis in Cremaster Microvessels. *Microcirculation* **2015**, *22*, 19–27. [CrossRef]
83. Wang, L.P.; Fan, S.J.; Li, S.M.; Wang, X.J.; Gao, J.L.; Yang, X.H. Protective Role of ACE2-Ang-(1–7)-Mas in Myocardial Fibrosis by Downregulating Kca3.1 Channel via ERK1/2 Pathway. *Pflug. Arch.* **2016**, *468*, 2041–2051. [CrossRef]
84. Shah, A.; Oh, Y.B.; Lee, S.H.; Lim, J.M.; Kim, S.H. Angiotensin-(1-7) Attenuates Hypertension in Exercise-Trained Renal Hypertensive Rats. *Am. J. Physiol. Heart Circ. Physiol.* **2012**, *302*, 2372–2380. [CrossRef] [PubMed]
85. Gava, E.; de Castro, C.H.; Ferreira, A.J.; Colleta, H.; Melo, M.B.; Alenina, N.; Bader, M.; Oliveira, L.A.; Santos, R.A.; Kitten, G.T. Angiotensin-(1-7) Receptor Mas Is An Essential Modulator of Extracellular Matrix Protein Expression in the Heart. *Regul. Pept.* **2012**, *175*, 30–42. [CrossRef]
86. Iwata, M.; Cowling, R.T.; Gurantz, D.; Moore, C.; Zhang, S.; Yuan, J.X.; Greenberg, B.H. Angiotensin-(1-7) Binds to Specific Receptors on Cardiac Fibroblasts to Initiate Antifibrotic and Antitrophic Effects. *Am. J. Physiol. Heart Circ. Physiol.* **2005**, *289*, 2356–2363. [CrossRef]
87. Grobe, J.L.; Mecca, A.P.; Lingis, M.; Shenoy, V.; Bolton, T.A.; Machado, J.M.; Speth, R.C.; Raizada, M.K.; Katovich, M.J. Prevention of Angiotensin II-Induced Cardiac Remodeling by Angiotensin-(1-7). *Am. J. Physiol. Heart Circ. Physiol.* **2007**, *292*, 736–742. [CrossRef] [PubMed]
88. Zeng, W.; Chen, W.; Leng, X.; He, J.G.; Ma, H. Chronic Angiotensin-(1-7) Administration Improves Vascular Remodeling after Angioplasty through the Regulation of the TGF-Beta/Smad Signaling Pathway in Rabbits. *Biochem. Biophys. Res. Commun.* **2009**, *389*, 138–144. [CrossRef] [PubMed]
89. Cunha, T.M.B.; Lima, W.G.; Silva, M.E.; Souza Santos, R.A.; Campagnole-Santos, M.J.; Alzamora, A.C. The Nonpeptide ANG-(1-7) Mimic AVE 0991 Attenuates Cardiac Remodeling and Improves Baroreflex Sensitivity in Renovascular Hypertensive Rats. *Life Sci.* **2013**, *92*, 266–275. [CrossRef] [PubMed]
90. McCollum, L.T.; Gallagher, P.E.; Tallant, E.A. Angiotensin-(1-7) Abrogates Mitogen-Stimulated Proliferation of Cardiac Fibroblasts. *Peptides* **2012**, *34*, 380–388. [CrossRef]
91. Marques, F.D.; Melo, M.B.; Souza, L.E.; Irigoyen, M.C.C.; Sinisterra, R.D.; de Sousa, F.B.; Savergnini, S.Q.; Braga, V.B.; Ferreira, A.J.; Santos, R.A. Beneficial Effects of Long-Term Administration of an Oral Formulation of Angiotensin-(1-7) in Infarcted Rats. *Int. J. Hypertens.* **2012**, *2012*, 795452. [CrossRef]
92. Romero, A.; San Hipólito-Luengo, Á.; Villalobos, L.A.; Vallejo, S.; Valencia, I.; Michalska, P.; Pajuelo-Lozano, N.; Sánchez-Pérez, I.; León, R.; Bartha, J.L.; et al. The Angiotensin-(1-7)/Mas Receptor Axis Protects from Endothelial Cell Senescence via Klotho and Nrf2 Activation. *Aging Cell* **2019**, *18*, e12913. [CrossRef]
93. Zhang, B.N.; Xu, H.; Gao, X.M.; Zhang, G.Z.; Zhang, X.; Yang, F. Protective Effect of Angiotensin (1-7) on Silicotic Fibrosis in Rats. *Biomed. Environ. Sci.* **2019**, *32*, 419–426.
94. Kangussu, L.M.; Melo-Braga, M.N.; de Souza Lima, B.S.; Santos, R.A.S.; de Andrade, H.M.; Campagnole-Santos, M.J. Angiotensin-(1-7) Central Mechanisms after ICV Infusion in Hypertensive Transgenic (Mren2)27 Rats. *Front. Neurosci.* **2021**, *15*, 624249. [CrossRef]
95. Stoyell-Conti, F.F.; Chabbra, A.; Puthentharayil, J.; Rigatto, K.; Speth, R.C. Chronic Administration of Pharmacological Doses of Angiotensin 1-7 and Iodoangiotensin 1-7 Has Minimal Effects on Blood Pressure, Heart Rate, and Cognitive Function of Spontaneously Hypertensive Rats. *Physiol. Rep.* **2021**, *9*, e14812. [CrossRef] [PubMed]
96. Flores-Munoz, M.; Work, L.M.; Douglas, K.; Denby, L.; Dominiczak, A.F.; Graham, D.; Nicklin, S.A. Angiotensin-(1-9) Attenuates Cardiac Fibrosis in the Stroke-Prone Spontaneously Hypertensive Rat via the Angiotensin Type 2 Receptor. *Hypertension* **2012**, *59*, 300–307. [CrossRef] [PubMed]
97. Sotomayor-Flores, C.; Rivera-Mejías, P.; Vásquez-Trincado, C.; López-Crisosto, C.; Morales, P.E.; Pennanen, C.; Polakovicova, I.; Aliaga-Tobar, V.; García, L.; Roa, J.C.; et al. Angiotensin-(1-9) Prevents Cardiomyocyte Hypertrophy by Controlling Mitochondrial Dynamics via Mir-129-3p/PKIA Pathway. *Cell Death Differ.* **2020**, *27*, 2586–2604. [CrossRef] [PubMed]

98. Norambuena-Soto, I.; Ocaranza, M.P.; Cancino-Arenas, N.; Sanhueza-Olivares, F.; Villar-Fincheira, P.; Leiva-Navarrete, S.; Mancilla-Medina, C.; Moya, J.; Novoa, U.; Jalil, J.E.; et al. Angiotensin-(1-9) Prevents Vascular Remodeling by Decreasing Vascular Smooth Muscle Cell Dedifferentiation through a Foxo1-Dependent Mechanism. *Biochem. Pharmacol.* **2020**, *180*, 114190. [CrossRef] [PubMed]
99. Mendoza-Torres, E.; Riquelme, J.A.; Vielma, A.; Sagredo, A.R.; Gabrielli, L.; Bravo-Sagua, R.; Jalil, J.E.; Rothermel, B.A.; Sanchez, G.; Ocaranza, M.P.; et al. Protection of the Myocardium against Ischemia/Reperfusion Injury by Angiotensin-(1-9) through an AT2R and Akt-Dependent Mechanism. *Pharmacol. Res.* **2018**, *135*, 112–121. [CrossRef] [PubMed]
100. Menasché, P. Cardioplegic Solution Challenges. *Ital. Heart J.* **2000**, *1*, S40–S42. [PubMed]
101. Reichert, K.; Carmo, H.R.; Lima, F.; Torina, A.G.; Vilarinho, K.A.; Oliveira, P.P.; Silveira Filho, L.M.; Severino, E.S.; Petrucci, O. Development of Cardioplegic Solution without Potassium: Experimental Study in Rat. *Rev. Bras. Cir. Cardiovasc.* **2013**, *28*, 521 530.
102. Ocaranza, M.P.; Lavandero, S.; Jalil, J.E.; Moya, J.; Pinto, M.; Novoa, U. Angiotensin (1 9) Regulates Cardiac Hypertrophy In Vivo and In Vitro. *J. Hypertens.* **2010**, *28*, 1054–1064. [CrossRef]
103. Gomes, E.R.M.; Lara, A.A.; Almeida, P.W.M.; Guimarães, D.; Resende, R.R.; Campagnole-Santos, M.J. Angiotensin-(1-7) Prevents Cardiomyocyte Pathological Remodeling through a Nitric Oxide/Guanosine 3′,5′-Cyclic Monophosphate-Dependent Pathway. *Hypertension* **2010**, *55*, 153–160. [CrossRef]
104. Oparil, S.; Sanders, C.A.; Haber, E. In-Vivo and In-Vitro Conversion of Angiotensin I to Angiotensin II in Dog Blood. *Circ. Res.* **1970**, *26*, 591–599. [CrossRef] [PubMed]
105. Rice, G.I.; Thomas, D.A.; Grant, P.J.; Turner, A.J.; Hooper, N.M. Evaluation of Angiotensin-Converting Enzyme (ACE), Its Homologue ACE2 and Neprilysin in Angiotensin Peptide Metabolism. *Biochem. J.* **2004**, *383*, 45–51. [CrossRef] [PubMed]
106. Ocaranza, M.P.; Jalil, J.E. Protective Role of the ACE2/Ang-(1-9) Axis in Cardiovascular Remodeling. *Int. J. Hypertens.* **2012**, *2012*, 594361. [CrossRef]
107. Xie, Y.; Shi, X.; Sheng, K.; Han, G.; Li, W.; Zhao, Q. PI3K/Akt Signaling Transduction Pathway, Erythropoiesis and Glycolysis in Hypoxia (Review). *Mol. Med. Rep.* **2019**, *19*, 783–791. [CrossRef] [PubMed]
108. Weeks, K.L.; Bernardo, B.C.; Ooi, J.Y.Y.; Patterson, N.L.; McMullen, J.R. The IGF1-PI3K-Akt Signaling Pathway in Mediating Exercise-Induced Cardiac Hypertrophy and Protection. *Adv. Exp. Med. Biol.* **2017**, *1000*, 187–210.
109. Yang, C.; Wu, X.; Shen, Y.; Liu, C.; Kong, X.; Li, P. Alamandine Attenuates Angiotensin II-Induced Vascular Fibrosis via Inhibiting P38 MAPK Pathway. *Eur. J. Pharmacol.* **2020**, *883*, 173384. [CrossRef]
110. Hekmat, A.S.; Navabi, Z.; Alipanah, H.; Javanmardi, K. Alamandine Significantly Reduces Doxorubicin-Induced Cardiotoxicity in Rats. *Hum. Exp. Toxicol.* **2021**, *40*, 1781–1789. [CrossRef]
111. Villela, D.C.; Passos-Silva, D.G.; Santos, R.A.S. Alamandine: A New Member of the Angiotensin Family: A New Member of the Angiotensin Family. *Curr. Opin. Nephrol. Hypertens.* **2014**, *23*, 130–134. [CrossRef]
112. Zhu, J.; Qiu, J.G.; Xu, W.-T.; Ma, H.-X.; Jiang, K. Alamandine Protects against Renal Ischaemia-Reperfusion Injury in Rats via Inhibiting Oxidative Stress. *J. Pharm. Pharmacol.* **2021**, *73*, 1491–1502. [CrossRef]
113. Angiotensin-(1-7) Cardiovascular Effects in Aging. Available online: https://www.clinicaltrials.gov/ct2/show/NCT05301192?term=NCT05301192&draw=2&rank=1 (accessed on 3 March 2023).
114. Angiotensin 1-7 in Obesity Hypertension. 2022. Available online: https://www.clinicaltrials.gov/ct2/show/NCT03604289?term=NCT03604289&draw=2&rank=1 (accessed on 3 March 2023).
115. Sampaio, W.; Nascimento, A.; Santos, R. Systemic and regional hemodynamic effects of angiotensin-(1-7) in rats. *Am. J. Physiol. Heart Circ. Physiol.* **2003**, *284*, 1985–1994. [CrossRef]
116. Donoghue, M.; Hsieh, F.; Baronas, E.; Godbout, K.; Gosselin, M.; Stagliano, N.; Donovan, M.; Woolf, B.; Robison, K.; Jeyaseelan, R.; et al. A novel angiotensin-converting enzyme-related carboxypeptidase (ACE2) converts angiotensin I to angiotensin 1-9. *Circ. Res.* **2000**, *87*, E1–E9. [CrossRef] [PubMed]
117. Cha, S.; Park, B.; Gao, S.; Kim, S. Stimulation of ANP by angiotensin-(1-9) via the angiotensin type 2 receptor. *Life Sci.* **2013**, *93*, 934–940. [CrossRef] [PubMed]
118. Shen, Y.; Liu, M.; Xu, M.; Xu, Z.; Na, Y.; Zhang, N.; Geng, F. Simultaneous determination of nine trace concentration angiotensin peptides in human serum using ultra high performance liquid chromatography with tandem mass spectrometry with sephadex LH-20 gel solid-phase extraction. *J. Sep. Sci.* **2019**, *42*, 2247–2254. [CrossRef] [PubMed]
119. Campbell, D.J.; Lawrence, A.C.; Towrie, A.; Kladis, A.; Valentijn, A.J. Differential regulation of angiotensin peptide levels in plasma and kidney of the rat. *Hypertension* **1991**, *18*, 763–773. [CrossRef] [PubMed]
120. The Safety, Tolerability, PK and PD of GSK2586881 in Patients with Acute Lung Injury. 2014. Available online: https://ClinicalTrials.gov/show/NCT01597635 (accessed on 11 December 2023).
121. Safety and Tolerability Study of APN01 (Recombinant Human Angiotensin Converting Enzyme 2). 2009. Available online: https://clinicaltrials.gov/study/NCT00886353?term=APN01&rank=1 (accessed on 11 December 2023).
122. Effect of C21 on Forearm Blood Flow. 2022. Available online: https://classic.clinicaltrials.gov/ct2/show/NCT05277922 (accessed on 11 December 2023).
123. Angiotensin-(1-7) in Peripheral Arterial Disease. 2 December 2022. Available online: https://www.clinicaltrials.gov/ct2/show/NCT03240068?term=NCT03240068&draw=2&rank=1 (accessed on 3 March 2023).

124. Wagener, G.; Goldklang, M.P.; Gerber, A.; Elisman, K.; Eiseman, K.A.; Fonseca, L.D.; D'Armiento, J.M. A Randomized, Placebo-Controlled, Double-Blinded Pilot Study of Angiotensin 1–7 (TXA-127) for the Treatment of Severe COVID-19. *Crit. Care* **2022**, *26*, 229. [CrossRef] [PubMed]
125. de Souza-Neto, F.P.; Silva, M.M.E.; Santuchi, M.C.; de Alcântara-Leonídio, T.C.; Motta-Santos, D.; Oliveira, A.C.; Melo, M.B.; Canta, G.N.; de Souza, L.E.; Irigoyen, M.C.C.; et al. Alamandine Attenuates Arterial Remodelling Induced by Transverse Aortic Constriction in Mice. *Clin. Sci.* **2019**, *133*, 629–643. [CrossRef]
126. TXA127 in Non-Ambulant Patients with DMD Cardiomyopathy. 2023. Available online: https://clinicaltrials.gov/study/NCT06013839?intr=ang-(1-7)&rank=4#study-plan (accessed on 22 December 2023).
127. Phase 2 Study of TXA127 in Post-Ischemic Stroke Patients. 2023. Available online: https://clinicaltrials.gov/study/NCT06135103?intr=ang-(1-7)&rank=7#study-plan (accessed on 21 December 2023).
128. Marfella, R.; D'Onofrio, N.; Mansueto, G.; Grimaldi, V.; Trotta, M.C.; Sardu, C.; Sasso, F.C.; Scisciola, L.; Amarelli, C.; Esposito, S.; et al. Glycated ACE2 reduces anti-remodeling effects of renin-angiotensin system inhibition in human diabetic hearts. *Cardiovasc. Diabetol.* **2022**, *21*, 146. [CrossRef]
129. Zhao, K.; Xu, T.; Mao, Y. Alamandine Alleviated Heart Failure and Fibrosis in Myocardial Infarction Mice. *Biol. Direct* **2022**, *17*, 25. [CrossRef]
130. Ocaranza, M.P.; Kogan, M.J.; Lavandero, S.; Chiong, M. Angiotensin-(1-9) Analogue Based on D-Aminoacids, Pharmaceutical Compositions and Uses Thereof. Patent Application PCT/IB2021/054074, 13 May 2021.

MDPI AG
Grosspeteranlage 5
4052 Basel
Switzerland
Tel.: +41 61 683 77 34

Biomedicines Editorial Office
E-mail: biomedicines@mdpi.com
www.mdpi.com/journal/biomedicines

www.ingramcontent.com/pod-product-compliance
Lightning Source LLC
Chambersburg PA
CBHW061554210926
51850CB00009B/2105